Service User Involvement in Social Work Education

In 2006, *Social Work Education* produced the first special edition (vol. 25, no. 4) on service user and carer involvement in social work education, with all of the articles coming from the United Kingdom. In 2015, a mixed group of service users and social work academics wondered how, and if, the field had moved on since 2006. This publication confirms that it has.

Since 2006, service user and carer involvement in social work education has become embedded internationally – this book contains contributions from Australia, Israel, Italy, Norway, Slovenia, the Republic of Ireland and Sweden, as well as all four nations of the United Kingdom. Many of the contributions are jointly written with service users and carers, highlighting the innovative practices which challenge social work academics, students, social workers and managers to think how we can all benefit from learning with, and from, service users and carers. This book ably demonstrates that service users and carers can be effectively involved in social work curriculum planning, delivery, assessment and management. This is not to say that these issues are not without their tension, challenges or struggles, but working with these helps to ensure that the social workers and managers of the future can practice more effectively, meeting service user and carer priorities and needs.

The chapters in this book were originally published as a double special issue of *Social Work Education*.

Hugh McLaughlin is Professor of Social Work at Manchester Metropolitan University, UK. His research interests include keeping service user involvement in social work education and research honest, critical professional practice and the co-creation of learning organisations. He is editor-in-chief of *Social Work Education: The International Journal*.

Joseph Duffy is a Lecturer in Social Work at Queen's University, Belfast, UK. He is particularly interested in the development of innovative approaches to advancing user- and carer-based knowledge in helping students understand challenging curriculum topics such as the impact of conflict, social work values and international social work.

Brendan McKeever is an independent user researcher and comes from a user background. He has been involved in user involvement issues for over 20 years and has written extensively on issues impacting families of disabled children.

June Sadd is an independent survivor consultant in research, training, education and user involvement/co-production. She works with many social work programmes in England, and with national organisations such as the Social Care Institute for Excellence and Mind, using long-term personal experience as a survivor, and 23 years of work experience in health and social care as a survivor activist.

Service User Involvement in Social Work Education

Edited by
Hugh McLaughlin, Joseph Duffy, Brendan McKeever and June Sadd

Routledge
Taylor & Francis Group
LONDON AND NEW YORK

First published 2018 by Routledge

2 Park Square, Milton Park, Abingdon, Oxfordshire OX14 4RN
52 Vanderbilt Avenue, New York, NY 10017

Routledge is an imprint of the Taylor & Francis Group, an informa business

First issued in paperback 2020

British Library Cataloguing in Publication Data
A catalogue record for this book is available from the British Library

ISBN13: 978-0-8153-7830-3 (hbk)
ISBN13: 978-0-367-59279-0 (pbk)

Typeset in MinionPro
by diacriTech, Chennai

Publisher's Note
The publisher accepts responsibility for any inconsistencies that may have arisen during the conversion of this book from journal articles to book chapters, namely the possible inclusion of journal terminology.

Contents

Citation Information

The chapters in this book were originally published in various special issues of *Social Work Education*. When citing this material, please use the original volume number, issue number, year of publication and page numbering for each article, as follows:

Introduction
Service user and carer involvement in social work education – where are we now? – Part 1
Hugh McLaughlin, June Sadd, Brendan McKeever and Joseph Duffy
Social Work Education, volume 35, issue 8 (2016) pp. 863–865

Introduction
Service user and carer involvement in social work education – where are we now? – Part 2
Joseph Duffy, Brendan McKeever, Hugh McLaughlin, June Sadd
Social Work Education, volume 36, issue 2 (2017) pp. 125–127

Chapter 1
Outcomes focused user involvement in social work education: applying knowledge to practice
Susan Levy, Rowan Aiton, Jade Doig, John P. L. Dow, Shireen Brown, Liz Hunter and Ryan McNeil
Social Work Education, volume 35, issue 8 (2016) pp. 866–877

Chapter 2
Lessons from a comparative study of user involvement
Carolyn Gutman and Shulamit Ramon
Social Work Education, volume 35, issue 8 (2016) pp. 878–891

Chapter 3
Belonging to the library: humanising the space for social work education
Robin Sen, Nora McClelland and Beverley Jowett
Social Work Education, volume 35, issue 8 (2016) pp. 892–904

Chapter 4
A journey of embedding mental health lived experience in social work education
Kate P. Dorozenko, Sophie Ridley, Robyn Martin and Lyn Mahboub
Social Work Education, volume 35, issue 8 (2016) pp. 905–917

Chapter 5

Involving People with Profound and Multiple Learning Disabilities in Social Work Education: Building Inclusive Practice
Nicki Ward, Christian Raphael, Matthew Clark and Vicki Raphael
Social Work Education, volume 35, issue 8 (2016) pp. 918–932

Chapter 6

The benefits of prisoner participation in interdisciplinary learning
Ben Raikes and Rachel Balen
Social Work Education, volume 35, issue 8 (2016) pp. 933–944

Chapter 7

Gaining by giving? Peer research into service user and carer perceptions of inclusivity in Higher Education
Joy M. Rooney, Peter F. Unwin and Nina Osborne
Social Work Education, volume 35, issue 8 (2016) pp. 945–959

Chapter 8

Being a service user and a social work academic: balancing expert identities
Joanna Fox
Social Work Education, volume 35, issue 8 (2016) pp. 960–969

Chapter 9

Role-played interviews with service users in preparation for social work practice: exploring students' and service users' experience of co-produced workshops
Sara Hitchin
Social Work Education, volume 35, issue 8 (2016) pp. 970–981

Chapter 10

Learning from service users' involvement: a research about changing stigmatizing attitudes in social work students
Elena Cabiati and Maria Luisa Raineri
Social Work Education, volume 35, issue 8 (2016) pp. 982–996

Chapter 11

The Meaningful Involvement of Service Users in Social Work Education: Examples from Belgium and The Netherlands
Kristel Driessens, Hugh McLaughlin and Lia van Doorn
Social Work Education, volume 35, issue 7 (2016) pp. 739–751

Chapter 12

Mend the gap – strategies for user involvement in social work education
Ole Petter Askheim, Peter Beresford and Cecilia Heule
Social Work Education, volume 36, issue 2 (2017) pp. 128–140

Chapter 13

Social work undergraduates and service users as co-learners and researchers
Merav Moshe Grodofsky and Carolyn Gutman
Social Work Education, volume 36, issue 2 (2017) pp. 141–153

Chapter 14

A critical examination of the knowledge contribution service user and carer involvement brings to social work education
Kieron Hatton
Social Work Education, volume 36, issue 2 (2017) pp. 154–171

Chapter 15

Expert by experience research as grounding for social work education
Petra Videmšek
Social Work Education, volume 36, issue 2 (2017) pp. 172–187

Chapter 16

From service-user to social work examiner: not a bridge too far
Hilda Loughran and Gary Broderick
Social Work Education, volume 36, issue 2 (2017) pp. 188–202

Chapter 17

What difference does it make? Findings of an impact study of service user and carer involvement on social work students' subsequent practice
Mel Hughes
Social Work Education, volume 36, issue 2 (2017) pp. 203–216

Chapter 18

Life at the other end: participatory film-making, power and the 'common third'
Yohai Hakak and Kevin Holmes
Social Work Education, volume 36, issue 2 (2017) pp. 217–222

Notes on Contributors

Rowan Aiton gained his master's in Social Work from the School of Education & Social Work, University of Dundee, UK.

Ole Petter Askheim is a Professor at the Department of Health and Social Work, Lillehammer University College, Norway.

Rachel Balen is an ex-Principal Lecturer at the School of Human and Health Sciences, University of Huddersfield, UK.

Peter Beresford is Emeritus Professor of Social Policy at Brunel University London, UK. He is also Honorary Lecturer at the University of Essex, UK.

Gary Broderick is Director of the SAOL Project, Ireland.

Shireen Brown is a member of the Carer and User Group, School of Education & Social Work, University of Dundee, UK.

Elena Cabiati is a Professor at the Department of Sociology, Catholic University of Milan, Italy.

Matthew Clark is the Personal Assistant to Christian Raphael and supports Christian in delivering training on the lived experience of living with epilepsy.

Jade Doig studied for her master's in Social Work at the School of Education & Social Work, University of Dundee, UK.

Kate P. Dorozenko is a Research Associate at the School of Occupational Therapy and Social Work, Curtin University, Australia.

John P. L. Dow is a member of the Carer and User Group, School of Education & Social Work, University of Dundee, UK.

Kristel Driessens is a Teacher at the Department of Sociology, University of Antwerp, Belgium.

Joseph Duffy is a Lecturer in Social Work at Queen's University Belfast, UK. He is particularly interested in the development of innovative approaches to advancing user- and carer-based knowledge in helping students understand challenging curriculum topics such as the impact of conflict, social work values and international social work.

Joanna Fox is a Senior Lecturer at the School of Education and Social Care, Anglia Ruskin University, UK.

Carolyn Gutman is a Lecturer at the Department of Social Work, Tel-Hai Academic College, Israel.

Yohai Hakak is a Lecturer in Social Work at the Department of Clinical Sciences, Brunel University, UK.

Kieron Hatton is a Principal Lecturer at the School of Health Sciences and Social Work, University of Portsmouth, UK.

Cecilia Heule is a Lecturer and PhD student at the School of Social Work, Lund University, Sweden.

Sara Hitchin is a Teaching Fellow of Social Work at the University of Stirling, UK.

Kevin Holmes is a Technical Advisor and Film Editor for the Social Work Inclusion Group, University of Portsmouth, UK.

Mel Hughes is a Senior Lecturer at the Faculty of Health & Social Sciences, Bournemouth University, UK.

Liz Hunter is a member of the Carer and User Group, School of Education & Social Work, University of Dundee, UK.

Beverley Jowett is a University Teacher in Social Work at the University of Sheffield, UK.

Susan Levy is a Lecturer in the School of Education & Social Work, University of Dundee, UK. She uses a socio-spatial lens in her research to explore issues at the intersections of diversity, identity, integration and well-being of marginalised groups within society.

Hilda Loughran is Associate Professor at the School of Social Policy, Social Work and Social Justice, University College Dublin, Ireland.

Lyn Mahboub is a Lecturer at the School of Occupational Therapy and Social Work, Curtin University, Australia.

Robyn Martin is a Senior Lecturer at the School of Occupational Therapy and Social Work, Curtin University, Australia. Her research interests include consumer and family led research approaches, homelessness, domestic and family violence, and recovery in mental health and service delivery approaches.

Nora McClelland is a University Teacher in Social Work at the University of Sheffield, UK.

Brendan McKeever is an independent user researcher and comes from a user background. He has been involved in user involvement issues for over 20 years and has written extensively on issues impacting families of disabled children.

Hugh McLaughlin is Professor of Social Work at Manchester Metropolitan University, UK. His research interests include keeping service user involvement in social work education and research honest, critical professional practice and the co-creation of learning organisations. He is editor-in-chief of *Social Work Education: The International Journal.*

Ryan McNeil studied for his master's in Social Work at the School of Education & Social Work, University of Dundee, UK.

Merav Moshe Grodofsky is Senior Lecturer at the School of Social Work, Sapir College, Israel.

Nina Osborne runs an independent training and consultancy service for social care.

Ben Raikes is a Senior Lecturer at the School of Human and Health Sciences, University of Huddersfield, UK.

Maria Luisa Raineri is a Researcher at the Department of Sociology, Catholic University of Milan, Italy.

Shulamit Ramon is a Professor at the School of Health and Social Work, University of Hertfordshire, UK.

Christian Raphael works as an independent consultant/advisor on matters relating to profound learning disabilities and complex needs. Christian delivers training based on his personal experience of living with epilepsy, across the UK.

Vicky Raphael is the co-director of Inclusion East and co-chair of the National Valuing Families Forum. Vicky helps to support her son Christian who delivers training based on his personal experience of living with epilepsy, across the UK.

Sophie Ridley is a PhD student at the School of Occupational Therapy and Social Work, Curtin University, Australia.

Joy M. Rooney is an Associate Lecturer at the Institute of Health and Society, University of Worcester, UK.

June Sadd is an independent survivor consultant in research, training, education and user involvement/co-production. She works with many social work programmes in England, and with national organisations such as the Social Care Institute for Excellence and Mind, using long-term personal experience as a survivor, and 23 years of work experience in health and social care as a survivor activist.

Robin Sen is a Lecturer in Social Work at the University of Sheffield, UK. All his research has been connected to issues in children and families practice, with particular emphasis on issues of safeguarding and work with looked-after children.

Peter F. Unwin is a Senior Lecturer in Social Work at the Institute of Health and Society, University of Worcester, UK. His teaching interests are in safeguarding, foster care and in hearing the voices of service users and carers.

Lia van Doorn is a Professor of Innovation in Social Services Provision at Utrecht University of Applied Sciences, the Netherlands.

Petra Videmšek is a Senior Lecturer at the Faculty of Social Work, University of Ljubljana, Slovenia.

Nicki Ward is a Lecturer at the Department of Social Policy and Social Work, University of Birmingham, UK. She is particularly interested in issues diversity, intersectionality and care ethics.

INTRODUCTION

Service user and carer involvement in social work education – where are we now? – Part 1

This journal was proud to produce the first special edition on service user involvement in 2006 (Vol25 No.4) with 11 pioneering articles from the UK. One of those authors contributing to the first special edition, June Sadd, is also one of the guest editors of this special edition.

Over the years, the journal has continued to publish creative and challenging articles on service user involvement in social work education, reflecting a commitment to promoting further understanding in this important and developing area of knowledge. Importantly also, the journal has retained two places on its main board for service users and carers who play a key role in its development. This special edition and its call for papers, have been developed jointly by a team of service users and academics who between them, have widely published and practiced in the area of service user and carer involvement in Britain and Northern Ireland. The editorial team, therefore, worked closely together on all aspects of production for this special edition.

As it is now the 10th anniversary of this first ground-breaking edition, the current special edition editors wondered, 'what has happened since 2006?' This is what this two part special edition seeks to answer. The first thing that stands out is that the involvement of service users in social work education is now much more established, not only in the UK where it is mandated by key relevant regulatory bodies as a requirement for programme registration, but internationally as well. In other countries, we see examples of how 'involvement' has become increasingly embedded within education, even though it is not a curriculum requirement as it is across the four nations of the UK. However, that does not mean that it is any worse or better or more inclusive. You, the reader can decide on that, as you read the contributions of the special edition Parts 1 and 2.

Back in 2006, all the contributors to the special edition were based in the UK. For this special edition, we originally had 45 abstracts submitted representing 13 different countries, hence our reasoning behind creating and devoting a double special issue to this important topic. Interestingly, none of these submissions came from North America, even though our North American colleagues regularly contribute to the journal. We do not know whether this is because we use different terminologies for the same things or if there is something more structurally inbuilt in North American social work education that has decided that service users/clients should not, or cannot, be involved as key partners in the process. This is something we will try and find out more about.

In this, the first part of a two part special edition, we have contributions from five countries: Australia, England, Israel, Italy and Scotland. We have had contributions from those self identifying as service users, service users and academics, and by academics who are also service users (Fox). This provides the reader with a rich diversity and multiplicity of challenging intersections and perspectives. As this special edition highlights, these identifiers are fluid and are not fixed for life, but can and do change. Today's academic may be tomorrow's service user and vice versa, whilst not forgetting it is also possible to be both at the same time. This special edition sees both perspectives as essential for the continuing development of effective social work education and practice. For example, Fox identifies her hybrid identity, both as a social work academic and as a service user, as a strength allowing her to draw on different types of knowledge including experiential, practice and academic knowledge. In particular, she focuses on the place of experiential wisdom and how it can be shared in social work education.

However, it is also acknowledged that the service user perspective has often been silenced, othered or trivialised with the nature of its tacit knowledge deemed to be inferior to academic knowledge. This special edition seeks to challenge this view and argues that a healthy social work needs both practitioners and academics to be in a continuous dialogue with service users and carers learning with and from each other. In this way, we can ensure that the next generation of social work students will be fit for purpose and that we would be happy for them to be visiting us, or our families, in our time of need.

Part 1 of the special edition involves a wide range of service user groups including articles focusing on service users who are older people (Gutman and Ramon) those with a mental health diagnosis (Dorozenko, Ridley, Martin and Mayhoub, women in prison (Raikes and Balen) and those with learning difficulties (Ward, Raphael(C), Clark and Raphael(V)). The other articles contain the experiences of a range of service users and carers. Gutman and Ramon undertook a comparative research study to evaluate the involvement of older service users in social work education in Israel and England. One of the interesting findings from this study was that that the Israeli students valued the involvement of service users more so than those in England. It is suggested that this is because service user involvement is a new development. Dorozenko et al. describe a project in Australia which went beyond the norm of guest lecturing for people with experience of mental health services. In particular, they highlight the processes and findings from their Valuing Lived Experience Project.

Ward et al. argue that people with learning disabilities have traditionally been excluded for involvement in social work programmes. They then describe how their university worked with a man with profound and multiple learning disabilities who was commissioned to design and deliver specialist teaching to qualifying social workers. From this experience, they argue that it is our lack of imagination and our assumptions and attitudes about people's capabilities that are the real barriers to inclusion. Cabiati and Raineri, from an Italian perspective, also discuss how stigmatizing attitudes form barriers to working with service users and carers. In seeking to reduce these barriers, they describe the results from their project of exposing students to service users and carers and measuring the student's attitudes pre and post involvement on an attitudes scale and through the use of a qualitative interview. The results suggested that social work students showed reduced stigmatizing attitudes after this contact.

Raikes and Balen also recount their experiences of working with another often excluded group, imprisoned mothers. They discuss the development and findings of an inter-professional workshop between social work, police and nursing students in the UK. As a result of the workshop, the students reported an increased understanding of the challenges facing children whilst their mother was in prison and the need for inter-disciplinary work to provide an effective service to these mothers.

This leads onto Sen, McLelland and Jowett's article on the running of four 'living libraries' in which the 'living books' of the lived experiences of carers and service users are used to promote a dialogue between carers, service users, students, practitioners and social work educators. They also discuss how the living libraries were established, the ground rules for their use and their potential to impact upon social work education.

The other articles contain a range of service user groups whist Levy describes the results of a three-year experiential study in Scotland involving student social workers spending 15 hours with a service user and/or carers. During this time, the students are expected to discuss two policy practice questions, whereby the placement becomes both a site of knowledge creation and knowledge application in practice. One reinforcing and challenging the other.

Rooney, Unwin and Osborne report on a service user and carer led research project into the professional training of social workers and the influence of service users and carers. This qualitative research found that there were significant benefits for service users and carers, not only in terms of increased self-development, but also in increased confidence in managing their own care needs. This suggests that the benefits of such involvement are more far reaching than previously thought whilst such involvement may also challenge the increasingly marketized higher education culture.

As you can see, the range of articles on service user and carer involvement in social work education in this Part 1 edition, not only describe the processes of this involvement, but also seek to evaluate if it has been effective or not. The evaluations though, tend to be module/workshop specific and, except for Levy, which covers a 3 year period, tend not to be longitudinal. There is also a bias within these articles of being primarily qualitative. When we come to write about the articles in the special edition Part 2, these are themes we will return to and discuss further.

We feel we have now answered an important part of our question for this special edition. Service user and carer involvement continues to grow and has blossomed in many ways into an established way of working in many social work education settings across the world. The popularity of the special edition, evidenced by the number of submissions we received, is testament to the fact that there is a wealth of interesting work going on which we take immense encouragement from. The next special edition will feature additional aspects of this important topic. For now, we hope you enjoy reading and learning from the work included in this first part of our two special editions.

Guest Editors
Hugh McLaughlin, June Sadd,
Brendan McKeever, Joseph Duffy

INTRODUCTION

Service user and carer involvement in social work education – where are we now? – Part 2

This second of our special editions features papers which are linked by the following themes: international examples of service user involvement, the nature of service user knowledge, service user involvement in research and an analysis of the impact of involvement on subsequent social work practice.

The first paper by Ole Petter Askheim, Peter Beresford & Cecilia Heule provides an important focus on ways of addressing the gaps between service users and professionals that can characterise and shape social work practice. By using examples from social work practice and education in both Scandinavia and the UK, these authors argue that their experiences of meaningful partnership working in social work education can shine an important light on analysing both the opportunities and challenges that need to be considered.

The second paper by Merav Moshe Grodofsky & Carolyn Gutman brings service users and social work students together in an international context to examine perceptions of human rights. Again, a similar theme emerges about partnership working and the ingredients necessary for this to work between professional staff as providers and service users on the receiving end. The common experiences of exclusion and marginalisation shared by students and service users about human rights issues highlight the fact that the experience of *othering* is not something solely experienced by service users.

The third paper by Kieron Hatton interrogates the nature of service user knowledge and provides a necessary critical analysis. The author contextualises this debate on knowledge within a partnership approach to social work curriculum design involving service users. The paper mirrors the social work practice requirements around social justice and social change by examining how these key aspects are also entwined within the fabric of meaningfully collaborating with service users in the educational setting.

The fourth paper by Petra Videmšek reports on the findings of a project where social work students and service users collaborated together to research the views of mental health service users living in group care settings. This paper raises questions and issues around the contribution to research of service users whose skills and insights are based on their own lived experience. In this way, again we see the theme of knowledge being interrogated and where service user knowledge can be positioned within the overall continuum of what counts as *knowing*.

The fifth paper by Hilda Loughran & Gary Broderick again positions service users in an important and elevated position as examiners in the assessment of a Masters level social work programme. Again, what we see is that the social work educational context can be a potentially transformative site for influencing and shaping the types of inclusive social work practice that service users want from social workers when they qualify. So therefore, whilst such partnership working is important in the learning and educational context, this will amount to little if social workers when they qualify don't follow through on these important messages about involvement in their day-to-day work with service users and carers.

The final paper in this collection by Mel Hughes links to this latter point in its focus on evaluating the impact of service user and carer educational involvement on social work students' practice when they qualify. This is becoming an emerging area of research given that service user and carer involvement has now been part of UK social work education for about fifteen years but there are to date too few studies focusing on impact. Interestingly, this paper highlights the individualistic nature of how service user involvement impacts on students when they are in practice and are reflecting back on their learning. This paper therefore points educators towards reflections on how service user and carer involvement can be developed in ways which will further augment the learning experience for students, thinking ahead to when they qualify.

Ideas in Action includes a first for the journal with an article on the issues involved in participatory film-making between experts by experience, social workers and therapists by Yohai Hakak and Kevin Holmes. This is in keeping with the special edition and identifies an alternative way in which service users can contribute to the development of social work education.

We also include a book review by a German foster carer Andrea Kuhn and the foster child's sister Madeline Kuhn reviewing, from their perspective, reviewing the messages for foster carers and social workers working with a traumatised foster child. We would welcome further book reviews by service users and carers.

Reflecting on the question we posed for these two special editions, we feel we can express confidence that progress has been considerable in regard to the expanding way in which service user and carer involvement have taken hold within social work education. In particular, we want to highlight how what was a peculiarly UK initiative is now an international one. We in the UK now have as much to learn from our international colleagues as they do from us. It is however interesting to note that whilst we had abstracts from 13 different countries there were none from the US or Canada. It should also be noted that this way of working is not without its challenges as various authors have identified in special editions part 1 and 2, it often brings challenges from colleagues, service users and carers, academics and students. It is not to be entered into lightly, but we would argue that the benefits can outweigh the costs. It is also a form of education that requires academics to accept that they do not have all the answers and that co-production in learning is a positive development. There is a need to be open to sharing power and learning from others whether they be service users, carers or students.

It was good to see that we can now demonstrate a wider range of involvement building on service user and carer testimonies. We can now point to a host of examples to show creative and imaginative ways in which this important knowledge has been incorporated to assist students in their learning and development of practice insights. Increasingly, what we now see from these examples is how the educational setting has become a very important learning arena for students to understand how their social work practice needs to respond in meeting the needs of service users and carers when they qualify. This arena is also important for service users and carers representing a site for affirming self-esteem and promoting social justice.

It is also welcome to see the development of theorising to develop our understanding of service user knowledge and where and how this fits alongside other types of knowledge that are necessary for social work students in their learning. This further enquiry is now increasingly evident not only in looking at the contribution of user knowledges to education but also to research. The routine evaluation of service user involvement in social work education, common to all of the papers in this second edition, adds considerably to developing the evidence base to support and promote the contribution of user knowledge to education and research. In this way, the status of user knowledge is enhanced through the provision of evidence which is regarded as objective, thereby challenging the criticism of service user knowledge being too individualistic and subjective.

There are however, still challenges to overcome; the major of these is the continuing need to build up a bank of outcome evidence. Much of this work is still short-term and process driven in nature and we need more longer term evidence to identify how the involvement of service users and carers in social work education, both qualifying and post-qualifying, impacts upon the outcomes for service users and the quality of social work practice. There is also a need to continue to show that service user and carer's meaningful involvement in social work education is not merely a micro issue of improving individual practice, but also a macro issue challenging the grounds on which groups become 'othered' and where notions of 'deserving' and 'undeserving' are constructed. This is needed more than ever in a globalised world, still suffering the material effects of austerity politics, the increasing privatisation of social life and the growth of the independent and for-profit sectors alongside increasing ideologically motivated attacks on social welfare. It is the view of these editors; service user, academic, academic and service user, service user and academic, academic and potential service user, that social work education is richer and more relevant when it includes and learns from the experiences of those who are on the receiving end of social work practice.

Guest Editors
Joe Duffy, Brendan McKeever,
Hugh McLaughlin, June Sadd

Outcomes focused user involvement in social work education: applying knowledge to practice

Susan Levy, Rowan Aiton, Jade Doig, John P. L. Dow, Shireen Brown, Liz Hunter and Ryan McNeil

ABSTRACT

This paper discusses an innovative approach connecting service user and carer involvement (SUCI) in social work education to social work practice. The research team, comprised service users, carers, social work students and module leader, worked collaboratively democratising the research process. At the University of Dundee, a core social work module facilitates students to spend 15 h with a service user and/or carer (host) gaining a unique insight into their everyday lives. During this time, hosts and students discuss two policy practice questions, responses to these questions are generating annual qualitative data, with study findings being disseminated at local and national level. The experiential learning students acquire from spending time with their host becomes the site of knowledge creation through involvement that is applied to practice. This paper reports on the narratives emerging from the longitudinal data (2012–2015, $n = 90$) on the changing landscape of social care in Scotland and the dissemination of project findings. We explore the intersection where the voices of service users and carers, student learning and social work practice coalesce. A model of outcomes focused SUCI is introduced as a template for meaningful, sustainable and outcomes-focused SUCI in social work education.

Introduction

Debate around service user and carer involvement (SUCI) in social work education is maturing as the process of involvement is problematised. The context of involvement is being revisited through calls to broaden the focus on the 'how' of involvement to also include the 'impact' of involvement on student learning, social work practice and, ultimately the lives of service users and carers. The genesis of the SUCI in social work education debate is threefold, located in the mandatory requirement for SUCI in social work education (Scottish Executive, 2003), epistemological debates around knowledge production and what is valued as knowledge for social work education and practice (Beresford & Boxall, 2012), and outcomes of involvement in practice. Robinson and Webber's (2013) review of the SUCI literature found no empirical evidence on outcomes in practice, however, a recent paper by Tanner, Littlechild, Duffy, and Hayes (2015) has begun to address this omission.

This paper will contribute to moving this debate forward by providing a model for outcomes-based SUCI in social work education, linking involvement to knowledge creation that is taken into practice. The model draws on data from work completed by social work students whilst spending time with service users and carers as part of a core module, Community Care and the Caring Experience (Caring Experience), MSc Social Work, University of Dundee, Scotland. The research team (module leader, three MSc Social Work students and three members of the university Carers and Users (CU) group) have worked collaboratively drawing on individual strengths to analyse and disseminate the study findings to local and national stakeholders involved in social care, and to write this paper.

The paper first situates the study within the literature on SUCI, the Caring Experience module and the study methodology. The findings are then discussed and connections made with student learning as a site of knowledge production that is disseminated in social work practice. Whilst this study is located within the policy and practice context of social work in Scotland, our model for knowledge creation through SUCI that is applied to practice provides a template for use in different professional and international contexts.

Literature context: SUCI in social work education

Over the last decade SUCI has moved from being a marginal activity, perceived as an innovative addition to students' learning, into the mainstream of social work education. Policy intervention can be identified as a primary catalyst for this change, and certainly making involvement mandatory on qualifying programmes in Scotland (Scottish Executive, 2003) and the rest of the UK (Department of Health, 2002) has been influential at a strategic level. However, the work of the disability movement and disability theorising can't be overlooked in laying the foundations in challenging expert knowledge and the value of other knowledges (Beresford & Boxall, 2012). This is coupled with the framing of social work education within a discourse of social justice, inclusion and anti-oppressive practice (Levin, 2004). In contrast, within the broader field of SUCI in social work practice and research, a managerialist/consumerist approach prevails.

The managerialist approach is embedded within the prevailing neoliberal discourse that has re-shaped social work over recent decades. It has utilised user involvement and partnership working as a means to sustain structures of oppression and marginalisation at the same time as cost cutting through austerity. Involvement framed within neoliberalism has failed to achieve meaningful redistribution of power, as the scope for individual service users to achieve a voice and respsonsibility in decision-making has been within narrowly defined boundaries. Involvment has been understood as a bureaucratic requirement rather than a meaningful redistribution of power. As McLaughlin (2009, p. 1106) argues, '[T]he act of involving service users has become more important rather than providing more effective services'. Thus, a culture has emerged that has valued a consumerist and procedural approach to practice over activism, change and social justice, leading to SUCI becoming a mechanism for sustaining, not challenging, the hegemonic discourse (Carey, 2009; Cowden & Singh, 2007; McLaughlin, 2010; Tanner et al., 2015).

Within social work education, a critical lens is beginning to problematise SUCI as the discussion and focus of involvement evolves and matures. The papers in a 2006 Special Issue of Social Work Education: The International Journal captured the infancy of the concept of SUCI with attention coalescing around the process of 'how' to involve people. A decade later, SUCI within social work education is becoming an essential norm in Scotland and the UK. This is creating a space for a new discourse on involvement, with attention focusing on whether it is 'meaningful' and 'effective'; including 'meaningful' to who: students, service users and carers or practitioners? and 'effective' where: student learning, social work practice, the everyday lives of service users and carers or policy? In doing so, the question has shifted from the 'how' of involvement to a focus on 'impact' and 'outcomes' (Irvine, Molyneux, & Gillman, 2015; Rhodes, 2011; Rummery, 2009). Robinson and Webber's (2013) literature review on SUCI in social work education used a modified version of Kirkpatrick's (1967) framework for the evaluation of training, making it relevant to social work education (Carpenter, 2011) and SUCI (Morgan & Jones, 2009) (Table 1). This review highlighted that current work continues to unite around the process of SUCI, but 'there are gaps in literature about SUCI that aims to add value to social work education rather than to empower service users and carers' (Robinson & Webber, 2013, p. 927).

Internationally, whilst the language used may vary, for example, 'consumer' in the USA, the concept of SUCI in social work education remains largely in the embryonic stages, and 'is still limited' in Nordic countries (Askheim, 2012; Schön, 2016). A series of papers on SUCI in social work education in Central Europe appeared in a Special Issue of Ljetopis Socijalnog Rada (Bašic, 2009; Bornarova, 2009; Brkić & Jugović, 2009; Džombić & Urbanc, 2009). These papers evidence the early stages of integrating involvement into social work programmes in Central European countries. The papers also engage in some of the fundamental epistemological challenges of involvement, of shifting accepted understanding of knowledge and knowledge creation towards recognising that service users and carers' experiential knowledge of policy, practice and services has value, and they are 'experts by experience' (Scheyett & Diehl, 2004; Stevens & Tanner, 2006). 'Traditionally service users have been left out of the process of theorizing and understanding their experiences, echoing their wider absence from the academy and processes of knowledge production' (Warren & Boxall, 2009, p. 281). Bašic's (2009) work in Bosnia and Herzegovina calls for social work education to move away from hegemonic ownership of knowledge and knowledge creation, and to open up a space for other knowledges including the voices of service users and carers to be valued in social work education, through the adoption of a broader view

Table 1. Framework for Evaluation of Educational Programmes (Robinson & Webber, 2013, p. 929).

Level 1a	Learner perceptions	Students' views on their learning experience and satisfaction with the training
Level 1b	Service user or carer perceptions	Service user or carer views on their involvement experience
Level 1c	Staff perceptions	Staff views on involving service user or carers
Level 2a	Modifications in attitude and perceptions	A measured change in attitudes or perceptions towards service users or carers, their problems, needs, circumstances or care
Level 2b	Acquisition of knowledge and skills	A measured change in understanding the concepts, procedures and principles of working with service users or carers, and the acquisition of thinking/problem solving, assessment and intervention skills
Level 3a	Changes in behaviour	Observation of whether the newly acquired knowledge, skills and attitudes are evident in the practice of the social worker
Level 3b	Changes in organisational practice	Observation of wider changes in the organisation/delivery of care, attributable to service user or carer involvement in an educational programme
Level 4	Benefits to users and carers	Assessment as to whether there is a tangible difference to the well-being and quality of life of service users or carers who receive social work services

of knowledge (Brown & Young, 2008). A critique of this 'broader view' is pertinent here to make sense of which voices are/aren't being heard in SUCI. Cowden and Singh (2007, p. 5) caution against 'professional users' those with the experience and knowledge of how the system works, in the language of Bourdieu (1992) those with cultural capital, becoming the privileged voice of service users to the exclusion of silent, hard to reach groups. A focus on the former risks perpetuating current hierarchies of knowledge rather than challenging the outcomes of neoliberalism on the lives of CU (Cowden & Singh, 2007; and Tanner et al., 2015). The question of the representativeness of SUCI is fundamental if there is a genuine openness to listen, learn and change, and to avoid service users being selected to 'fit' and conform to existing knowledge, language and structures (Stickley, 2006).

The links between epistemology and SUCI are now visible in the literature and current social work education, the logical next step is to apply service user and carer knowledge, as well as the knowledge students' acquire from spending time with service users and carers, to practice, and to the lives of the people that social workers work with (Levels 3 and 4, Table 1). In a recent Swedish study, Schön (2016) explored the reasons why service users and carers participate in social work education. The paper concludes that the main reasons for participation are to share their lived experience, to help improve services and to obtain respect for their own personal knowledge and experience. Service users and carers clearly envisioned their involvement having an impact on practice. Yet Robinson and Webber (2013) found in their literature review, that 'no studies evaluated its (SUCI) effect on social work practice' (pp. 925, 926). Whilst progress is being made in SUCI, Campbell's (1996) argument that involvement can appear tokenistic and lacks meaningful outcomes has retained its relevance over two decades (Brkić & Jugović, 2009; Burrows, 2011; Carey, 2009; Sadd, 2011). McLaughlin (2009) and Robinson and Webber (2013) have called for greater SUCI in social work education that explicitly engages with outcomes in practice (Levels 3 and 4, Table 1). This paper begins to fill this lacuna through introducing a model of outcomes based SUCI that takes knowledge, created through social work students spending time with service users and carers, to practitioners and policy-makers.

Outcomes-based SUCI in social work education: community care and the caring experience module

The Framework for Social Work Education in Scotland (Scottish Executive, 2003) has been salient in driving change in SUCI. The framework introduced a 'requirement' for SUCI in social work education, where previously it had been 'desirable'. In response to this change, a CU group was established at the University of Dundee. The group is active across the BA (Hons) and MSc Social Work qualifying programmes, including in the admissions process, teaching, role play and the chairing of the Programme Board. A key area where the CU group has 'real influence' is the MSc core module, Community Care and the Caring Experience (Caring Experience). The module involves students spending a minimum of 15 h with a carer or service user (host family) to observe and to learn from them. The module was initially entitled 'Making Sense of the Caring Experience' (Gee, Ager, & Haddow, 2009) and facilitated for students to spend 24 h (across a number of weeks) with a carer. Over time, the module has evolved in response to the changing policy and practice landscape of social care, including being renamed the 'Community Care and the Caring Experience', students spending 15 h instead of 24 h with their host family, and hosts, whilst initially only carers, are now both carers and service users. These changes have retained the kernel of the module; of enabling students to learn first-hand about the day-to-day lives of service users and carers in a safe environment where they can ask questions and learn from the experiential knowledge of their host.

Host families comprised members of the CU group as well as service users and carers connected to local organisations. The module leader works closely with local organisations to identify individuals and families who would be interested in participating in the module, and people volunteer to participate. Experienced hosts lead on introducing new hosts to the module and the role of the host. Feedback from our hosts highlights that they value the opportunity of participating in the module and that it enables them to respond to the question:

> How can we share our real life experience of receiving services and supporting those who require services with students who will, after graduation, be the very professionals we will rely upon to deliver the services we require? (Member, Carers and Users Group)

Methodology

This study has used participatory forms of inquiry with the module leader working collaboratively with three members of the CU group and three MSc Social Work students. Creative methodologies for SUCI (Duffy, Das, & Davidson, 2013) have been used with qualitative data collection being integrated into students' assessment; a formative assignment written as a response to two policy practice questions (Figure 1). The policy practice questions were written by the CU group and were designed to capture discussions between hosts and students. The responses to the policy practice questions (n = 90) represent a narrative on the lived experience of social care policies and service provision.

The policy practice questions were introduced to the Caring Experience module in 2012–2013, data used for this paper cover the three-year period: 2012–2013, 2013–2014 and 2014–2015. Over the three years, 90 students have completed the Caring Experience module, with each submitting a response to the two policy practice questions (500 words per question). Twenty-eight hosts have welcomed students into their home over the 3 years, seven hosts have been involved in the module each year, three for two of the three years, leaving 18 who were involved for one of the 3 years. Ethical approval for the study was received by the University of Dundee's ethics committee. The responses to the policy questions have two different functions: as a formative assignment for the Caring Experience module as well as research data. This difference was explained to the study participants (students and hosts) and consent was received separately and specifically for using the data for research

Qu. 1 If your host family could give a message to policy makers in your local authority/health board about the services and supports they require, what would that message be?

Qu. 2: As practitioners of tomorrow and after having experienced this module, are there issues or concerns that you or your host family would like to see highlighted for future practice development?

Figure 1. Policy practice questions.

purposes. Both students and host families were given the option to request that any data pertaining to them be removed from the data-set. All participants gave their consent for inclusion in the study.

The responses to the questions were written by MSc social work students, however, they were co-constructed, where possible, with their hosts. Our hosts volunteer to support students and are keen to take an active role in the students' learning journeys. As such, students discussed the questions and their responses with their hosts. There was inevitably variation amongst hosts with regard to the level of engagement, understanding and interest each had in the specific questions, and students were responsive to this when working on their assignments.

On submission of the students' assignments, the responses were anonymised and grouped together under each question. The module leader worked with members of the CU group to analyse all of the data (2012–2015), and MSc social work students joined the research team for the analysis of the 2013–2015 data. Regular team meetings and email exchanges ensured an ongoing dialogue between researchers at each stage of analysis and writing. The researchers used thematic analysis to identify dominant and prevailing themes in the data. This was achieved through members of the research team analysing sections of the data separately and then coming together to share identified themes allowing for the cross-checking of emerging themes to add rigour to the process. Once themes were agreed, they were divided between team members for further analysis. The findings presented in this paper cover some of the key themes that are threaded through the data (Table 2), full coverage of the findings can be found in the bi-annual reports (Levy, Hunter, Dow, & Dowson, 2014; Levy et al., 2016).

Findings

The findings below explore the everyday lives and challenges of service users and carers and the knowledge they have acquired through these personal experiences. The quotations are the words of MSc social work students that have captured the social care experiences of their host family.

Working with this longitudinal data has allowed for the temporal context of emergent themes and knowledge creation to be explored. This has revealed how the themes of 'communication, information and relationships' resonate over time as well as being reinterpreted over time by our host families. The following section explores these themes along with the interconnections between them. First, the quotations below provide an insight into the positive impact that SUCI has had on students' learning.

> the caring experience above all has made an indelible mark on my social work practice. (2012–2013)

Table 2. Key themes.

2014 Report	2016 Report
Communication	Communication
Information	Information and access to services
Services	Relationships and partnership working
Choice	Austerity
Transitions	

> One important experience gained from this module by both hosts and the students is that working together in a sensitive and respectful manner is vital not only in this module, but also in wider practice. … it enables the practitioners of tomorrow to gain an insight into service users' lives. (2013–2014)

> It made me realise how hard it must be for families to allow two complete strangers into their lives and to pass over very personal information. (2014–2015)

In contrast to the students' accounts of their experience of user invovlement, host families talked of feeling distant and remote from the decision-making process in relation to the services they receive. With tokenisitc involvment compunding feelings of disempowerment.

> Service users deserve input into the services that they receive. This ensures service users are in an empowered position. They can identify who and what works well for their own needs. Services which are user led enable control, choice and empowerment. (2014–15)

> Lack of communication from professionals and not being informed of up to date information about services was a key issue within my host family. (2013–2014)

A tension appeared to emerge between hosts' expectations of what involvment ought to mean and the reality of their experiences. This connects to the juxtaposition between what appears to be offered by the involvment discourse, and the reality of its limitations within the prevailing neoliberal context (Cowden & Singh, 2007).

Communication, information and relationships

Communication and information are contested concepts that resonate across the three years of data collection. These concepts appear to be contingent on external variables such as the policy context which is leading to them being re-interpreted and redefined over the years by our host families. A prevalent and persistent narrative in the data is that social workers need to listen to service users and carers more and involve them in decisions affecting their lives and the lives of the people they care and support.

> … all involved with working with carers and service users need to communicate more and improve their communication skills. (2012–2013)

> There isn't enough communication or enough time spent to understand the lives of carers and service users. They are more than tick boxes and pieces of paper. (2012–2013)

> As a practitioner of tomorrow and having experienced this module I think it is essential that everyone takes away the important message of good communication and listening to everyone involved. (2014–2015)

In the 2014–2015, data-set new issues started to emerge related to communication, in particular, inter-professional communication and professionals being pro-active in communicating and providing information. Students noted how their host families were frustrated with having to repeat the same information to numerous professionals, time and again, and they couldn't understand why there isn't better communication between different professionals involved in their care. There was however, optimism for change with the integration of health and social care heralding new integrated working practices from April 2016 in Scotland (Public Bodies (Joint Working) (Scotland) Act 2014).

Over the three years of the data, host families articulated a need for social workers to be more pro-active in initiating conversations, asking questions and in providing relevant and up-to-date information. However, a transition appears to be emerging with regard to the type of information our host families are expecting to access. In the earlier data, interest centred on information about the different services that were available to them, with practitioners seen as the gatekeepers, the 'care managers' of these services. In the most recent data, the narrative appears to have shifted towards accessing information that will assist service users and carers to make decisions about activities that are more holistic than narrowly defined social care services. This connects with the current policy discourse of personalisation and outcomes-based approaches. Access to information can now mean information on personal social care services, but it may also mean information on inclusive yoga classes and/or information on training courses to develop skills to prepare for employment. This increased appetite for information relates to our hosts wanting to exercise their right to greater choice and control in their lives. Without information, they are unable to make informed decisions about the services they receive and opportunities to lead a life that they value (Sen, 2009). The tensions between our hosts' changing expectations and their lived experiences were quite marked with families identifying limited professional knowledge and the ways that information is gathered and shared as barriers to them accessing information.

> They felt that their local authority doesn't provide enough information and feel that the reason the council can't provide it is that the information hasn't been properly pulled together. (2014–2015)

> A lot of the services are not very well publicised and therefore more effort needs to go into making the public more aware of the support they could be offered... social media could be used in a more positive way to promote services and available support. (2014–2015)

The centrality of personalisation and relationships within the changing social care policy context in Scotland requires a fundamental shift in the social work role and how social workers interact with service users and carers (Lymbery, 2014). The data highlight how our host families are interpreting and re-defining relationships that are meaningful to them. They articulated the need for social workers to recognise service users and carers' knowledge (other knowledges), to work closely with service users and carers to empower them to be active partners in decision-making and to allow their voice to be valued and heard.

> ... professionals need to invest the time in order to gain knowledge and more importantly an understanding of each individual's unique situation. This therefore highlights the importance of professionals working in partnership with users of services and carers in order to allow experiences to be shared and to allow for a deeper, perhaps, more emotional understanding of an individual's needs. (2012–2013)

> Building trusting relationships requires the investment of time and the rejection of the position of the distant professional. My host describes bad practice as a worker who is 'clock watching'. He suggests the worker ask themselves: 'Did I put myself in their position?' This talks of empathy and stresses the importance of understanding the service users' perspective. (2013–2014)

Outcomes focused SUCI in social work education: applying knowledge through involvement to practice

Through spending time with their host family, students gained from a unique learning experience and developed their understanding of the everyday lives and challenges of service users and carers. This experiential knowledge is relevant to students at an individual level, for their own personal and professional development; this knowledge also has the potential to be relevant at an organisational and policy level for influencing change in social work practice. It is at the organisational level that this study contributes to building new evidence on outcomes-based SUCI in social work education impacting on practice. The findings discussed above provide an insight into some of the issues that have emerged in our data over the last three years, issues that are timely and relevant to the prevailing discourse on social care policy and practice. We have used these findings to start to bridge the current divide between SUCI in social work education and social work practice (Robinson & Webber, 2013), between knowledge creation through SUCI with social work practice (Beresford & Boxall, 2012) and to respond to the expectations of service users and carers that their participation in social work education will impact on practice (Schön, 2016). Our first report (Levy et al., 2014) was distributed to stakeholders involved in social care at local and national level. These stakeholders ranged from local authorities and voluntary organisations, to the Scottish Social Services Council, NHS Education for Scotland and the Scottish Government. Some organisations communicated that they would be using the report for planning purposes and some uploaded it onto their website. However, the research team agreed that more creative and interactive ways of disseminating the findings would have the potential for greater impact and wider reach. For 2016, the findings report and its distribution to stakeholders has been retained (Levy et al., 2016) but complemented with face-to-face dissemination through a knowledge exchange workshop at a national social work conference and the presentation of the findings at local authority practitioner forums. These dissemination events have allowed for knowledge exchange between practitioners, academics, policy-makers, service users, carers and student social workers. Discussions have been structured around applying the study findings to practice and the sharing of knowledge and experience, a process that is generating new knowledge that can be applied to social work practice and education. The dissemination of the study findings at these face-to-face events and the opening up of space for discussion, re-interpretation and application to practice is developing more meaningful and a more nuanced engagement with the concept of outcomes-based SUCI. It replaces a unidirectional process of knowledge transfer between social work education and social work practice, i.e. the dissemination of a findings report (Levy et al., 2014), with a cycle of knowledge creation and knowledge exchange through SUCI in social work education (Figure 2). Figure 2 highlights the key elements of our four-stage relational model of outcomes-focused SUCI in social work education. Stage 1: SUCI in Social Work Education. The Caring Experience module facilitates for social work students to spend time with service users and carers. This shared experience leads to Stage 2: Knowledge Creation. A student assignment becomes data that are analysed collaboratively (module leader, service users, carers and social work students) and prepared for dissemination. Stage 3: Applying Knowledge to Practice. This is achieved through sharing and discussing findings with relevant stakeholders and importantly, facilitates for the voices of service users and carers to be represented in practice. Stage 4: Knowledge Exchange, through opening up a dialogue between academics, service users, carers and students with stakeholders involved in policy and practice, the process of applying knowledge to practice itself creates new knowledge that can be introduced into Stage 1. This model is a framework for sustainable SUCI in social work education that makes user involvement functional and fully integrated into student learning. However, it is premised on the basis that service user

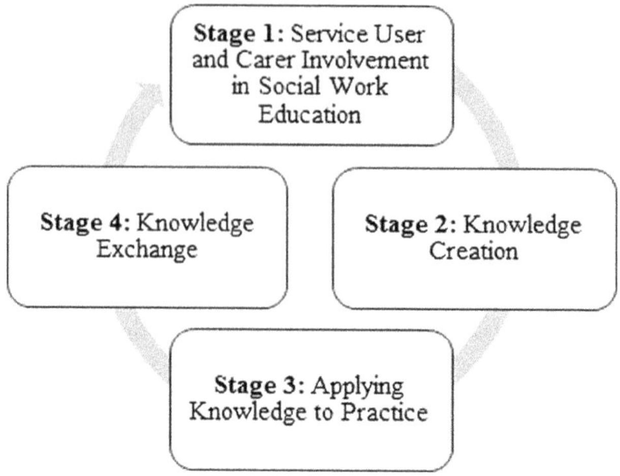

Figure 2. Outcomes focused service user and carer involvement in social work education: applying knowledge through involvement to practice.

and carer experiences are conceptualised and valued as knowledge that can be applied and is relevant to social work education and practice.

Conclusion

SUCI in social work education needs to retain its focus on the process of involvement and the building of evidence on the impact of involvement on student learning. There is also the need to evidence work that is challenging the hegemonic ownership of knowledge and knowledge creation (Bašic, 2009; Beresford & Boxall, 2012), as well as developing evidence on applying knowledge through SUCI to practice. This three pronged approach to SUCI suggests a maturing in the debate around involvement. Whilst this must be acknowledged, Campbell's (1996) claim, that SUCI in social work education lacks meaningful outcomes, still resonants today. This was confirmed in Robinson and Webber's (2013) literature review that highlighted the absence of evidence on outcomes-based SUCI in social work education being applied to practice. Our outcomes-based model begins to connect with Levels 3 and 4 of Robinson and Webber's (2013) framework for the Evaluation of Educational Programmes (Table 1). Whilst we acknowledge that we are in the early stages of understanding the impact of our findings on practice, the process is in place and further empirical work will be completed.

Meaningful and effective SUCI in social work education introduces epistemological challenges to established understandings of what is knowledge, what knowledges are valued and specifically, what is valued as knowledge within social work education and social work practice. For this to happen, a broader lens on knowledge is required that isn't confined to 'expert' knowledge, but embraces and utilises experiential knowledge that is inclusive of marginalised and silent voices. This approach unsettles the prevailing neoliberalist and manageralist discourse and refocuses the lens of social work on communication and relationship-based practice (Henderson & Forbat, 2002; Smith et al., 2012), of getting to know service users and carers at a personal level, and working with them to elucidate agreed outcomes for their lives. Working collaboratively to reach these ends, requires valuing service users and carers as individuals and valuing the knowledge and experience they have of living with a disability and/or as a carer. The Caring Experience module creates opportunities for students to learn through experience about personalisation and other fundamentals of social work practice in the twenty-first century. There is a logic in applying this experiential knowledge to practice, and this study evidences how student learning through SUCI becomes the site of knowledge production taken into practice. This process becomes a vehicle for the voices of service users and carers to be represented in practice. The outcomes-based model to SUCI used in this study is premised on social justice and operates at the intersection where the voices of service users and carers, student learning and social work practice interconnect to develop meaningful, sustainable and outcomes focused SUCI in social work education. It is hoped that this study will open up a space for future dialogue and that the model will be used as a template for SUCI in social work and other professions elsewhere in Scotland as well as internationally.

Funding

No funding was received for this project.

ORCiD

Susan Levy http://orcid.org/0000-0001-6556-5043

References

Askheim, O. (2012). 'Meeting face to face creates new insights': Recruiting persons with user experiences as students in an educational programme in social work. *Social Work Education, 31*, 557–569.

Bašic, S. C. (2009). Service user involvement in social work practice, education and research in the federation of Bosnia Herzegovinia. *Ljetopis Socijalnog Rada, 16*, 241–267.

Beresford, P., & Boxall, K. (2012). Service users, social work education and knowledge for social work practice. *Social Work Education, 31*, 155–167.

Bornarova, S. (2009). User involvement in social work education: Macedonian perspective. *Ljetopis Socijalnog Rada, 16*, 279–298.

Bourdieu, P. (1992). *An invitation to reflexive sociology*. Cambridge: Polity Press.

Brkić, M., & Jugović, A. (2009). Experience of service user involvement in the education of social workers in Serbia. *Ljetopis Socijalnog Rada, 16*, 469–481.

Brown, K., & Young, N. (2008). Building capacity for service user and carer involvement in social work education. *Social Work Education, 27*, 84–96.

Burrows, H. M. (2011). Evaluation of the involvement of service users in post-qualifying social work education. *Social Work and Social Sciences Review, 15*, 44–56.

Campbell, P. (1996). The history of the user movement in the United Kingdom. In T. Heller, J. Reynolds, R. Gomm, R. Muston, & S. Pattison (Eds.), *Mental health matters* (pp. 218–225). Basingstoke: Macmillan.

Carey, M. (2009). Happy shopper? The problem with service user and carer participation. *British Journal of Social Work, 39*, 179–188.

Carpenter, J. (2011). Evaluating social work education: A review of outcomes measures, research designs and practicalities. *Social Work Education, 30*, 122–140.

Cowden, S., & Singh, G. (2007). The 'User': Friend, foe or fetish? A critical exploration of user involvement in health and social care. *Critical Social Policy, 27*, 5–23.

Department of Health. (2002). *Requirements for social work training*. London: Author.

Duffy, J., Das, C., & Davidson, G. (2013). Service user and carer involvement in role-plays to assess readiness for practice. *Social Work Education, 32*, 39–54.

Džombić, A., & Urbanc, K. (2009). Involvement of persons with disability in the education of social work students. *Ljetopis Socijalnog Rada, 16*, 375–394.

Gee, M., Ager, W., & Haddow, A. (2009). The caring experience: Learning about community care through spending 24 hours with people who use services and family carers. *Social Work Education, 28*, 691–706.

Henderson, J., & Forbat, L. (2002). Relationship-based social policy: Personal and policy constructions of 'care'. *Critical Social Policy, 22*, 669–687.

Irvine, J., Molyneux, J., & Gillman, M. (2015). 'Providing a link with the real world': Learning from the student experience of service user and carer involvement in social work education. *Social Work Education, 34*, 138–150.

Kirkpatrick, D. L. (1967). Evaluation of training. In R. L. Craig, & L. R. Bittel (Eds.), *Training and development handbook* (pp. 87–112). New York, NY: McGraw-Hill.

Levin, E. (2004). *Involving service users and carers in social work education* (Report No. 4). London: Social Care Institute for Excellence.

Levy, S., Aiton, R., Doig, J., Dow, J., McNeil, R., Brown, S., & Hunter, L. (2016). *Social care in Scotland: Learning from the real life experiences of services users, carers and social work students* (Report No. 2). Dundee: University of Dundee.

Levy, S., Hunter, L., Dow, J., & Dowson, E. (2014). *Social care in Scotland: Learning from the real life experiences of services users, carers and social work students* (Report No. 1). Dundee: University of Dundee.

Lymbery, M. (2014). Understanding personalisation: Implications for social work. *Journal of Social Work, 14*, 295–312.

McLaughlin, H. (2009). What's in a name: 'Client', 'Patient', 'Customer', 'Consumer', 'Expert by Experience', 'Service User' – What's next? *British Journal of Social Work, 39*, 1101–1117.

McLaughlin, H. (2010). Keeping service user involvement in research honest. *British Journal of Social Work, 40*, 1591–1608.

Morgan, A., & Jones, D. (2009). Perceptions of service user and carer involvement in healthcare education and impact on students' knowledge and practice: A literature review. *Medical Teacher, 31*, 82–95.

Rhodes, C. (2011). User involvement in social work education: A concept analysis. *Nurse Education Today, 32*, 185–189.

Robinson, K., & Webber, M. (2013). Models and effectiveness of service user and carer involvement in social work education: A literature review. *British Journal of Social Work, 43*, 925–944.

Rummery, K. (2009). Healthy partnerships, healthy citizens? An international review of partnerships in health and social care and patient/user outcomes. *Social Science and Medicine, 69*, 1797–1804.

Sadd, J. (2011). *'We are more than our story': Service user and carer participation in social work education* (Report No. 42). London: Social Care Institute for Excellence.

Scheyett, A., & Diehl, M. J. (2004). 'Can we talk?': Using facilitated dialogue to positively change student attitudes towards persons with mental illness. *Journal of Teaching in Social Work, 24*, 39–54.

Schön, U. K. (2016). User and carer involvement in social work education: Reasons for participation. *Scandinavian Journal of Disability Research, 18*, 154–163. doi:10.1080/15017419.2015.1063539

Scottish Executive. (2003). *The framework for social work education in Scotland*. Edinburgh: The Stationery Office.

Sen, A. (2009). *The idea of justice*. London: Harvard University Press.

Smith, M., Gallagher, M., Wosu, H., Stewart, J., Cree, V. E., Hunter, S., ... Wilkinson, H. (2012). Engaging with involuntary service users in social work: Findings from a knowledge exchange project. *British Journal of Social Work, 42*, 1460–1477.

Stevens, S., & Tanner, D. (2006). Involving service users in the teaching and learning of social work students: Reflections on experience. *Social Work Education, 25*, 360–371.

Stickley, T. (2006). Should service user involvement be consigned to history? A critical realist perspective. *Journal of Psychiatric and Mental Health Nursing, 13*, 570–577.

Tanner, D., Littlechild, R., Duffy, J., & Hayes, D. (2015). 'Making it real': Evaluating the impact of service user and carer involvement in social work education. *British Journal of Social Work*, 1–20. doi: 10.1093/bjsw/bcv121.

Warren, L., & Boxall, K. (2009). Service users in and out of the academy: Collusion in exclusion? *Social Work Education, 28*, 281–297.

Lessons from a comparative study of user involvement

Carolyn Gutman and Shulamit Ramon

ABSTRACT
Grounded in the context of the significant differences in service user involvement in social work education and research between the UK and Israel, a joint project between Anglia Ruskin University in the UK and Tel-Hai College in Israel was developed. Its aim was to develop a comparative research methodology to evaluate the outcomes of service user involvement in social work education. A main tenet of our research methodology consisted of partnering with a group of older people who used health and social care services as co-researchers from each country. This co-researching methodology together with the evaluation tools worked effectively in the two respective countries. The key findings highlight that while students in both countries valued the involvement of service users in their training, this occurred more so in Israel, where this is a very new development. Students in both countries developed rich concept maps illustrating the complexity of such an involvement. Yet, while the responses of both groups to vignettes describing user involvement scenarios reflected the positive impact of such an involvement, the UK students focused on the negative impact of potential risk more so than the Israeli students.

This paper looks at service users' involvement (SUI) in social work education within a comparative action research project conducted cross-nationally between an English and an Israeli university (Anglia Ruskin University (ARU) in the UK and Tel Hai College in Israel). Consistent with our belief in the value of recognizing and incorporating the service user perspective into social work education, this project aimed to evaluate students' views of SUI in social work education and to engage service users as co-researchers. The collaboration between the two sites was developed in the hope that such a cross-national comparison may lead to a deeper understanding of these relatively new types of involvement in both countries (Hantrais, 1998).

The paper will first outline the rationale behind the involvement of service users in social work education, conceptually and developmentally in the two countries. It will then focus on the research process and methodology, describing the comparative evaluation tools and evaluation framework, and the involvement of older service users as co-researchers. Key findings will be presented together with lessons to be learned from such a study.

Service user involvement

Client participation in the intervention process lies at the heart of all aspects of social welfare practice, in which service providers should enhance service users' self determination to secure their active involvement as part of a more effective shared work between them and social workers (Allan, Pease, & Briksman, 2003). The professional codes of ethics in both the UK and Israel state that workers are expected to aspire to clients' optimal collaboration in the intervention process. While in the UK the first steps in this direction have been in place for more than a decade, in Israel this professional focus is just beginning.

In Israel, the generally accepted term for those who use health and welfare services is client—emerging from a neoliberal discourse—whereas in the UK they are referred to as 'service users' (Beresford et al., 2006). While recognizing that the term service user is not clear-cut and may limit us in viewing 'the totality of the person through the prism of their service user status' (McLaughlin, 2015, p. 154), it has been adopted in this paper to assure consistency in our collaboration, and refers to people who 'have or have had long-term experience of health and social care services or would qualify to receive such services' (Beresford et al., 2006, p. 4).

Service user involvement in social work education

In the UK, SUI has been a formal feature of social work education since the early 2000s (Levin, 2004), originating in the social model of disability (Oliver, 1997), where the body of professional knowledge in social work (and other helping professions) was enriched with service users' experiential knowledge (Beresford & Wallcraft, 1997). Formally recognized through the adoption of General Council of Social Care regulations in 2003, this involvement requires the inclusion of service users in the planning and delivery of social work programs (Levin, 2004). In practice, this often translates into service user involvement in the teaching of courses, involvement in the admissions process, development of the course curriculum and marking. However, the involvement of service users in research on social work practice and social work education is a more recent, non-mandatory, development (Ramon, 2003).

The problematic aspects of this innovation include the considerable ambiguity of the terms used (McLaughlin, 2009a), the difficulties encountered in maintaining meaningful user involvement in training and especially in research (McLaughlin, 2009b), and the claim that, while not aiming to do so, it serves a primarily neoliberal ideology (Carey, 2009). Due to space limitations, these issues cannot be addressed here, but the authors do recognize that they are helpful in identifying concerns that deserve further attention. Nevertheless, SUI has the potential to contribute to reducing power differentials and promote more collaborative relationships between service users and workers in both social work education and research, through recognition of the knowledge service users bring to social work and its value. Key potential barriers to meaningful and respectful SUI were identified at the outset of this project and addressed (e.g. accepting co-researchers' chosen titles, pay at the same rate as qualified researchers).

In contrast to the UK, service user involvement in welfare training in Israel is still in its infancy; there is no formal recognition of service users' contribution to social work education and research. Influenced by the British model and recognizing the value of service user involvement for students, Tel Hai college had established two third-year undergraduate social work courses that include ongoing pedagogic contributions of service users as part of the curriculum: The first of these two courses is in gerontological social work that includes older adults as participants (Hantman, Ben-Oz, Gutman, & Criden, 2013), while the second is a disability course, in which a national disability movement activist serves as an ongoing co-teacher throughout the year together with the first author (Gutman, Kraiem, Criden, & Yalon-Chamovitz, 2012). In both countries, the evaluation of the contributions of user involvement in social work education is still in its early stages, despite the recognition of its necessity (Burrows, 2012).

Service users as researchers

The emerging UK discourse about service users' participation in the research process is characterized by an increasingly complex array of terms such as service user research, emancipatory research, user-led research and user co-researchers (Beresford, 2002), each highlighting a different focus for the role of the service user in the research process and representing a continuum of involvement in research. They also refer to different levels of training for undertaking research roles and tasks. This new approach challenges traditional positivist perceptions of the creation of knowledge by uninvolved researchers, supporting the value of alternative types of research for knowledge building (McLaughlin, 2009b). It also enables people with limited formal knowledge of the research field to undertake specific research tasks, as may be the case with co-researchers.

The involvement of older people as co-researchers

While mental health and physically disabled service users have led the way in service user research (Ramon et al., 2014), additional user groups, such as older people are now showing interest. Existing ageist stereotypes may hinder such involvement, together with concerns about the possible additional time and costs incurred when involving them meaningfully in the research process (Dewar, Jones, & O'May, 2004).

Despite these reservations, there is increasing evidence that collaboration with older researchers in social research offers a significant tool to 'improve the relevance, quality, and impact, and thus the social value, of the research' (Delman & Lincoln, 2009, p. 140), resulting in richer and more relevant methodologies (Littlechild, Tanner, & Hall, 2015).

Systematic reviews conclude that the benefits of such an involvement include increased knowledge, awareness and confidence, meeting others in similar situations, empowering older people to become active in their community, improving community capacity for addressing needs of marginalized groups (Blair & Minkler, 2009). However, this type of participation may also give rise to dilemmas of power imbalances and interpersonal dynamics between the 'researcher' and the 'researched' (Ray, 2007, p. 80)

The study context

The two universities differ not only in being situated in different societies with different traditions of SUI, but also in that ARU is a large new university based in two urban centres, while Tel Hai is a municipal new college, based in a rural area near the northern border of Israel.

To the best of our knowledge, this is the first study attempting to compare user involvement in social work education on a cross-country basis. Such a comparison would highlight the shared components of SUI, as well as the context-specific components of this innovation, while indicating key process issues. This study was not aimed at increasing students' readiness to implement SUI in their future practice, rather focused on evaluating their attitudes to SUI and their knowledge about it.

Ethical approval was given prior to commencing the study by each university's ethics committee, according to each country's ethics regulations.

Methodology

We aimed to establish a comparative research methodology that evaluates students' views of service users' and carers' engagement on their respective courses, enabling their active involvement in research, while developing valid and feasible comparative tools.

The participatory action research model (PAR) (Reason, 1994) provided the study methodological framework, fitting well the inclusion of older people who use health and social care services as co-researchers. Earlier evaluations of user involvement carried out by the ARU team were valuable in assisting in the process (Anghel, Fox, & Warnes, 2010), as was its extensive experience in employing older people as co-researchers (Munn-Giddings, McVicar, Boyce, & O'Brien, 2009).

The co-researchers

ARU had previously developed a training course focusing on research skills for older people in health and social care. A number of graduates of this course established an independent research cooperative titled the Why Not Co-operative (Munn-Giddings et al., 2009) and four members of this group were commissioned by ARU to participate as co-researchers in the current study.

The Israeli group of older co-researchers was drawn from those who had participated in the third year gerontology course and expressed an interest in continuing their involvement with academia. At the outset, this group comprised eight members (Gutman et al., 2014).

The co-researchers in both groups were ambivalent about their title as service users, illustrated by the Israeli group's preference for being addressed as 'older adults', claiming that the term 'service users' was associated with frailty and dependency, whereas 'older adults' suggested maturity and wisdom.

The students

The evaluation was conducted with graduating students at the two sites: the UK group included third-year undergraduate students as well as those from the final year of the MA course. The Israeli students were third-year undergraduate students. These groups were selected because they had received more cumulative exposure to user involvement on their courses and because as final year students in all three programmes, they were about to embark on a social work career.

The tools

As stated, we aimed to create a comparative research methodology to evaluate the students' attitudes following service user involvement in their social work courses. To achieve a valid comparison between the sites, it was important that the evaluation methods be relevant to both cultures, with their different history of user involvement. Given that social work education is focused on preparing social workers to become qualified practitioners, the evaluation had to include a measure of students' readiness to implement such an involvement in their future practice. A formative evaluation was conducted, employing a blend of a multiple embedded case study (MECS) (Yin, 2002) within a PAR framework. The MECS approach focuses on triangulation of evidence from different data sources. Data were collected through the application of two tools, concept mapping and responses to a vignette.

Concept mapping is grounded in cognitive psychology, enabling visual organization of knowledge in a particular area, allowing the identification of what was learned, inclusive of gaps in knowledge. Originally developed for quantitative analysis and summative evaluation (Novak & Gowin, 1984), this method was used as a qualitative method in our project. This decision suited the formative purpose of the evaluation based on previous research conducted by the UK partner that applied concept mapping to the evaluation of social work education outcomes (Anghel et al., 2010), and adopted as the means to evaluate the interpretive nature of social work knowledge. The concept map task was open-ended to allow the students to respond by addressing concepts they considered most relevant to SUI in social work practice (Stoddart, Abrams, Gasper, & Canaday, 2000).

The students were asked to illustrate in a map format the key features of service user involvement in social work and their interrelationships, to demonstrate their meaningful learning of SUI, and how they conceptualize it in their practice.

Drawing on the UK partner's experience (Ramon, 2003), vignettes were chosen as the second tool. These are hypothetical scenarios often used in social work teaching, practice and research as a tool for considering likely responses to complex situations (Wilkes, 2004).

These short descriptions of real-life situations, followed by questions have been used to explore perceptions, beliefs meanings and likely course of practice regarding a particular situation in a variety of settings (Wilkes, 2004). They offer a helpful technique for evaluating outcomes relating to attitudes and perceptions as well as knowledge acquisition (MacIntyre et al., 2011) and for assessing the impact of practice learning on students' ability to integrate theory and practice (Fook, Ryan, & Hawkins, 2000). However, these responses may be only at the declarative and hypothetical level. Responses to vignettes may also offer the opportunity to compare different groups' interpretations of a situation (Charles & Manthorpe, 2009).

The vignette developed at ARU described a mental health-themed scenario in which the students would receive input in class from a recovering psychiatric survivor involved in paid peer support and then work with a client with a mental ill health diagnosis looking for employment during his recovery process. It aimed to highlight the potential of service users to use their experience to benefit other service users, as well as the issues involved in enabling such a development. The Tel Hai researchers then translated and adapted the vignette to reflect the key issues in the two electives they offer, namely gerontology and disability, taking into account the social work practice context in Israel.

Students in both countries were asked to specify how they would apply the learned values, skills and knowledge about SUI to the particular hypothetical client, and about their understanding of how such a context impacts on this specific case.

Co-researcher training

The ARU co-researcher group members had completed training in research methods two years ago, and since engaged in several research projects for the local authority and health trusts. The group selected which of its members would work in this project. In addition, they underwent a specific training with the project's research officer in the use of the study's comparative tools, namely c-maps and vignettes.

The Israeli co-researchers, who had joined the study with no previous research knowledge, participated in a training module in research methods, comprising two workshops led by the researchers from ARU together with the local team: the first addressed the objectives of the research project and the rationale behind service user involvement in academic research and learning, and the second introduced the co-researchers to interview skills for conducting face-to-face pilot interviews with a sample of third-year students as part of their training. This was followed by group meetings which focused on the rationale and process of analysing vignettes and c-maps.

Throughout the training, the Israeli co-researchers expressed their ambivalence about participation in the study. During the early stages, they expressed their satisfaction and sense of self-efficacy: but some were less enthusiastic about the concept maps and vignette analysis and spoke of the repetitiveness of working alone at home. This resulted in the re-establishment of group meetings led by the project coordinator to encourage the co-researchers' continued participation.

Data collection and analysis

All third-year students on the undergraduate social work degree at ARU as well as those in the second year of the MA social work degree course and all of the Tel Hai students who participated in the electives that included SUCI in their programmes were invited to participate in the study. Each student was requested to provide a c-map and responses to the vignette.

A total of 67 students participated in the study with 43 from Tel Hai and 28 from ARU. A larger percentage of the Tel Hai students participated in the study (70%) than of ARU students (20.5%), and more from the disability elective group. There were no indications that the students who participated in the study differed in any significant way from those who did not.

Tel Hai students completed c-maps and responses to the vignettes for the second time at the end of the academic year. Due to the differential structure of fieldwork in the UK whereby students are largely absent from college in the final semester of their training, this group was not available to complete the second stage of the study.

All c-maps and vignettes were analysed first locally by the co-researchers, researchers and lecturers. A sample of the Israeli data was analysed jointly by the English and Israeli researchers, and later together with the UK co-researchers, to ensure inter-researcher reliability and validity of the analysis. An Israeli researcher participated in the data analysis of a sample of the UK material together with the UK co-researchers for the purpose of improved reliability and validity of the analysis.

The responses to the questions asked in the vignettes were analysed thematically, following the widely used thematic analysis approach developed by Braun and Clarke (2006, 2014). Thus, references to each theme indicated in the questions were systematically grouped together for each respondent, then per each group of respondents, each country and finally compared at the cross-countries level.

Key findings

ARU students

The majority of ARU third-year BA students created elaborate and rich c-maps. Overall, they perceived SUI as offering a unique and valuable addition to their training which contributed to a fuller understanding of the complexity of the operational context of social work. As one student emphasized, this type of practice is *consistent with the core values of social work*. They perceive this involvement as being connected to client empowerment, making *service users feel empowered and in control*, promoting new and unique contributions to professional knowledge, framed in terms of *working with* or *alongside* the client, indicating a more equal power base in the relationship. A student identified the social worker's ability to be *open and honest* as making the *working together equal*. Another emphasized in her map *the service users are the ones who know themselves best* and that this type of practice focuses on *keeping the client at the centre*. Many students identified SUI as a non-academic practice, even though they had mostly encountered it in the college setting.

However, several of the Cambridge MA students provided elaborate maps focused on viewing SUI critically as a form of political manipulation aimed at neoliberal cost reduction, and as representing no more than a *buzz word*. This subgroup viewed SUI as practice that could potentially cause ethical dilemmas.

Tel Hai students

In the first stage, students from both courses created rich and complex c-maps that were more grounded in the emotional aspects of this type of involvement than conceptual ideas. However, there were differences between the two groups. The students in the old age elective focused on the relevance of SUI to the therapeutic relationships they were seeking to develop with their clients. This was reflected in terms of how SUCI enabled them as future social workers to become more accomplished professionals by overcoming their prejudices and perceiving the client's potential. One student identified *enriching knowledge* through *raising memories of elderly people in my life* and another *through looking at the old person in the context of all of his past*. Surprisingly, their emphasis on the worker–client relationship did not lead them to address the outcomes of SUCI for the client. Perhaps the emphasis on the one-to-one relationships in this course masked the students' perception of the collective role of service users.

The students in the disability course focused more on the need to eradicate stigma and to develop policies that would further client empowerment and the place of *social responsibility*.

They too found the experience of sharing the elective with service users very rewarding, allowing for an *authentic dialogue with both sides listening*, even though the service user involvement model differed between the two classes. This group of students viewed SUCI as an improved model of social welfare work, in which client dependency could be greatly reduced and resources better employed. For example, one of the students pointed to the fact that often *there are many bodies that provide parallel services to people with disabilities* and that *sometimes the services work in opposition to each other*.

Follow-up phase

In the old age elective, the enthusiasm for SUI continued to be largely expressed at the emotional level of its benefits for both workers and clients. However, the conceptual aspect continued to be less developed, perhaps due to the course's emphasis on experiential knowledge. The students seemed to use SUI as a tool with which to resolve tensions that emerged in their relationships with clients and in the context of the negative stereotypes in wider society of older people, and continued to be less concerned about the value of SUI for people who use services. Most of their c-maps remained at the descriptive level.

Likewise, in the disability elective, the enthusiasm for SUI continued, but took a different focus. The c-maps were much more elaborate than at the baseline stage, and included a mixture of concepts and links. They found the class experience exciting and viewed it as a model of good practice to be implemented in social work as a way of resolving some key barriers. A growing respect of service users' experiences and abilities was expressed, together with the wish for closer dialogue and mutual learning. Like the students in the old age elective, they too perceived experiential knowledge to be more important than theoretical knowledge, including concepts such as *authenticity* and *reciprocal learning* as part of their c-maps. Hence, for both groups, the follow-up phase highlighted an improved ability to produce more complex maps, but without significant changes in content.

The map below (Figure 1) illustrates several of the points raised above. For example, it specifies which theory is of relevance in the context of SUI and mentions the disability rights movement as a source, further linking it to social justice and social work values. The government and its regulatory body appear in the map and each is linked differently to

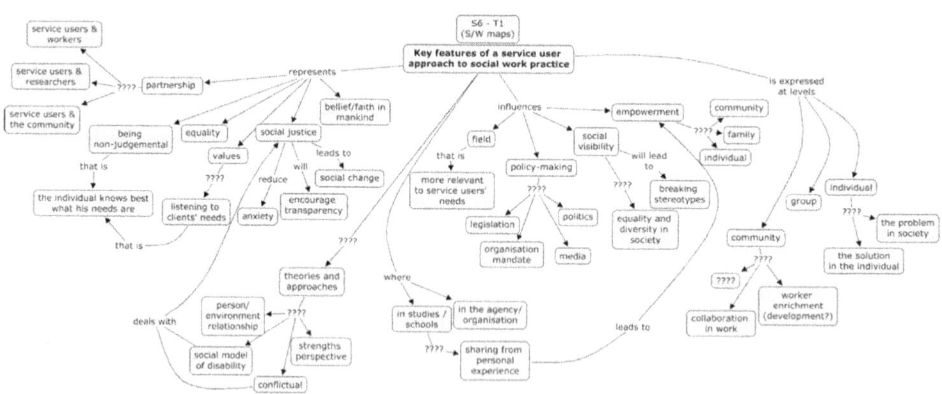

Figure 1. An example of a good c-map.

the concept within it (e.g. the General Social Care Council to professional guidelines, and government policy to lack of resources), thereby presenting a multi-layered description.

Responses to the vignette

Most of the respondents positively received the talk given by the service user activist, and valued its relevance to the client: *I felt upbeat about the talk because she (the user activist) was upbeat.* On the whole, the Israeli students were more enthusiastic than the UK students about the positive potential impact of this talk for the students' work with the hypothetical client in the future. As one student commented: *Now I see that people need to be in a power position for their wellbeing, through moving between a position of receiving to that of giving.* And another summed up by asserting that *service user led organizations are the future of social work practice*!

A minority of students in both countries did not like the negative comments made by the service user in the vignette about professional contributions to casework, where *service users' work with their peers was more important than that of the professionals, including social workers, and has the potential to radically change mental health services.* One student asserted: *It could have you feel less confident about yourself as a professional if Angela (from the vignette) and other service users can basically do your job;* and other students claiming that the comment was uncalled for and unjustified: *I would challenge the importance of service user work with peers....*

Both groups proposed that work with the client in the vignette should start with an assessment of the client's situation, abilities and difficulties, while attentively addressing his wishes. They then suggested acquiring more information about the proposed training programme referred to by the service user in the vignette before considering whether to support their client's request to apply to work with the peer support group. Some of the Israeli students considered arranging a meeting between the client and the user activist in order to help their client learn more about the peer programme before making a decision.

The UK students were more cautious in applying the principles of user involvement to the client and in following his wish to become a service giver, arguing that the risks involved have to be carefully considered. As one UK student surmised: *I would worry because of his refusal to take medications and because he has not attended the local mental health centre.* Some of the Israeli students also expressed their uncertainty about the client's readiness for this type of involvement, but did not phrase it so strongly in risk language.

A minority among students from both countries would have liked more information about the speaker's background as *she had provided no insight into her own circumstances or history of mental health,* while others stated that they would have liked to bombard her with questions.

Nearly all of the Israeli students mentioned the strengths approach as the key theory to rest their practice upon, together with the ecological approach. Yet relatively few of the English students mentioned specific theoretical frameworks to rely on; those who did, applied relevant approaches, such as IPS (Individual Placement Scheme) or brief solution therapy which are often developed outside the social work profession. Overall, key values mentioned included adhering to an equal opportunities policy and adoption of a nonjudgmental, non-oppressive, person-centred, respecting and empowering approach.

No differences were noted between the responses of the Tel Hai students in the two electives or in their responses at the beginning and end of the academic year.

Discussion

The project aimed to compare the evaluation of SUCI by social work students in both the UK and Israel using a PAR design that involved older people as co-researchers.

The data on the students' perceptions of SUCI were obtained through completion of c-maps and responding to questions on vignettes. Consideration of the co-researchers' experience was noted throughout the different stages of the project and reviewed during a summing-up focus group meeting.

Tools

The value of the chosen methodology was reflected in the ease of understanding the required tasks by the majority of the respondents, as well as the richness of the data collected, highlighting both the cross-cultural similarities and differences between the two populations studied.

The c-maps produced a rich, yet complex, understanding of the students' perceptions of SUI in both sites. They not only successfully illustrated the multiple variables and their interconnections reflecting the different cross-country cultural nuances, but also the different emphases of the different courses, i.e. mental health in the UK, and disability and ageing in Israel. Both teachers and students alike were enthusiastic about the possibilities of using the c-map as a tool in different aspects of social work training, including in the practice setting, such as with supervisors and clients.

The vignettes were also positively received by the students as offering the opportunity to think through the impact of SUI on practice. The vignette design comfortably crossed cultures and effectively mirrored the different practice setting in both countries.

Students' views

The similarities between the students in both sites included the positive view of user involvement, perceiving it to be an enriching and essential element of social work education and their future practice. A minority of students in both sites reacted defensively to critical comments made by the service user speaker in the vignette scenario, a finding that replicates the previous ARU evaluation study (Anghel & Ramon, 2009).

Perhaps this was viewed as a threat on their professional integrity, as well as anxiety about their professional identity and readiness for completing their studies and entering the workforce as a social work professional.

Another similarity between the two sites was the students' ambivalence between receiving detailed information about the user speakers, and their hesitation to ask them questions. This point touches not only on the encounter between service users and students, but also between students and their clients, regarding the ethical boundaries of respecting privacy as set out in the profession's code of ethics. As Kadushin and Kadushin (2013) warn, 'the line between interest and curiosity is thin' (p. 109).

Concepts of risk perception and its management were addressed to varying degrees in both sites. However, in the UK, this theme was more clearly viewed as impacting professional behaviour. Here, the students reflected the professional view that risk avoidance overrides key social work values such as self-determination. These students appear to view negative risk-taking (i.e. preventing risk to self and to others, as well as preventing failure) as being the practitioner's responsibility to ensure that action taken will not harm anyone.

They also overlooked the benefits inherent in positive risk-taking as key to further personal and collective growth (Ramon, 2005; Soyer, 1963). Perhaps the UK students reflected the local professional viewpoint, prevalent particularly in child protection and the mental health arena (Karban, 2011), which focuses on risk avoidance management at the expense of promoting social work's humanist values.

Furthermore, the difference between the two sites may be also be explained by the specific study context in each country. While in the UK, professional training and practice is embedded in a risk management discourse, this is not so apparent in the Israeli context, as reflected in the two Israeli courses.

The overall warm endorsement of SUI within both training and practice by most students, as indicated by their responses to the vignettes, highlighted how natural it seemed to them to have service users involved in a socially inclusive and empowering way in their training.

Was the data analysis enriched by the inclusion of co-researchers? As outlined above, the data analysis was carried out in groups of co-researchers together with qualified researchers. The professional researchers found the contribution of the co-researchers refreshing, as it focused on aspects of the responses previously taken for granted (Cotterell, 2008). For example, in exploring a concept map theme of *social work knowledge of service users,* the Israeli co-researchers proposed the inclusion of knowledge of family, history and self-identity, as necessary to create a portrait of the client as a unique person. The English co-researchers contributions focused on potential human rights issues and risk management thinking in their responses to the vignettes, thereby aligning themselves with the position of the service user activist.

As mentioned above, both co-researcher groups did not wish to be addressed as service users, although they were receiving health and social care services. While previous work suggests that the term restricts the individual's identity by identifying one aspect of their life (McLaughlin, 2015), our interpretation of this finding is that they did not identify with the prevailing stigmatizing cultural image of people receiving social welfare support as vulnerable and poor.

Limitations

The much smaller number of students from ARU who opted to participate in the study in comparison to the Israeli number represents a major limitation of this study. We believe that the UK students' college assignments and practice placement requirements in this their final year impacted on their willingness to participate in the study, together with the demeaning attitude to research that is often expressed by practitioners.

Another explanation may relate to the fact that the Israeli students who participated in the project were also involved in the classroom with the service users and felt a personal involvement in the project. Furthermore, service user involvement is an innovative project at Tel Hai College, and the course teachers' enthusiasm and investment in developing this type of participatory classroom was also reflected in the students' responses.

The differences between the views of the two groups of co-researchers may be explained by the prolonged vs. brief training, viewing the new role as one-time or long-term and importantly the significance of being part of a group rather than a collection of individuals.

Finally, while responses to vignettes may reflect how new knowledge may be integrated into practice situations, we recognize that there may be a gap between what the students say and how in reality this new knowledge is acted upon in the field.

Conclusions

On the basis of our work in this cross-cultural study of students' perceptions of SUCI, we believe that there is a compelling case for service user participation in social work education, service training and research. Our experience highlights clients' abilities and strengths, and sheds lights on a previously under-researched area in social work education, namely the contributions of service user involvement to students' training. Furthermore, we have seen that this type of participation increases the students' ability to not only connect to the world of the service user but also their ability to recognize the value of the contributions service users can make to their training and to professional practice. Highlighting the client's perspective and abilities offers not only an optimistic stance (Saleeby, 2009), but also supports the current tentative literature on the value of partnership with our clients for bringing about positive outcomes changes in their lives. However, following Cameron, Lart, Bostock, and Coomber's (2012) challenge that more research is needed to sharpen and broaden our understanding of the potential outcomes of such partnerships with service users, the current study highlights the need for additional empirical research on the outcomes of service user involvement in social work education for all stakeholders.

This project has reinforced our vision for social work education. This vision includes the place of older people as well as other service user groups, who will routinely be involved in the planning of learning goals and experiences for the students, in defining curriculum and coursework contents and promoting integration between the field and the academic courses. We have added another dimension—evaluating the students' level of competency in the social work course as it relates to understanding and applying the new knowledge of user involvement in social work education and in social work practice.

Acknowledgements

We should like to acknowledge our appreciation to the contributions of our research team, especially the service user co-researchers in both countries.

Funding

This work was supported by The British Council [grant number 50263].

References

Allan, J. M., Pease, B., & Briksman, L. (2003). *Critical social work: An introduction to theories and practices*. Crows Nest: Allen Unwin.

Anghel, R., Fox, J., & Warnes, M. (2010). An exploration of concept mapping as a method of evaluating student learning in social work. In H. Burgess & J. Carpenter (Eds.), *The outcomes of social work education: Developing evaluation methods* (pp. 34–50). Southampton: Higher Education Academy SWAP.

Anghel, R., & Ramon, S. (2009). Service users and carers' involvement in social work education: Lessons from an English case study. *European Journal of Social Work, 12*, 185–200.

Beresford, P. (2002). User involvement in research and evaluation: Liberation or regulation? *Social Policy & Society, 1*, 95–105.

Beresford, P., Branfield, F., Taylor, J., Brennan, M., Sartori, A., Lalani, M., & Wise, G. (2006). Working together for better social work education. *Social Work Education, 25*, 326–331.

Beresford, P., & Wallcraft, J. (1997). Psychiatric system survivors and emancipatory research: Issues, overlaps and differences. In C. Barnes & G. Mercer (Eds.), *Doing disability research* (pp. 67–87). Leeds: The Disability Press.

Blair, T., & Minkler, M. (2009). Participatory action research with older adults: Key principles in practice. *The Gerontologist, 49*, 651–662.

Braun, V., & Clarke, V. (2006). Using thematic analysis in psychology. *Qualitative Research in Psychology, 3*, 77–101.

Braun, V., & Clarke, V. (2014). What can "thematic analysis" offer health and wellbeing researchers? *International Journal of Qualitative Studies on Health and Well-Being, 9*. doi: 10.3402/qhw.v9.26152. Retrieved from http://doi.org/10.3402/qhw.v9.26152

Burrows, H. (2012). Evaluation of the involvement of service users in post-qualifying social work education: Expected and unexpected results. *Social Work & Social Sciences Review, 15*, 44–56. doi: 10.1921/095352212X655339

Cameron, A., Lart, R., Bostock, L., Coomber, C. (2012). *Factors that promote and hinder joint and integrated working between health and social care services*. London: Research Briefing 41. London: Social Care Institute for Excellence

Carey, M. (2009). Happy shopper? The problem with service user and carer participation. *British Journal of Social Work, 39*, 179–188.

Charles, N., & Manthorpe, J. (2009). An exploratory qualitative study of equity and the social care needs of visually impaired older people in England. *British Journal of Visual Impairment, 27*, 97–109.

Cotterell, P. (2008). Exploring the value of service user in data analysis: Our interpretation is about what lies below the surface. *Educational Action Research, 16*, 5–17.

Delman, J., & Lincoln, A. (2009). Service users as paid research workers: Principles for active involvement and good practice guidance. In J. Wallcraft, B. Schrank, & M. Amering (Eds.), *Handbook of service user involvement in mental health research* (pp. 139–152). Oxford: Wiley.

Dewar, B., Jones, C., & O'May, F. (2004). *Involving older people: Lessons for community planning*. Edinburgh: Scottish Executive Social Research.

Fook, J., Ryan, M., & Hawkins, L. (2000). *Professional expertise: Practice, theory and education for working in uncertainty*. London: Whiting and Birch.

Gutman, C., Hantman, S., Criden, W., Ben-Oz, M., Anghel R., & Ramon, S. (2014). Involving service users in social work education: Developing a bi-national participatory action research framework. *Educational Gerontology, 40*(3), 186–197.

Gutman, C., Kraiem, Y., Criden, W., & Yalon-Chamovitz, S. (2012). Deconstructing hierarchies: A pedagogical model with service user co-teachers. *Social Work Education, 31*(2), 202–214.

Hantman, S., Ben-Oz, M., Gutman, C., & Criden, W. (2013). Bringing older adults into the classroom: The sharing community model. *Gerontology and Geriatrics Education, 34*, 135–149.

Hantrais, L. (1998). *Cross national research methods*. New York: Bloomsbury.

Kadushin, A., & Kadushin, G. (2013). *The social work interview* (5th ed.). New York, NY: Columbia University Press.

Karban, K. (2011). *Social work and mental health*. Cambridge: Polity Press.

Levin, E. (2004). *Involving service users and carers in social work education*. London: Social Care Institute for Excellence.

Littlechild, R., Tanner, D., & Hall, K. (2015). Co-research with older people: Perspectives on impact. *Qualitative Social Work, 14*, 18–35.

MacIntyre, G., Green Lister, P., Orme, J., Crisp, B., Manthorpe, J., Hussein, S., … Sharpe, E. (2011). Using vignettes to evaluate the outcomes of student learning: Data from the evaluation of the new social work degree in England. *Social Work Education, 30*, 207–222.

McLaughlin, H. (2009a). What's in the name? "Client", "patient", "customer", "expert by experience", "service user" – What's next? *British Journal of Social Work, 39*, 1101–1117.

McLaughlin, H. (2009b). Keeping service user involvement in research honest. *British Journal of Social Work, 39*, 1–8.

McLaughlin, H. (2015). Alternative futures for service user involvement in research. In P. Staddon (Ed.), *Mental health service users in research* (pp. 137–157). Bristol: Policy Press.

Munn-Giddings, C., McVicar, A., Boyce, M., & O'Brien, N. (2009). Older people as researchers – Why not? *Working with Older People, 13*, 16–19.

Novak, J., & Gowin, D. (1984). *Learning how to learn*. Cambridge: Cambridge University Press.

Oliver, M. (1997). Emancipatory research: A realistic option or an impossible dream. In C. Barnes & G. Mercer (Eds.), *Doing disability research* (pp. 15–31). Leeds: The Disability Press.

Ramon, S. (Ed.). (2003). *Users researching health and social care: An empowering agenda?* Birmingham: Venture Press.

Ramon, S. (2005). From risk taking to risk avoidance in multidisciplinary mental health work. In J. Tew (Ed.), *Social perspectives in mental health: Developing social models to understand and work with mental distress* (pp. 184–199). London: Jessica Kingsley.

Ramon, S., Hantman, S., Anghel, R., Gutman, C., Criden, W., & Ben-Oz, M. (2014). Learning from a cross country evaluation of serivce users' involvement in social work education and research. In A. L. Matthies & L. Uggerhoj (Eds.), *Participation, marginalisation and welfare services: Concepts, politics and practices across european countries* (pp. 255–273). Farnham: Ashgate Publishing.

Ray, M. (2007). Redressing the balance? The participation of older people in research. In M. Bernard & T. Scharf (Eds.), *Critical perspectives on aging societies* (pp. 73–88). Bristol: The Polity Press.

Reason, P. (Ed.). (1994). *Participation in human inquiry*. London: Sage.

Saleeby, D. (Ed.). (2009). *The strengths approach in social work* (3rd ed.). London: Longman.

Soyer, D. (1963). The right to fail. *Social Work, 8*, 72–78.

Stoddart, T., Abrams, R., Gasper, E., & Canaday, D. (2000). Concept maps as assessment in science inquiry learning – A report of methodology. *International Journal of Science Education, 22*, 1221–1246.

Wilkes, T. (2004). The use of vignettes in qualitative research into social work values. *Qualitative Social Work, 3*, 78–87.

Yin, R. K. (2002). *Case study research, design and methods* (3rd ed.). Newbury Park, CA: Sage.

Belonging to the library: humanising the space for social work education

Robin Sen, Nora McClelland and Beverley Jowett

ABSTRACT

This article describes the running of four Living Libraries on a UK postgraduate social work course. A Living Library is a metaphoric remodelling of a conventional library where people, as authors of their experiences, provide specialist knowledge based on authorial areas of expertise. In the Living Libraries discussed here, 'Living Books' carried stories of social work—their narratives were of lived experiences as people using social care services; as carers in personal relationships with others who use social care services; or, as social work practitioners. The focus of this article is on those Living Libraries involving the participation of the first two of these groups. Drawing on social psychology, phenomenology and human geography, we propose that a Living Library can act as a connective space within social work education by engendering a discursive forum where all participants—people with experiences of services, students, practitioners and social work educators—are given both the freedom and obligation to talk openly about their differential experiences, fears and hopes for social work. Through this process, opportunities are created to consider how improvements that meet all stakeholders' interests may be achieved.

Introduction

In this article, we describe the running of four Living Libraries on a UK postgraduate MA in social work course. Two of the libraries were thought of as 'generalist' where people with experience of social work services[1] in any capacity were invited to take part, and two were 'specialist' libraries, themed around particular experience—in these instances newly qualified social workers (NQSWs) and young people with experiences of social care services:

- Library 1, Generalist Living Library I, September 2014
- Library 2, Generalist Living Library II, October 2015
- Library 3, Specialist Living Library, The Experience of The First Year in Social Work Practice, June 2015
- Library 4, Specialist Living Library, Young Person's Living Library, October 2015

While we draw on our experience of running all four libraries, the focus here will be on Libraries 1 and 4. We outline a vision for the Living Library as a connective space within social work education where students join people with various experiences of practice to hear different stories of social work. By exploring these narratives, participants can develop more nuanced constructions of relationships in social work that can start to accommodate the needs of different partners, including the professional responsibilities of social workers and the interests of people using social work services. The article starts by providing an overview of what a Living Library is. It then explores the rationale for developing a Living Library in the university setting for social work, drawing on ideas from social psychology, phenomenology and human geography. Thirdly, the running of the Living Libraries is examined in more detail. Finally, the operation of the libraries is reviewed, drawing on participant feedback, and some future possible developments are considered. A short film was made about Living Library 4 which is available online alongside some other materials relating to the different Living Libraries which have been run (The Living Library Repository, 2016, http://www.shef.ac.uk/socstudies/prospt/ppt/masocialwork/livinglibrary).

An overhead still of the library

A Living Library is a metaphoric remodelling of a conventional library where people, as authors of their experiences, provide specialist knowledge based on authorial areas of expertise. In our Living Libraries, Living Books all carry stories of social work—their narratives are of lived expertise as people using social care services; as carers in personal relationships with others who use social care services; or, as social work practitioners. Just like a conventional library, students may borrow a Living Book to read for a period of time, but in the Living Library reading is confined by the time and space of the classroom. As the author, the Living Book decides on their book title, has control over the content of their book and decides which chapters of their book they will share and discuss with their student Readers. Reading is a small-group interaction in the Living Library: Readers listen and talk with their Living Book, and in talking Readers also share their stories about their own experiences of social work with their book. The story exchange in a Living Library is comparable to a book-club meeting with the author who, after reading a chapter of their book aloud, opens up a discussion about their book with the audience. In turn, the audience share their stories about their reading the book and discuss what meaning the issues raised have for them. Before a Living Library closes, there is always an open plenary space where Readers and Living Books share their learning from their experience with everyone who has participated in the library.

The library metaphor works well as it identifies a place that most of us are familiar with. A recent report on the library service in England described libraries as providing safe places for literacy and learning (Sieghart, 2013, p. 5). In the USA, libraries are recognised by the Federal Emergency Management Agency (FEMA) as essential community organisations. When a disaster happens in a community people take shelter, seek advice and exchange stories in the public library. Narratives of what happened—sense making around profoundly difficult experiences—are developed within the library space which thereby serves as one where people 'reinforce social bonds and … establish norms of helping, cooperation, and reciprocity' (Veil & Bishop, 2014, pp. 18, 44). As with all metaphors, there are limits to the fit of the comparison. Birdi, Wilson, and Cocker (2008) provide a salutary insight that as much as community libraries are inclusive in policy and strategy, this can mask more socially exclusionary practices. However, the strength of the metaphor lies precisely in the normative assertion that the library can be a powerful place of communal meaning that we can all join and belong in together.

Libraries are also central places of learning in universities, repositories of knowledge, stored in books and other media, which any member can access. In the Living Library, expert knowledge is 'stored' in the stories of lived experiences told by the Living Books. Students access this specialist knowledge through reading with the Living Books in the Living Library space. Living Books do not substitute for academic or other practice-based sources of information, but they are accorded similar status to the academic texts and journals that social work educators direct students to read during the programme. The Living Library provides an additional repository of knowledge that broadens and enriches the range of knowledge available for students to read and learn from.

Within the library vaults: the challenge of the other

The original Living Library (The Human Library) was designed in Denmark as a means through which stereotypes and prejudices that undermine people's capacity to connect with fellow human beings could be openly examined and challenged (Abergel, Rothemund, Titley, & Wootsch, 2005). The core assumptions underpinning a Living Library are that when people meet and talk with each other they confront the beliefs or fears they have about the other. Their face-to-face encounter provides them with knowledge and greater understanding, which increases their capacity to empathise with others (Abergel et al., 2005). These ideas are rooted in the classic social psychology theory (Allport, 1954) which indicates that to have best effect the encounter needs to be experienced as real: participants in the Living Library are not role playing, they are together in the Library as themselves, and they are engaged together in a shared purposeful activity.

In considering the rationale for a Living Library, we also draw on Levinas' (1969) claims regarding the privileged opportunity which the face-to-face encounter with another human being presents. Away from the co-present encounter Levinas (1969) argues our conception of 'the Other' may be reduced by positioning them as objects within our own framework of understanding, necessarily delimiting their otherness. The intensity—the pleasure, the simultaneous proximity and distance, sometimes the sheer awkwardness—of the face-to-face encounter demand a recognition of the alterity of the other, and from this also a recognition of our ethical obligations to them as a being separate from and different to us (Levinas, 1969). Some connection may be seen between this strand of Levinas' work and Merleau-Ponty's (1962/2013 edition) focus on the embodied nature of human experience. Critiquing the traditional dualist separation between mind and body, particularly the exaltation of cognitive thought, Merleau-Ponty asserts that the body is the means through we are, act and know the world. For Merleau-Ponty (1962/2013), therefore, embodied experience is the basis for our engagement in the world and for reflective thought. For Levinas (1969), the face-to-face encounter is the basis for our engagement in the world, where the face may be viewed as the 'corporeal emblem of the other' (Waldenfels, 2002, p. 63). While there is an ongoing debate as to how far communication mediated by digital technology may simulate or replace face-to-face communication (Sen, 2015), the Living Library is unashamedly premised on the power of the co-present, embodied, encounter with another being who is different to us and from whom we are ethically obliged to learn. The Living Library places a demand on Readers to recognise, explore and reflect on the otherness of both the Living Books they encounter and their fellow Readers. Through this, it reinforces their obligations to take account of the insights of the lived experiences of social work practice which Living Books and fellow Readers hold.

The initial suggestion of running a Living Library on our course was made by a person with experience of services who was assisting us to review the MA course. We were concerned to examine how particular formulations of the involvement of people with experience of services could create barriers to envisioning the multitude of different partnership arrangements there might be between people who use and provide services in social work. Too often this involvement can be limited by oversimplified constructions that constrain the interactions that people with experience of services and students have in the classroom. We want our students to be curious and to develop a range of skills for communication and critical thinking. But, in the classroom, our shared experience had been that students listened politely and rarely questioned, or got into meaningful discussion, with people with experience of services about their own understandings of social work, particularly when it appeared these might hold alternative constructions of what social workers' roles and responsibilities should be. It was as if the stories of people with experience of services were sacrosanct in the classroom.

We agree with many, like Gupta and Blewett (2008, p. 469), that people with experience of social work services are 'essential ingredients' for social work education but it does seem that we only talk about their involvement as teachers for social work in classroom settings (*learning about practice*). Explicit recognition of their role as teachers in practice placements is missing in the literature and research in this area (Anghel & Ramon, 2009; Beresford & Croft, 2004; Robinson & Webber, 2013; Sadd, 2011). We have also noticed students' acknowledgement of this role is often missing in their discussions about practice-based experiences where discourse is principally about learning to 'do' social work. Students' focus in placement tends to be on establishing a professional identity and developing knowledge of the roles and responsibilities they will have as social workers (*doing practice*). Concern to achieve a professional social work identity seems to obscure the educative role people with experience of services actively play in students' practice, and their contribution to students' learning becomes primarily defined in relation to social workers' *doing of* the practice. This separation erects a barrier to the development of meaningful partnerships with people with experience of services. As alternative, primarily employer-based, training models for social work are privileged in England through Government sponsorship, there is a challenge for universities to maintain a connective space for social work education. If *teaching about* social work goes on in the academy and *learning to do* social work goes on in practice placement then the university space for social work education needs to better connect these two domains. The involvement of people with experience of services is central to this ambition.

How to develop the authentic involvement of people with experience of services is a constant challenge. Fox (2011) considers if and how people with experience of services can be treated as equals in the academic community whilst also having their needs considered. To form meaningful partnerships for practice, we all need to be freed up to articulate our own views of what social work is, and might be, and examine the differences—the 'otherness' (Levinas, 1969)—there may be between us as potential partners. As Jenkins

(2008, p. 102) implies identity entails establishing the things that might separate us as well as the commonalities that can unite us, for 'defining us involves defining [...] thems'. The Living Library attempts to achieve this by establishing a connective space, to which we now turn in more detail.

Spanning boundaries in and out of the university: the library as connective space

Research from human geography highlights how space can undermine or enhance particular inequalities through the ways in which people who occupy it are identified, and the status they are accorded within a given space according to that identity (Valentine, 2007). A core transformative aim of the Living Library is as a space which develops the possibility of different, multiple, constructions of the identities and relationships social workers and people who use social work services have. Discursive exchange in the Living Library also helps us to think about how these identities and relationships span the boundaries of the spaces which social work occupies. To take an illustration, some of our students bring prior or current experiences of using services to the libraries, while some with experience of using social work services who have been involved in teaching on our course also carry experience as social work practitioners. Over and above these particular instances of multiple role identities, the Living Library can provide a connective space by engendering a discursive forum where 'we'—people with experiences of services, students, practitioners, social work tutors—are given both the freedom and obligation to talk openly about our differential experiences, fears and hopes for social work. Through this process, opportunities are created to consider how improvements that meet all stakeholders' interests may—or may not—be achieved. While participants have different roles as Living Books, Readers and Librarians (social work tutors) all are accorded equal status. This is underpinned by an interdependence and interconnectedness for the purpose of knowledge production and exchange within the Living Library space: Readers need Books, Books need Readers, Libraries require Librarians and Librarians need good Books and enthusiastic Readers. This embodied interconnectedness is comparable to social work practice where there is an interdependence between the people who use social work services and the people who provide them. Indeed, the relational co-construction of knowledge in the Library resonates with the (re)turn to relational engagement and embodied ways of knowing within contemporary social work practice (Broadhurst & Mason, 2014).

It would be naïve to think that membership of the Library space overcomes the multiple layers of social exclusion those with experience of services encounter within and outside the academy (see Warren & Boxall, 2009). However, nor is the accessing of social space trivial, both reflecting social relations and helping produce/reproduce them in ways that help or hinder how different people interact and influencing how they identify themselves and others (Hopkins, 2011; Valentine, 2007). The running of the libraries has made us consider how the university space can be more genuinely opened up to those with experience of services. Some Living Books have told us that they felt they did not previously have permission to enter the university buildings where we have held the Living Libraries. Our university, like many others, was set up by community subscription so that people in the community could benefit through the different ways—educational, cultural and economic—a university can contribute to community life. The buildings are key landmarks in the community landscape. Many applicants to our programme have told us how the university architecture, the buildings they walked past as children, influenced their aspirations to study here. Yet, though these buildings might meaningfully be said to belong to the community, the pulls of the university teaching and research excellence agendas are exclusionary, delimiting membership to those who may be deemed to 'excel' in given ways. While the narratives of those with experience of services may be reified during teaching inputs in the university classroom, outside of these selective times the university space can reinforce their exclusion. For this reason, several social work education projects have chosen to instead work in the community settings where service users live (see Duffy & Hayes, 2012).

Our choice to undertake the Living Libraries within the university is deliberate—we wanted to recognise the university as part of the place where people live and grow up, and therefore part of their identity (Valentine, 2007). We have envisaged the Living Libraries as spaces which are meaningfully shared by different stakeholders who are connected through a relationship of mutual interest and investment in social work education. This has brought us to consider how open the university space is to those with experiences of services beyond the temporal and spatial boundaries of the Living Libraries themselves. Although a small symbol of our wish to open up our own university space, we were able to facilitate university library access for two people who wanted to use them, following their participation as Living Books. One later told us of her surprise and pleasure when, reading in one of the university libraries, she was recognised by a social work student she had previously met in the Living Library and, just as two people meeting might do, they had a conversation. The experience is related here to represent the way in which the Living Library may be part of a process of opening up the borders of social work education: it can create possibilities for multidimensional experiences of fellow human beings that go beyond the restricted constructions we might hold of each other arising from the single role identity bestowed through provision or receipt of social work services.

Glancing inside the library doors

Library 1 was a full-day event involving, at different points in the day, students joining the course and students starting their second year following completion of a first period of assessed practice. Living Books were recruited by email circulated through a range of different networks and follow-up telephone conversations. The opportunity to narrate experiences of social work in person clearly appealed as we had a good response (see *Book Titles* below), including people who had not, to our knowledge, ever previously been involved in social work education. The format appears to be one through which we might therefore foster greater inclusion and diversity in our partnerships with people. Living Books who participated had a range of expertise through experiences of mental distress, learning difficulties, physical disabilities, non-verbal communication, surviving childhood trauma, life at older age, foster care and caring for a partner through terminal illness. It was made explicit to all members of the Living Library that it was a place where every Living Book had full control over the story they wished to share, their book title, and the time they wanted to spend in the library. Some people chose to bring supporters with them, some decided to spend a half day and others a whole day. Living Books also had the freedom to restrict Readers' questions to certain areas of their experience if they wished, though most felt comfortable responding to all that were posed. We are aware that a Living Library requires Living Books to narrate personal, and often difficult, experiences to groups of people they do not know. Amongst other things, this could reawaken feelings associated with those experiences. We are mindful of providing appropriate support to Living Books before a Library so they are aware of what to expect during an event. We also ensure we 'check in' with Living Books soon after a Library to get a sense of how they experienced it. However, we have also taken a deliberate stance that we do not vet Living Books. The decision on whether to participate is left to a Living Book to take, sometimes in discussion between them and their supporters.

In Library 1, all the Living Books were authored by adults. Our reflections on this led to Library 4. We recognised that young people with experience of services are often poorly represented within our university space, as they tend to be within social work education more generally. There are complex dynamics affecting which social groups access particular spaces (Valentine, 2007) but a very practical barrier to younger young people's engagement with the university space is the overlap between the university teaching calendar and school or college timetables. Consequently, we arranged to run Library 4 in the school half-term week and worked with a local partner organisation to identify young people with experiences of social work who might wish to take part. We were conscious of the potential spatial dynamics of young people accessing an unfamiliar place (Hopkins, 2011): some young people who were interested in participating might have reservations about being in a space traditionally restricted to adults, particularly perhaps those who did not see themselves going to university or have family members who had done so. We therefore chose to limit this library to our second-year students and two of us met with the young people a week before the event in a space familiar to them, a venue used by the organisation we were working with. This meeting allowed us to explain how the process of 'authoring' a Living Book could work and provide a short embodied example of a Living Library exchange in which one of us (RS) was the Living Book, and the other (NM) the curious Reader.

In the Living Library, student Readers are allocated into small reading groups of between four and seven students, with reading group exchanges taking between 45 minutes and an hour each time. The interaction in reading groups may be thought of as student-led small group teaching (Dennick & Exley, 2004) guided by a Living Book. Tutors' primary role is to ensure each reading group is set up and working, and to facilitate the plenary session at the end of the Living Library. Students know they must complete reflective tasks after the exchanges and this may help structure their questions, but discussions are also fluid and open-ended, facilitating the exploration of different perspectives. In Library 1, we gave students a particular focus according to their stage of learning on the programme. First years were asked to think about what people who have experience of using services find helpful and unhelpful about social workers and to later record their reflections. Second years were asked to undertake and present a 'Living Book review' to their Living Book at the plenary session at the end of the day. The plenary sessions add a workshop element (Dennick & Exley, 2004) to the small group collaboration evident in reading groups, facilitating the sharing of learning between all Library participants.

In Library 1, we also asked second-year students to create something tangible and personal to give to their Living Book—a letter, picture, piece of creative writing or whatever else they decided was most appropriate. We construed this as a gift created and given by the students to the Living Books in return for the gift of knowledge the Living Books had given them, reflecting the ethos of exchange and reciprocity within the Library. We felt we could enhance the reciprocal exchange further and so, in Library 4, we arranged an undergraduate student-led tour of the university for the young people taking part in the Living Library. The tour highlighted the university space as one they might choose to access afterwards, either as local residents or as potential future students. As another aspect of the exchange, after the young people had presented their experiences as Living Books, some of our MA students became Living Books, articulating their own narratives in choosing to study social work, with both fellow students and the young people as Readers within the small reading groups. The library thereby constituted a knowledge exchange where social work students learned from young people's experiences of services, and young people had the opportunity to develop insights into why someone might choose to pursue a career in social work, and how life experience might have influenced that decision.

The voluntary exchange of experience was one of the essential principles of the original Human Library: participation is a gift from which both Living Books and Readers derive benefit (The Human Library, 2015). While our course normally offers payment to people with experience of services for their involvement in teaching, we have explicitly not done so for participation in Living Libraries for this reason. We have offered any financial support that was needed to facilitate participation—mainly transport costs (taxis, bus fares, petrol and parking) and the payment of costs for any support Living Books required to attend. We were also committed to making the libraries welcoming and hospitable spaces, so refreshments have been available throughout the days. In Library 1, due to budgetary constraints, refreshments were only available to Living Books and we excluded students. During discussions with Living Books afterwards, it dawned on us that, to our embarrassment, this created a division which was contrary to the spirit of equality and interconnectedness within the Living Library. We managed to access funds to offer refreshments to all in Libraries 2 and 3 and in Library 4 we adopted the practice of 'Jacob's Joints', whereby tutors and students each brought some food in to share for lunch and everyone—the young people, their supporters, tutors, social work students and undergraduate students who had led the university tour—ate together before the Living Library commenced.

Book titles from Living Libraries 1 and 4 are given below by means of an illustration. It should be borne in mind that some titles may give an indication of what the stories might be about while others do not:

Living Book titles Living Library 1

- Life after trauma
- My marbles and how I lost them. Volume two: The wilderness years. Containing special Limited Edition bonus chapters
- I'm a lunatic
- Right then! what's next?
- A person centred life
- Recovery: Fighting back
- Saved from closure
- Living with anxiety
- Living with disability in a normal world
- If I were a book
- Leap of faith
- My life as a carer

Living Book titles from Living Library 4

Authored by young people

- Uncertainty and Joy
- Live and Let Live
- For Those Who Care
- Diaries of a Self-Confessed Moron
- Changes and Shape Shifters
- An Old Shoe & a Used Tampon: Diaries of a Boss Ass Bitch
- Don't Judge a Book by its Cover

Authored by social work students

- 360°: Turning (–) into (+)
- 4's the Charm
- Great Expectations
- Choices
- Why am I here?
- A Series of Unfortunate Events … Ends in a Rainbow
- Forgiveness
- Behind enemy lines
- Social Work? You must be crazy!

Several Living Book authors chose titles that appear to play with negatives stereotypes and labelling they had encountered. The possibility of 'non-derogatory in-group use' of language as a progressive form of re-appropriation has been documented (Croom, 2013). But, such language can also serve as a source of tension and discomfort when its use extends across the boundaries of a given 'in-group' and 'out-group', and because it seems to jar with values which social work education seeks to promote around the challenging of discriminatory labelling. Such potential tensions, though, precisely illustrate the expectation to engage in dialogical exchange which the Living Library provokes. Questions around the differential use of language, and the experiential basis for it, can start to be explored and unpicked. Though this is not without its challenges for all involved, it is part of what makes the embodied encounters in the Living Library meaningful, real and developmental.

Surveying the library

We did not set out to undertake a formal evaluation of the libraries. Rather, we took stock of their operation by primarily considering information that was already available to us. This consisted of the following:

- Feedback from those with experiences of services or their supporters shortly after the Libraries on their experience of being a Living Book in Libraries 1, 2 and 4 (n = 13).[2]
- A review of students' mandatory written reflections on Libraries 1, 2, and 4 undertaken shortly after the Libraries (n = 204).

Additionally, six months after Library 1 and two months after Library 4, we made a request to students to provide us with:

- Any further reflections they had on the impact of the libraries, if they wished to provide them. We received a modest number of responses to the request ($n = 21/152$).

A thematic analysis of the comments and reflections was undertaken (Braun & Clarke, 2006) and brief excerpts are used below to illustrate three core themes. Permission to use comments was provided by their authors. Though there were some suggestions for improvement (see below), their overwhelming tenor suggested the Living Library experience had been developmental for Living Books and Readers. The Living Libraries are nonetheless a small part of the curriculum and, in the absence of more robust longitudinal data, we acknowledge that is no certainty such feedback has translated into better practice, and consequently, better outcomes for the people our students will work with. While, as Carpenter (2011) argues, this final consideration is the ultimate arbiter of social work education, the challenges in clearly establishing that any educational input has indubitably met it are manifold, and educators often have to gauge whether teaching will positively affect students' future practice on less than full information. Alongside our own insights from running the events, the comments and reflections collected on the Living Library experience do sustain a reasoned belief that it carries the potential to positively influence participants' approaches to social work practice.

The first theme, from the feedback from Living Books and their supporters, was a view that narrating experiences in the Library had made a difference. This was in two ways—Living Books felt that students Readers valued and respected their stories, and connected to this, that the exchanges were thereby influencing future practice:

> Pleasure to be involved, I prefer smaller groups of students ... more chance of good interaction, and from a service user viewpoint, you get a better feel for how they are in and around the people they will be working with. It's not just the professional that is assessing things, service users also do it to a lesser degree, "Can I work with this person, do I feel comfortable, and more to the point, can I trust them?" (Living Book, Library 1).

> It's definitely worth taking part as these people are going to be the social workers of the future, it is the perfect medium in which to articulate your concerns to shape social work practice in the coming years. (Living Book, Library 4).

For student Readers, the power of accessing direct narratives about good and poor social work practice resonated strongly. The embodied face-to-face encounter with the other (Levinas, 1969; Merleau-Ponty, 1962/2013) meant the messages conveyed were persuasive and compelling:

> Continuity and consistency are vital. You are a stranger going into someone's home, you must build a relationship with them. You are dealing with human beings, not the problem on its own. (1st Year Reader, Library 2, Immediate feedback on one thing they had learnt from a Living Book).

> Being able to ask the foster carer's honest opinion was the most valuable experience. Normally when working with service users it's not always appropriate to question them in such depth or with such freedom! (1st Year Reader, Library 1, Immediate Feedback).

The proportion of students who provided comments some months after the libraries was small, and it is unclear how well they reflect the overall cohorts' thoughts. In the comments which were provided, however, the power of the first-hand narratives of social work practice in the Living Library exchanges remained a salient theme. This suggested the possibility of their enduring influence:

> What has stayed with me is how people have been affected both positively and negatively by social workers. I always knew this was the case, however hearing it first-hand has more of an impact. (2nd Year Reader, Library 1, 6 Months After).

> The Living Library was an exceptional opportunity to see how social workers were perceived through the eyes of a young service user. The most significant learning point was to understand how social workers' dishonesty created feelings of distrust, anxiety and oppression (2nd Year Reader, Library 4, 2 Months After).

There were also indications that some students carried learning from the Library exchanges into their subsequent practice placements, providing illustrative support for the contention that the Library can function as a connective space between the *learning about* and the *doing of* social work:

> My book's belief that her being labelled as diagnosis X involved a barrier to good practice, in that she was treated *as* a diagnosis, was interesting. Later informed my understanding of the medical model being less person-centred. (1st Year Reader, Living Library 1, 6 Months After).

> I asked [the foster carer] how she felt when she had brought up a girl from a matter of weeks old and she was adopted when she was 18 months and the de-attachment not only for the child but for the foster carer. This made me think about how parents dealt with the issue of loss when their child has been taken away, and that there are no real services for that biological parent once the child has been removed. (1st Year Reader, Living Library 1, 6 Months After).

Suggestions for improving the Living Library experience focussed on practical aspects of their running. Getting the right physical space is a challenge. Feedback highlighted the importance of a venue that allows for the intimacy required for sensitive small group work and can also accommodate a larger plenary session and accessibility needs. It is a challenge we have better met in the later libraries but given the demand for university space in peak teaching times it remains an ongoing one. Some students indicated they wanted greater freedom in Living Book selection, and the opportunity to read more Living Books. Following Library 1, students have had the opportunity to read two Living Books and Readers' access to two different, sometimes differing, narratives on social work practice has been valuable, requiring the navigation of a path to understanding them together. There are though limitations to how much choice, and how many Living Books, we can offer Readers in one Library session. We have discovered that conversations between students after the Library are also a good means of sharing learning from the different reading experiences, as well as a mechanism for supporting the translation of learning from the Library to practice. This has brought focus onto developing exercises after a Living Library which encourage Readers to share experiences between them, as well as reflect on them individually.

Architects' plans for new developments

We are currently developing an online 'archive' of the libraries. The archive does not seek to directly record or replicate the Living Library exchanges themselves which are private and dependent on embodied dialogic interaction. Rather, it has been conceived of as an eclectic mix of objects which, between them, should provide a core record of each Library which has taken place, as well as some additional insights into how particular libraries have run. So far it consists of a record of each of the Book titles within every library there has been, a video of footage from Library 4 and two audio interviews with Living Books undertaken after Libraries 1 and 3.

We are seeking to establish partnerships to sustain the Living Library model and intend to run Generalist Living Libraries as part of our student introduction programme each year. Many of the Living Books from Library 1 returned for Library 2, which reflects their commitment to conveying their experiences to student social workers, as well as their positive experience of Library 1. At the same time, we want to ensure opportunities for new Living Books to participate. We also want to develop further specialist Living Libraries around particular service areas or groups of people using social care services, particularly those with experience of services who may be less well represented within social work education. Current embryonic thoughts are for libraries involving those with experiences of mental distress, parents with experience of child protection services and young people with disabilities.

If anyone is considering developing a Living Library, we would be happy to hear from you.

Notes

1. While 'service users and carers' is current mainstream terminology, we are aware of grassroots discontent with the term 'service user'. Therefore, where possible, we use 'people with experience of services' or 'people with expertise of services' to refer collectively to both 'service users' and 'carers'.
2. In addition to these 13, we received feedback from all the NQSWs who were Living Books in Library 3 but, given the focus of the article, do not consider this here.

Acknowledgement

Thank you to all those whose have enriched our Living Libraries as Living Books and Readers.

Funding

This work was supported by a University of Sheffield Engaged Curriculum Award, 2014.

References

Abergel, R., Rothemund, A., Titley, G., & Wootsch, P. (2005). *Don't judge a book by its cover! The living library organiser's guide*. Budapest: Council of Europe, Directorate of Youth and Sport.

Allport, G. W. (1954). *The nature of prejudice*. Reading, MA: Addison-Wesley.

Anghel, R., & Ramon, S. (2009). Service users and carers' involvement in social work education: Lessons from an English case study. *European Journal of Social Work, 12*, 185–199. doi:10.1080/13691450802567416

Beresford, P., & Croft, S. (2004). Service users and practitioners reunited: The key component for social work reform. *British Journal of Social Work, 34*, 53–68. doi:10.1093/bjsw/bch005

Birdi, B., Wilson, K., & Cocker, J. (2008). The public library, exclusion and empathy: A literature review. *Library Review, 57*, 576–592. doi:10.1108/00242530810899568

Braun, V., & Clarke, V. (2006). Using thematic analysis in psychology. *Qualitative Research in Psychology, 3*, 77–101. doi:10.1191/1478088706qp063oa

Broadhurst, K., & Mason, C. (2014). Social work beyond the VDU: Foregrounding co-presence in situated practice – Why face-to-face practice matters. *British Journal of Social Work, 44*, 578–595. doi:10.1093/bjsw/bcs124

Carpenter, J. (2011). Evaluating social work education: A review of outcomes, measures, research designs and practicalities. *Social Work Education: The International Journal, 30*, 122–140. doi:10.1080/02615479.2011.540375

Croom, A. M. (2013). How to do things with slurs: Studies in the way of derogatory words. *Language and Communication, 33*, 177–204. doi:10.1016/j.langcom.2013.03.008

Dennick, R., & Exley, K. (2004). *Small group teaching: Tutorials, seminars and beyond*. London: Routledge Falmer.

Duffy, J., & Hayes, D. (2012). Social work students learn about social work values from service users and carers. *Ethics and Social Welfare, 6*, 368–385. doi:10.1080/17496535.2012.654497

Fox, J. (2011). The view from inside: Understanding service user involvement in health and social care education. *Disability and Society, 26*, 169–177. doi:10.1080/09687599.2011.544057

Gupta, A., & Blewett, J. (2008). Involving services users in social work training on the reality of family poverty: A case study of a collaborative project. *Social Work Education: The International Journal, 27*, 459–473. doi:10.1080/02615470701380261

Hopkins, P. (2011). Young people's spaces. In P. Foley & S. Leverett (Eds.), *Children and young people's spaces: Developing practice* (pp. 25–39). Basingstoke: Palgrave Macmillan.

The Human Library. (2015). Retrieved from http://humanlibraryuk.org/human-library/the-methodology/

Jenkins, R. (2008). *Social identity* (3rd ed.). London: Routledge.

Levinas, E. (1969). *Totality and infinity: An essay on exteriority* (A. Lingis, Trans.). Pittsburgh, PA: Duquesne University Press.

Merleau-Ponty, M. (1962/2013). *The phenemonology of perception* (D. A. Landes, Trans.). London: Routledge.

Robinson, K., & Webber, M. (2013). Models and effectiveness of service user and carer involvement in social work education: A literature review. *British Journal of Social Work, 43*, 925–944. doi:10.1093/bjsw/bcs025

Sadd, J. (2011). *We are more than our story: Service user and carer participation in social work education* (Report 24). London: Social Care Institute for Excellence.

Sen, R. (2015) Not all that is solid melts into air – care experienced young people, friendship and relationships in 'the Digital Age'. *British Journal of Social Work*. Advanced Access. doi:10.1093/bjsw/bcu152

Sieghart, W. (2013). An independent review of E-lending in public libraries in England. Department of Media Culture and Sport. Retrieved September 1, 2015, from https://www.iwight.com/azservices/documents/2791-E-Lending%20in%20Public%20Libraries.pdf

Valentine, G. (2007). Theorising and researching intersectionality: A challenge for feminist geography. *The Professional Geographer, 59*, 10–21. doi:10.1111/j.1467-927.2007.00587.x

Veil, S., & Bishop, B. W. (2014). Opportunities and challenges for public libraries to enhance community resilience. *Risk Analysis, 34*, 721–734. doi:10.1111/risa.12130

Warren, L., & Boxall, K. (2009). Service users in and out of the academy: Collusion in exclusion? *Social Work Education: The International Journal, 28*, 281–297. doi:10.1080/02615470802659464

Waldenfels, B. (2002). Levinas and the face of the other. In S. Critchley & R. Bernasconi (Eds.), *The Cambridge companion to Levinas* (pp. 63–81). Cambridge: Cambridge University Press.

A journey of embedding mental health lived experience in social work education

Kate P. Dorozenko, Sophie Ridley, Robyn Martin and Lyn Mahboub

ABSTRACT

The value of learning from mental health lived experience is widely acknowledged, however, the nature of lived experience involvement in Australian social work education seldom extends beyond guest lecturing. Further, few opportunities exist that build the capacity of people with lived experience to become educators within tertiary settings. In this paper we present the Valuing Lived Experience Project (VLEP), an initiative led by a Lived Experience Academic (LEA) that seeks to systematically and meaningfully embed lived experience into the social work curriculum at a Western Australian university by providing significant opportunities for the capacity building of both individuals with mental health lived experience and academics. Given the relative infancy of service user involvement in Australian social work education, the VLEP offers a number of opportunities for reflection and consideration. A long-standing partnership between a LEA and Social Work Academic is described, the activities and key learnings of the VLEP to date are outlined, and we offer our reflections on challenges encountered throughout the journey. We hope that our experiences and learnings can be drawn upon to progress lived experience participation in tertiary settings and further legitimise lived experience involvement in the education of social workers.

Introduction

There is widespread consensus that the involvement of people with lived experience (PLE)[1] in the education of social workers and other mental health professionals represents good practice (Bell, Whitehead, Aslani, Sacker, & Chen, 2006; Duffy, Das, & Davidson, 2013; Happell et al., 2015). Learning from lived experience provides students and practitioners with unique insights that facilitate professional compassion, expand understanding, challenge negative and stigmatising attitudes, and facilitate skill development (Bell et al., 2006; Beresford & Boxall, 2012; Happell & Roper, 2003; Irvine, Molyneux, & Gillman, 2015).

Research exploring the views of university academics, reports that the form of expertise that is brought by Lived Experience Educators can challenge some academics (Basset, Campbell, & Anderson, 2006; Felton & Stickley, 2004). As a consequence of this, it has been argued that academic staff may 'gate keep' lived experience involvement in education

(Happell et al., 2015). These points draw attention to the role of power relations within academia and the potential for Lived Experience Educators to unsettle these structures and dynamics (Beresford & Boxall, 2012; Felton & Stickley, 2004). Knowledge derived from medicalised epistemology (and the associated notions of pathology and reduced competency) pervades mental health education, reinforcing beliefs that PLE of mental distress are unreliable, dangerous and lack the capacity to occupy esteemed roles such as educator (Basset et al., 2006; Felton & Stickley, 2004). Finally, some academics have argued that formal processes and clear guidelines which preserve service user autonomy and avoid tokenistic involvement are needed to progress lived experience education (Happell et al., 2015).

In considering the views of PLE, a lack of training has been identified as a significant issue, resulting in PLE feeling unsupported and unprepared for their role (Basset et al., 2006). Historically and typically, Australian service users and family members provide guest lectures sharing their experiences of 'mental illness' and the mental health system, with little attention paid to building capacity prior to educational involvement (Happell & Roper, 2009; Happell et al., 2014). This ad hoc approach often leaves individuals needing to 'learn on the job' (Basset et al., 2006). This suggests that a change in culture within universities and academia is needed (Felton & Stickley, 2004; Happell et al., 2015).

Where PLE are involved in tertiary education, several limitations have been noted in the literature. First, studies from the discipline of nursing tend to dominate; 73% of studies compared to 7% in social work (Happell et al., 2014), which raises questions about the transferability of these findings to social work. Second, student and academic perspectives pervade, while the voices of PLE are comparatively muted (Happell et al., 2014; Meehan & Glover, 2007). Third, within the literature, the empowerment of PLE is often emphasised as a reason for lived experience inclusion in social work education, yet their involvement is considered an 'added extra'; rather than essential, if funding permits (Felton & Stickley, 2004; Robinson & Webber, 2013). This can lead to tokenistic involvement, whereas the primary objective should be to harness the expertise of lived experience to progress social work education (Robinson & Webber, 2013). Fourth, there is a dearth of studies which deeply explore the underlying assumptions, values and attitudes that drive resistance and receptiveness to mental health service user involvement (Felton & Stickley, 2004; Happell, 2014; Happell et al., 2014). Finally, studies which document the process of how lived experience can be systematically embedded within the curricula and offer reflections on successes, tensions and challenges are not readily available to guide practice (Felton & Stickley, 2004).

The act of meaningfully involving PLE in social work education directly mirrors the professions' values of respect, partnership and self-determination (Scheyett & Diehl, 2004). A study conducted by Duffy and Hayes (2012) reported that first year social work students' interactions with service users and family members representing a variety of fields were the most significant influential factor in the students' knowledge and values development. More locally, a small-scale Western Australian study found that learning from lived experience is essential to the development of critically informed understandings of mental distress (Ridley, Martin, & Mahboub, in press). It has been argued that dominant views of mental distress and associated practices that are informed by biomedical understandings need to be problematised within social work education in order to avoid obscuring alternative frameworks of understanding (Beresford & Boxall, 2012). Furthermore, it is essential that students see and hear from people who can share their stories of recovery from mental ill health and come to understand first-hand that people can and do recover.

The inclusion of PLE in social work education also reflects national and international policy directives which tout personal recovery approaches. It is, however, important to note that despite gaining prominence in political rhetoric, 'personal recovery' as a concept has been problematised by some as being ambiguous, value-laden and dependent on notions of deficit (Beresford, 2015; Harper & Speed, 2012). It has also been argued that the emphasis on the individual in personal recovery marginalises those collective, structural experiences of inequity and injustice that contribute to mental distress (Beresford, 2015; Harper & Speed, 2012). We agree that the co-option of personal recovery to serve neoliberal aims, and the subsequent invisibility of structural factors that underlie many experiences of mental distress, must be continually interrogated within social work curriculum, learning and teaching.

In Australia, social work education is based on a four-year Bachelor of Social Work or a two-year qualifying Master of Social Work university-based degree. While social work is not a registered profession, the Australian Association of Social Workers' accredits the course work and 1,150 h of supervised fieldwork placement within educational programmes. Mental health service user involvement in the planning and delivery of social work education is recommended, but not mandated, by the Australian Association of Social Workers (2008). While the value of learning from lived experience has been widely acknowledged, the nature of service user and family involvement in Australian health sciences education seldom extends beyond guest lecturing (Happell et al., 2015; Moxham, McCann, Usher, Farrell, & Crookes, 2011). In contrast to the Australian context, service user and family involvement in social work education in the United Kingdom is said to be an 'established feature' (Duffy & Hayes, 2012, p. 368) and includes active involvement in design, management, delivery, monitoring and evaluation of social work programs (Duffy & Hayes, 2012). However, it is important to note that there is debate and contestation about what constitutes meaningful involvement of PLE in social work education (Robinson & Webber, 2013).

The relative infancy of service user involvement in Australian social work education offers a number of opportunities for reflection and consideration. A key point is the importance of lived experience involvement being deeply valued and avoiding tokenistic attitudes and approaches (Beresford & Boxall, 2012; Scheyett & Diehl, 2004). The meaningful involvement of PLE in tertiary education settings requires a reconsideration of the relationships between service users and academics, and the unsettling of existing power structures within academia (Felton & Stickley, 2004; Happell & Roper, 2009). Involvement as a Lived Experience Educator can provide significant opportunities for capacity building and development of both service users and academics, and holds promise for service system improvements (Meehan & Glover, 2007).

This paper describes an ongoing project which is attempting to embed lived experience into social work curriculum in Curtin University. We begin by reflecting on the partnerships underpinning the initiative, called the Valuing Lived Experience Project (VLEP), which aims to systematically and meaningfully embed lived experience education into social work and occupational therapy curriculum in the first instance. While detailing the activities of the project, we offer our reflections on the challenges and achievements. Finally, we share our key learnings, goals and plans for the VLEP.

The foundations

The VLEP emerged from the long-standing partnership between two academics; one employed as a Lived Experience Academic (LEA) and one as a Social Work Academic (SWA) in the School of Occupational Therapy and Social Work (the School) at Curtin University. The LEA and SWA first met in 2007 when they attended a five-day, live-in, recovery training programme. From this meeting, their work together grew, starting with the LEA being invited by the SWA to engage in paid employment as a guest lecturer and share her lived experience, critical understandings of 'madness', and the hearing voices approach with final-year social work students in a mental health and recovery unit. The two academics then worked with other academics from occupational therapy, nursing and psychology, to develop a Masters of Mental Health. While different standpoints were adopted in relation to 'mental illness' and mental distress within this group, the value of lived experience was held as central by the LEA and SWA. The postgraduate programme was taken up by students with both lived and professional experience from a variety of disciplines. Due to staff changes, the LEA and SWA developed and delivered the majority of teaching in the course. Consequently, privileging lived experience came to be central in the teaching.

During this time, the LEA's position was cemented and extended beyond the Masters programme. Within both the Masters and undergraduate social work teaching, this involved; coordinating units, creating unit outlines, developing and delivering lectures and workshops (including simulated learning on topics such as hearing voices), developing student assessments, marking student assessments and negotiating with industry partners to coproduce student learning and assessments. From the LEA's perspective, the journey from invited guest lecturer to equal partner has been an enriching and inclusive adventure, largely due to the partnership she had with the SWA. In this partnership, the LEA and SWA were able to share power, embrace each other's assets and blur the boundaries between the diverse knowledge that they each brought to the table.

While the LEA had a history in tertiary education (as both student and tutor), she had limited exposure to the full range of teaching and learning activities involved in a unit or course. At the request of the LEA, the SWA provided mentoring and support to the LEA in these areas. As a result, the partnership between the LEA and SWA grew and in turn, provided professional and personal development opportunities for the SWA. Particularly, it provided the SWA with a deep, rich and contextual understanding of the opportunities and challenges associated with embedding lived experience into social work curriculum. As a consequence of the work undertaken together and a deep respect for each other's world view, values and philosophy, the LEA and SWA frame their working partnership as a peer relationship.

Another activity the LEA and SWA coproduce is the supervision of research students, extending activities beyond the classroom into the research space. One successful research project examined the impact of learning from lived experience on social work students' practice during their first fieldwork placement (Ridley et al., in press). Findings suggested that learning from lived experience promotes social work practice which honours lived experience expertise and privileges personal recovery approaches. Students also identified ways in which lived experience learning influenced their ability to resist dominant biomedical cultures and disempowering practices.

This project extended and broadened the LEA and SWA's understanding of the place of lived experience in the social work curriculum.

Despite the cessation of the Masters programme, the School committed to the LEA role which led to the development of the VLEP. Underpinning the VLEP is the desire to create opportunities for other PLE to be involved in education within the School. Led by the LEA, the VLEP is founded on, and guided by, principles of coproduction (Slay & Stephens, 2013). The VLEP aims to carry out an array of activities and events which build capacity of PLE (both individuals and family members) and academics within the School and broader university. This capacity building involves creating the conditions for PLE to become educators within tertiary settings, and creating the conditions under which academics can privilege and centre lived experience in their teaching, learning and research activities.

In addition to the LEA, a project officer, the SWA and a mental health recovery researcher provide the backbone to the VLEP. Financial support has been garnered from the School, Curtin University (a non-government mental health recovery service provider), and a university teaching and learning grant. The support by leaders and staff from within the School has been invaluable, providing encouragement and communicating their belief in the significance of the project and most importantly, in the value of lived experience. The LEA and SWA have sound networks and connections with service users and service providers, and the project is well regarded within the Western Australian mental health sector.

Activities of the VLEP

The following section describes the activities of the VLEP to date (see Figure 1) and the challenges encountered by the team on the journey to embedding lived experience in the School. The principles and values of participatory action research and coproduction have guided this project, facilitating the empowerment of those involved and enabling change and improvements to be made to the project. This also enabled a reflective approach which contained feelings of uncertainty and anxiety in what is new and unchartered territory for the VLEP team. Without guidelines to follow, much of our learning has been through trial and error. It is expected that planned activities will change as the project progresses and evolves, and that this reflects the dynamic approach which is central to the project.

Discussion forum on lived experience involvement in education

In July 2015, PLE were invited to attend a discussion forum hosted by the School. The forum sought to gauge community interest in lived experience involvement in tertiary education, create a space for dialogue and networking, and showcase the work of PLE already involved in the education of professionals. Thirty-eight people attended the event, and PLE were invited to be involved in the VLEP, future events and educational opportunities. The atmosphere of the forum was one of excitement, enthusiasm, and robust discussion. Importantly, the forum offered an encouraging environment where lived experience was legitimated and categorised as expertise. Further, all who attended the forum were convinced of the value of lived experience involvement in education and shared a passion and commitment to enact change in the university and mental health contexts. Following this event, more than 65 PLE, service providers, academics and researchers expressed interest in the project and receive newsletters providing updates on VLEP activities, achievements and opportunities to be involved in the project.

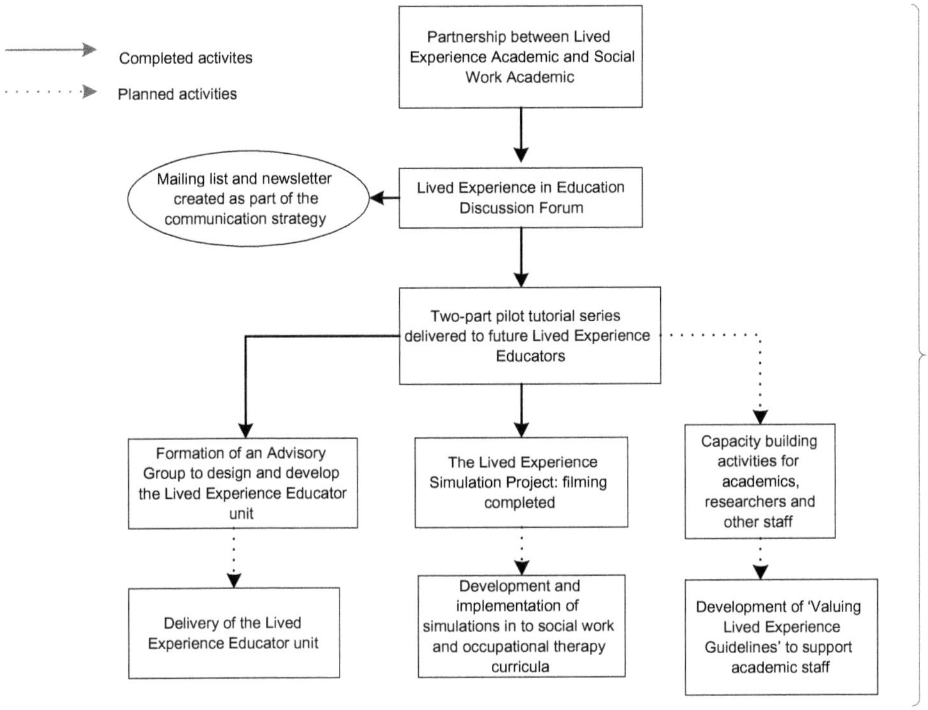

Figure 1. The Valuing Lived Experience Project map showing completed and planned activities.

Pilot tutorial series

Following on from the discussion forum, a two-part pilot tutorial series was designed and delivered by the LEA to 12 individuals who expressed an interest. The aim of this tutorial series was to capitalise on the interest generated from the discussion forum and provide an introduction to those wanting to pursue a future in lived experience education. It was also anticipated that the feedback provided from the participants would inform the development of a larger capacity-building unit to upskill future Lived Experience Educators. The tutorials were facilitated by the LEA and topics presented and discussed within the group included the history of the service user movement in mental health, different frameworks of understanding 'madness', and personal recovery. One of the tutorials elicited critique of the term 'madness', which then produced a rich discussion of the Mad Pride Movement, of which some participants were unaware. This example highlighted the importance of understanding history from a critically informed stance as it underpins and legitimates a Lived Experience Educator role. Tutorial participants reported that the content was useful and particularly valued the critical thinking elements, provision of resources and the knowledge and skills of the LEA who delivered the tutorial series.

The formation of an advisory group

Following the forum and pilot tutorial series an advisory group was formed in October 2015 to guide the design and development of a unit of study on becoming a Lived Experience Educator. On completion of the unit participants will be able to offer strategic input into curriculum development; plan and deliver lectures, tutorials, workshops and laboratories; develop and mark student assessments; and work in partnership with university academics to create opportunities for lived experience teaching and learning. While the initial focus of the VLEP is lived experience in mental health, it is anticipated that this will be broadened across a range of sites of social work practice such as domestic and family violence, older people, children and young people, disability, culturally specific practices and families.

Recruitment to the advisory group was by expression of interest, and individuals were required to outline; their consultancy experience and educational experience, knowledge of the service user and family movement, understanding of personal recovery (as differentiated from clinical and social recovery), and to demonstrate a critically informed view of 'mental illness'. Shortlisted applicants attended a brief interview with the LEA and were required to demonstrate that they could attend all five meetings. The advisory group comprised the LEA as project lead, seven Lived Experience Consultants, four SWA staff and one occupational therapy student. The Lived Experience Consultants who sat on the advisory group had a wealth of knowledge and experience in the areas of mental distress, service delivery, training, and personal recovery. Many of the Consultants also had qualifications in teaching and education, training, and social work. Consultants were paid an industry standard rate for their involvement.

In order to coproduce a safe and trusting environment in the advisory group, a number of strategies were employed. In addition to the collaborative development of a group safety agreement, a co-chair was appointed to ensure sharing of power and promote openness in meeting facilitation, and multiple opportunities for feedback were created. Lived Experience Consultants were invited to remain for a debriefing session after the meeting. At the last meeting, a brief survey was given to advisory group members inviting feedback on the process. This data was collated by the project officer and analysed. Overall, members reported that they experienced the advisory group process as safe, respectful and as validating of their experiences and knowledge. Members credited this largely to the strong leadership and skilled facilitation of the LEA and the shared vision of the group.

On completion, the advisory group had established four learning outcomes (or education priorities) for the Lived Experience Educator unit (Table 1). The focus or themes of the six learning modules that comprise the unit were also developed (Table 2). In their feedback, advisory group members commented that they were impressed by what was achieved in just five meetings and attributed this productivity to the clear assignment of tasks and strong sense of accountability within the group.

The issue of eligibility for the unit was raised by a number of advisory group members and stimulated robust discussion. Some argued that only individuals with prior teaching experience, pedagogical knowledge and skills, and confidence using technology should

Table 1. The learning outcomes developed by the advisory group for the Lived Experience Educator unit.

Learning outcomes of the Lived Experience Educator unit
Describe the history of the consumer and family movement and the current concepts of involvement, participation and co-production in the lived experience involvement.
Apply contemporary mental health concepts of personal recovery, mental distress and 'madness' from a critically informed perspective, taking into account the global context and diverse frameworks of understanding.
Demonstrate application of self-awareness, self-reflection and self-care skills required of the Lived Experience Educator role.
Demonstrate and apply the relevant academic concepts and practices that provide the context and inform the role of Lived Experience Educators within the School.

Table 2. Learning modules for the Lived Experience Educator unit.

Module	Examples of material covered
Introduction to the unit, the unit objectives and assessments	• Co-creating safety and trust • What is a Lived Experience Educator? • Introduction to critical thinking and frameworks of understanding in relation to 'madness'
History, current context, participation, involvement and coproduction	• Our elders and histories of consumer and recovery movements • Differences and similarities between individual and family needs • Wearing two hats: Can you advocate for both consumer and family/carer perspectives at once?
Self-care, self-awareness, story and voice	• Strategic use of story • Self-compassion, self-nurture, resilience, dealing with triggers • Stepping into leadership
Critical thinking	• Critical thinking applied to diagnosis • The language of 'power' and 'empowerment' • Critical thinking applied to language • Language and power
Recovery	• Differentiating between personal, social and clinical recovery • Critical thinking applied to 'recovery' • Maintenance, risk aversion and rescue
Understanding academia, practical matters, teaching and learning skills	• Marking rubrics • Unit outlines • Learning outcomes • Assessment guidelines • Skills audit • Creating a professional plan

participate in the unit. Others contended that eligibility for the unit should be broadened to be inclusive of all with an interest in the education of future mental health professions. While consensus on the issue was not reached, the discussion demonstrated that individuals may have different motivations for undertaking training to become a Lived Experience Educator. The advisory group agreed that given the nature and trajectory of individual recovery journeys, some people undertaking the unit may require scaffolding to support 'unit readiness'.

The lived experience simulation project

Running parallel to the advisory group was the lived experience simulation project. While competitive funding was initially obtained for the project, contract and ownership requirements imposed by the national funding body led the VLEP team to decline this grant funding (discussed later). Fortunately, the School funded the simulation project. Simulation is an educational tool that enables students to learn and develop skills in a safe and controlled environment (Alinier, Hunt, Gordon, & Harwood, 2006). Simulation resources are often video-recorded clips which feature people who act or simulate different situations that the students can then learn from.

Modelled on the work of Orr, Gallagher, Stein-Parbury, Gill, and Heffernan (2015), the lived experience simulation project produced four video-recorded vignettes featuring people with mental health lived experience. The LEA participated in one of the simulations and the SWA interviewed people on their lived experience. Topics discussed by the PLE in the simulations included lived experience of 'mental illness', service delivery experiences, recovery journeys and best practice approaches. This simulated learning tool will provide a powerful experiential learning opportunity and a useful introduction to mental health lived experience, particularly in disciplines where fieldwork placements occur much later in the course. These vignettes will be trialled and evaluated in the School initially, and then made available to all other health science disciplines. Learning activities to accompany the simulations are currently being developed.

Unlike the majority of simulation tools, the people featured in the vignettes were not paid actors, but PLE of mental distress. By way of initialising support, significant attention was paid to discussing, exploring and unpacking what would happen before, during and after filming. As a result of these conversations, one person elected to not continue prior to filming. While this created some disruption in project plans, it was viewed by the VLEP team as a sign of informed choice by the individual. Academic and lived experience colleagues from another Australian university who had previously produced lived experience simulations provided input and support prior to commencing filming. Particular issues raised in this consultation by the Lived Experience Educator included having conversations about a person's right to self-censor and share what they were comfortable with; confidentiality; role and identities in different contexts (such as being a service user in one context and a student supervisor in another); creating a safe environment; and the importance of debriefing following the live simulation.

With this feedback in mind, the issues of confidentiality and anonymity were explored with simulation participants at length and formed the employment contract. Participants had the option of having their face shown or pixilated, and of using a pseudonym. The prompt questions were provided in advance, and it was emphasised that they were not obliged to answer questions that were uncomfortable or revealing. Participants were advised that they would receive a copy of the final product; and while the University retained ownership of the resource, the participant could use it for non-commercial purposes.

Tensions and key learnings

In this section, we present some issues encountered during the VLEP activities and subsequent key learnings.

During the pilot tutorial series, notions of potential co-option into academia were explored when the feeling of not wanting to be 'turned into an academic' was expressed. Underpinning this was the potential discomfort with the perceived elitism and prestige associated with the role and how this can collide with one's identities or positioning as a non-academic. It was also argued that as a Lived Experience Educator one should not be required to pay lip service to the mental health system or self-censor one's lived experience to make it more palatable to an audience of university students and academics. This sentiment is underscored by Felton and Stickley (2004) who reported that lecturers did not want service users to become too 'professionalised' and expressed aversion to service users being trained as educators. These lecturers argued that 'career service users' were too distanced from their experiences and did not represent individuals with 'mental illness', and as such would be of little value to students. Paradoxically, service users who were still actively engaged in services or receiving treatment were also considered problematic by lecturers who suggested they may be too vulnerable or too unpredictable to participate in teaching (Felton & Stickley, 2004). We agree with Happell and Roper (2009) that it is essential for service users' involved in tertiary education to be afforded genuine autonomy and the safety to share the 'service user perspective'. We feel (and this is also echoed by many PLE involved in education) that adequate preparation for all is crucial to ensuring that lived experience is valued and respected in this space.

Another issue encountered related to the payment of PLE who were employed as Consultants in the advisory group. Concerns surfaced within the advisory group that the payment of sitting fees had the potential to interfere with welfare and income support payments (also found by Basset et al., 2006). Duffy and Hayes (2012) drew attention to the irony of this situation, stating that service user remuneration is '... not helped by a benefits system which mitigates against their working as social work educators despite government rhetoric about personalization and co-production' (p. 371). To circumvent this issue, some PLE involved in the VLEP opted to be paid with vouchers for major retailers. Tew, Gell, and Foster (2004) offer other practical strategies to ensure that service users are renumerated for their contribution, such as spreading payments over a longer time period so that the earnings threshold is not exceeded.

Finally, issues arose when creating an employment contract for the PLE involved in the simulation project that met the requirements of the research grant (particularly around intellectual property), while being accessible for service users. The VLEP team developed a contract that clearly described reciprocal responsibilities that was concise and utilised accessible language. This contract was then sent to the University legal section for approval. Following conversations between the legal team and the simulation grant funding body, the contract developed by the VLEP was rejected. To meet the grant requirements, a new contract was produced that was full of jargon, complicated, lengthy and required professional indemnity and public liability insurance, which made the Lived Experience Consultants ineligible. To the disappointment of the team, the simulation grant funding body adopted a risk-averse stance and was unwilling to modify this contract. The team felt strongly about maintaining the integrity of the project and honouring lived experience, so rather than adopting this contract, the decision was made to forgo the grant funding and seek funding elsewhere. This issue highlighted to the VLEP team how bureaucracy and complex and inflexible systems can be not only distancing for service users but also discriminatory. This exemplified the need to affect change at a systemic level.

Next steps and anticipated challenges

The VLEP team were successful in securing a grant to work with Lived Experience Consultants in developing specific content, learning approaches and activities for the Lived Experience Educator unit. This unit will commence in July 2016. The team feel that it is important that those individuals who participate in the Lived Experience Educator unit are formally recognised for this learning. The unit will require a significant time and emotional investment from participants. Participants may also wish to use the skills and knowledge developed in this unit within the broader mental health community as Consultants and Trainers. Achieving accreditation for this unit would allow participants to seek recognition of prior learning enabling pathways to higher education, while further legitimising the expertise of service users and family members. Finding pathways to accreditation for the unit is something the VLEP team will pursue.

The team will also develop 'Valuing Lived Experience Guidelines' to support academic staff who wish to embed lived experience education into existing curricula. Central to these guidelines will be a focus on preparing students to learn from lived experience and debriefing for the Lived Experience Educators. To accompany these guidelines, a conversation hub will be established within the School to provide the opportunity for academics, researchers and other staff members to discuss the place, purpose and impact of lived experience learning across all units. Although most university academics broadly agree that service user and family involvement in education is valuable (Happell et al., 2015), a range of reasons for not advancing service user and family involvement in tertiary education are put forward. Some of the cited barriers include the so-called 'attributes' of people with mental health issues and the degree of 'representativeness' of views expressed by PLE (Felton & Stickley, 2004). We believe that many of these perceived barriers can be overcome through the education and capacity building of academics, and supporting them through the provision of resources and tools. For academics to fully engage in this initiative, more than a superficial or fleeting interest in lived experience education is needed. A transformation of thinking and a change in culture is required (Felton & Stickley, 2004; Happell, 2014).

In 2016, the simulations featuring service users and family members will be rolled out within the School, which also includes the discipline of occupational therapy. The team have already received request from another School to use these simulations, and while we are appreciative of this interest and enthusiasm, we are committed to ensuring the integrity of the learning tool when it is used across disciplines. To address this concern, briefing, monitoring and mentoring will be provided by the LEA and SWA to other disciplines who choose to share the simulations with students. In addition, coproduced learning materials and activities will be developed to accompany the simulated learning tool.

Research and evaluation of the VLEP will be ongoing. In 2016, the team will conduct research exploring the experiences of participants who undertake the Lived Experience Educator unit. We also plan to further explore the experiences of Lived Experience Consultants involved in the advisory group for quality improvement. Future research will evaluate the impact of the lived experience simulations on student learning as well as the experience of the academics who implement the teaching tool. The VLEP journey will continue to be documented and disseminated. It is our hope that providing honest accounts of the tensions and challenges faced and the achievements and outcomes realised will assist others to meaningfully include lived experience in the curriculum.

Perhaps the greatest challenge faced by the team is ensuring the longevity and sustainability of the VLEP into the future. For the momentum of the lived experience education movement to continue it must be truly embedded in the curriculum and School and university processes. To do this, securing funding through nationally competitive grants and forming strategic partnerships with other universities and organisations is key. Communication with two other universities has commenced in regard to potential partnerships, along with organisations which champion mental health recovery, leading policy-makers, and governing mental health bodies. Ultimately, we would like to extend lived experience education beyond the area of mental health to include service users and family members with lived experience of child protection services, homelessness, substance misuse, disability and the criminal justice system as others (e.g. Duffy & Hayes, 2012) have done. Further, we would like to expand lived experience education beyond the discipline of social work to include other health science disciplines such as psychology, occupational therapy and nursing.

Conclusion

We argue that the idea of supporting people to become Lived Experience Educators' legitimises the role and highlights their expertise by experience, while simultaneously arming them with information about academic processes and protocols to enable deeper involvement. It is true to say that in Australia, PLE are involved in education and training in an array of ways across the mental health sector, however, we believe that providing resources and materials to build capacity of individuals seeking to be involved at an academic level can only enhance other areas of involvement that individuals are engaged in. We propose that part of this capacity building is also to challenge existing structures within universities, and strengthen the ability of academics to work with lived experience in broad and value-based ways.

Note

1. The term 'people with lived experience' includes both individuals and their family members who have lived experience of mental distress and/or mental illness and/or mental health recovery. The term 'family' will be used in this paper as opposed to 'carer', as the term 'carer' is often contested as it implies a relationship of dependency and excludes other chosen identities (Stanbridge & Burbach, 2007). 'Family' encapsulates whomever a service user may claim as family.

Acknowledgements

We would like to thank the Lived Experience Consultants involved in the Valuing Lived Experience Project for their time and expertise. We also acknowledge Richmond Wellbeing, the School of Occupational Therapy and Social Work and Curtin University's Teaching and Learning for their ongoing support.

Funding

This work was supported by the Richmond Wellbeing, the School of Occupational Therapy and Social Work and Curtin University's Teaching and Learning.

References

Alinier, G., Hunt, B., Gordon, R., & Harwood, C. (2006). Effectiveness of intermediate-fidelity simulation training technology in undergraduate nursing education. *Journal of Advanced Nursing, 54*, 359–369. doi:10.1111/j.1365-2648.2006.03810.x

Australian Association of Social Workers. (2008). *Practice Standards for Mental Heath Social Workers.*

Basset, T., Campbell, P., & Anderson, J. (2006). Service user/survivor involvement in mental health training and education: Overcoming the barriers. *Social Work Education, 25*, 393–402. doi:10.1080/02615470600593675

Bell, J. S., Whitehead, P., Aslani, P., Sacker, S., & Chen, T. F. (2006). Design and implementation of an educational partnership between community pharmacists and consumer educators in mental health care. *American Journal of Pharmaceutical Education, 70*(2).

Beresford, P. (2015). From 'recovery' to reclaiming madness. *Clinical Psychology Forum, 268*, 16–20.

Beresford, P., & Boxall, K. (2012). Service users, social work education and knowledge for social work practice. *Social Work Education, 31*, 155–167. doi:10.1080/02615479.2012.644944

Duffy, J., Das, C., & Davidson, G. (2013). Service user and carer involvement in role-plays to assess readiness for practice. *Social Work Education, 32*, 39–54. doi:10.1080/02615479.2011.639066

Duffy, J., & Hayes, D. (2012). Social work students learn about social work values from service users and carers. *Ethics and Social Welfare, 6*, 368–385. doi:10.1080/17496535.2012.654497

Felton, A., & Stickley, T. (2004). Pedagogy, power and service user involvement. *Journal of Psychiatric and Mental Health Nursing, 11*, 89–98. doi:10.1111/j.1365-2850.2004.00693.x

Happell, B. (2014, November). *Consumer participation in the education and training of mental health nurses*. Queensland Mental Health Commission. Retrieved from http://www.qmhc.qld.gov.au/wp-content/uploads/2015/05/Consumers-and-Mental-Health-Nurse-Education-Issues-Paper.pdf

Happell, B., Byrne, L., McAllister, M., Lampshire, D., Roper, C., Gaskin, C. J., … Lakeman, R. (2014). Consumer involvement in the tertiary-level education of mental health professionals: A systematic review. *International Journal of Mental Health Nursing, 23*, 3–16. doi:10.1111/inm.12021

Happell, B., & Roper, C. (2003). The role of a mental health consumer in the education of postgraduate psychiatric nursing students: The students' evaluation. *Journal of Psychiatric and Mental Health Nursing, 10*, 343–350. doi:10.1046/j.1365-2850.2003.00599.x

Happell, B., & Roper, C. (2009). Promoting genuine consumer participation in mental health education: A consumer academic role. *Nurse Education Today, 29*, 575–579. doi:10.1016/j.nedt.2008.01.004

Happell, B., Wynaden, D., Tohotoa, J., Platania-Phung, C., Byrne, L., Martin, G., & Harris, S. (2015). Mental health lived experience academics in tertiary education: The views of nurse academics. *Nurse Education Today, 35*, 113–117. doi:10.1016/j.nedt.2014.07.006

Harper, D., & Speed, E. (2012). Uncovering recovery: The resistable rise of recovery and resilience. *Studies in Social Justice, 6*, 9–25.

Irvine, J., Molyneux, J., & Gillman, M. (2015). 'Providing a link with the real world': Learning from the student experience of service user and carer involvement in social work education. *Social Work Education, 34*, 138–150. doi:10.1080/02615479.2014.957178

Meehan, T., & Glover, H. (2007). Telling our story: Consumer perceptions of their role in mental health education. *Psychiatric Rehabilitation Journal, 31*, 152–154. doi:10.2975/31.2.2007.152.154

Moxham, L., McCann, T., Usher, K., Farrell, G., & Crookes, P. (2011). Mental health nursing education in preregistration nursing curricula: A national report. *International Journal of Mental Health Nursing, 20*, 232–236. doi:10.1111/j.1447-0349.2010.00735.x

Orr, F., Gallagher, I., Stein-Parbury, J., Gill, K., & Heffernan,T. (2015). *"Making it real": Facilitating recovery-focused nursing practice through consumer participation in the development of innovative and technology-rich learning experiences for final year nursing students*. Paper presented at The Mental Health Services Conference, Canberra.

Ridley, S., Martin, R., & Mahboub, L. (in press). *Learning from mental health lived experience and the influence on students' practice*. Manuscript submitted for publication.

Robinson, K., & Webber, M. (2013). Models and effectiveness of service user and carer involvement in social work education: A literature review. *British Journal of Social Work, 43*, 925–944. doi:10.1093/bjsw/bcs025

Scheyett, A., & Diehl, M. J. (2004). Walking our talk in social work education: Partnering with consumers of mental health services. *Social Work Education, 23*, 435–450. doi:10.1080/0261547042000245035

Slay, J., & Stephens, L. (2013). *Co-production in mental health: A literature review*. London: New Economics Foundation.

Stanbridge, R., & Burbach, F. (2007). Developing family-inclusive mainstream mental health services. *Journal of Family Therapy, 29*, 21–43. doi:10.1111/j.1467-6427.2007.00367.x

Tew, J., Gell, C., & Foster, S. (2004). *Learning from experience: Involving service users and carers in mental health education and training*. Nottingham: Higher Education Academy/National Institute for Mental Heath in England/Trent Workforce Development Confederation.

Involving People with Profound and Multiple Learning Disabilities in Social Work Education: Building Inclusive Practice

Nicki Ward, Christian Raphael, Matthew Clark and Vicki Raphael

ABSTRACT
Service user and carer engagement is a foundational requirement of social work education. Despite this, questions remain about how diverse experiences are represented and who might be excluded from involvement. This paper focusses on one group of people who it is suggested are excluded from involvement, people with profound and multiple learning disabilities. Evidence is presented which demonstrates the extent to which this group have been marginalised and excluded from processes of involvement. The paper then provides a case study of one universities' experience of developing work in this area, when a man with profound and multiple learning disabilities was commissioned to design and deliver specialist teaching for a group of qualifying social work students. We argue that the main barrier to inclusive involvement for people with profound and multiple learning disabilities is the attitudes and assumption of others about what they are capable of. We demonstrate how involvement in social work education helps to address these barriers by challenging the assumptions of students, the academy and society more broadly.

Introduction

Service user and carer involvement in public services is developing a significant history; its profile having been raised by policy initiatives and legislative change (Bamford, 2015; Cairney et al., 2006; Cowden & Singh, 2014; McLaughlin, 2009, 2010). The concept of involvement has many definitions, which may be focussed on levels of involvement (House of Commons Health Committee, 2007), areas of involvement (Tew, Gell, & Foster, 2004) or processes of involvement from more tokenistic forms of consultation through to citizen control (Arnstein, 1969). The language of involvement is also evolving and is perhaps reflective of our changing understanding moving from client and consumer through to service user, survivor and expert by experience (see e.g. Fawcett, Fillingham, River, et al., in press; McLaughlin, 2009).In this article, we consider involvement from the perspective of people with profound and multiple learning disabilities defined here as people who have more than one disability, the most significant of which is a profound learning disability (PMLD Network, n.d.).

The paper focusses on building inclusive practice considering this in the context of social work education, the experience of social work students and inclusive practice in the lives of people with profound and multiple learning disabilities. Drawing on the literature, the paper begins by considering the extent to which people with profound and multiple learning disabilities have been involved and what barriers might exist to prevent involvement. Drawing on a case study, we then report our experience of working together when Christian, was commissioned to design and deliver specialist teaching on working with people with learning disabilities on qualifying social work programmes. Student evaluations inform the findings on the value of this experience for their learning and development, whilst discussions with Christian and his supporters consider the experience from their perspective and how this informed their advocacy work with others. We conclude by arguing that all of the stakeholders in social work education need to question their own attitudes and assumptions when developing inclusive involvement for this group.

Before developing this paper, further we would like to introduce ourselves in order to personalise and contextualise the discussion which follows.

Christian Raphael has worked as an independent consultant/adviser on matters relating to people with profound learning disabilities and complex needs for a number of years. This has included work for the Department of Health and NHS England. In addition to this, Christian is a representative on the National Forum for People with Learning Disabilities. In 2016, he was awarded the MBE in recognition of his work.

Matthew Clark has supported Christian for the last 10 years, in both all aspects of his day to day life, as well as specifically in his work. Prior to working for Christian, Matt worked extensively in nursing, health and social care in a number of settings.

After a career in academia, Vicki Raphael spent time teaching in the special education system before becoming mum to Christian. In recent years, as well as continuing to directly support Christian, Vicki has worked tirelessly on a voluntary basis as a prominent figure of the inclusion movement. She is currently chair of the National Valuing Families Forum.

Nicki Ward is a social work lecturer at the University of Birmingham. Before joining academia Nicki worked for over 20 years with adults with learning disabilities in a variety of settings. This continues to influence her work as an academic through both her research and teaching.

Empowerment, Involvement and People with Profound and Multiple Learning Disabilities

Service user involvement in social work education has a long history which pre-dates policy requirements for involvement (Cairney et al., 2006). It is widely accepted as a foundational requirement of social work education, a principle reinforced in successive policy frameworks (The College of Social Work [TCSW], 2014; Department of Health [DoH], 2002; General Social Care Council [GSCC], 2005; Health and Care Professions Council [HCPC], 2009). Whilst much of this policy is focussed on the UK, specifically England, there is also growing emphasis on service user involvement internationally (International Federation of Social Workers [IFSW], 2004; Zaviršek & Videmšek, 2009). Nevertheless, important questions remain about the success of these developments, particularly how inclusive service user and carer involvement is (Cairney et al., 2006). Within social work, service user involvement is particularly important as it reflects the practice of anti-discriminatory and anti-oppressive approaches which are enacted through inclusion and challenging structural oppression.

Service user involvement aims to give voice to those who are oppressed and validate the voices of those who have been marginalised. However, whilst there have been significant developments in this area, the evidence on involvement of people with learning disabilities, as demonstrated below, suggests that we still have a way to go in furthering this aim. Research on involvement demonstrates that there are many whose voices are 'seldom heard' (Carr, 2004; Hernandez, Robson, & Sampson, 2010) and who are more likely to be excluded from processes of involvement (Beresford, 2007). In a recent text which sought to rethink Anti-discriminatory and Anti-oppressive practice, Green and Featherstone draw on the work of Judith Butler to consider the notion of 'normative violence' which it is suggested occurs through routine activities such as 'not allowing particular voices to be heard because they are not considered legitimate' (2014, p. 31). This is a useful concept when considering service user involvement as it prompts questions about whose voices are heard and whose voices are omitted from the increasingly dominant discourse of service user involvement in social work education? We would argue that people with learning disabilities, and particularly those with profound and multiple learning disabilities are regularly subjected to this 'normative violence' by not having their voices included and legitimated. It is important therefore to focus not only on involvement but on inclusive involvement (Bollard, Lahiff, & Parkes, 2012).

People with learning disabilities are amongst the most excluded within our society (DoH, 2001; Public Health England, 2014), and amongst them people with profound and multiple learning disabilities are likely to be more excluded still (HM Government, 2009). Research conducted for this paper would suggest that this extends to a lack of inclusion within professional education. A systematic search of six databases[1] which included the search terms learning disability/difficulty or profound learning disability/difficulty, AND involvement AND professional education generated minimal results. The literature that explicitly discusses the involvement of people with learning disabilities in academia tends to be located within medical and nursing studies (Bollard et al., 2012; Maestri-Banks, 2013; McClimens, Lewis, & Brewster, 2012) or research (Boxall, 2011; Gilbert, 2004; McClimens & Allmark, 2011; Tuffrey-Wijne & Butler, 2010). A keyword search of this journal uncovered one document which involved the experience of a person with a learning disability in social work education (Pendred & Chettle, 2006). None of this literature included people with profound and multiple learning disabilities.

Research by Shaping Our Lives supports the argument that participation in service user involvement initiatives is still rare for some groups; including people with learning disabilities and people who communicate differently (Beresford, 2013), which would suggest that involvement of those with profound and multiple learning disabilities is likely to be particularly difficult to secure. Research focussed specifically on inclusion and involvement for people with learning disabilities consistently finds that people with profound and multiple learning disabilities are more likely to be excluded (Abbott & McConkey, 2006; Clement & Bigby, 2009; Mencap, 2004).

As the case study considered here involved employing Christian as a visiting lecturer, this is also an important area to consider. Employment is seen as a valued social role (Priestley, 2003) and a route to securing inclusion (Ward, 2009) but it is a field which people with learning disabilities are routinely excluded from. In 2012, only 7% of people with learning disabilities of working age were in paid employment—mostly part time. A similar proportion undertook unpaid voluntary work (Public Health England, 2014). Amongst people with profound and multiple learning disabilities examples of employment are extremely rare (Commission for Social Care Inspection [CSCI], Mental Health Act Commission, & Healthcare Commission, 2009). For many the biggest barrier to employment is not their knowledge and skills but the attitudes and assumptions of others. As 'Valuing People Now' (2009) noted the 'lack of understanding and aspiration about what can be achieved sometimes leads to an assumption that people will be passive recipients of care throughout their lives as opposed to people who can … live as empowered citizens in our society' (HM Government, 2009, pp. 38, 39). Such assumptions about ability not only limit the opportunities available to people with learning disabilities but can also further exclude them by failing to recognise and value the contributions they do make (Ward, 2011, 2015).

Attitude change towards those who have a learning disability is particularly important. Scior and Werner (2015) conducted a review of evidence on approaches to attitude change. They found that contact with those whose lives challenge negative stereotypes, (including beliefs that people with learning disabilities are childlike or in need of protection), was more effective in improving attitudes than other methods. The report emphasises the importance of balancing this so as not to deny the needs of those 'people with severe and profound disabilities who may be at risk of being further marginalised' (Scior & Werner, 2015, p. 16). The beliefs and assumptions which are held about what people with complex needs can achieve and what they are capable of is a significant barrier to inclusive involvement. An evidence review on advocacy for people with high support needs found that attitudes and cultures were particularly important:

> the challenge is changing the mindset and creating an atmosphere where people with PMLD are involved as actively as possible and are seen (and see themselves) as equals. (Lawton, 2009, p. 46)

The teaching initiative described and evaluated below aimed to do both of these things; challenging the attitudes and beliefs of student social workers about the potential of people with profound and multiple learning disabilities, whilst also offering Christian an opportunity to develop his own skills in relation to employment and inclusion.

The Teaching—Working with People Who Have a Learning Disability

Baldwin (2013), notes that the key to challenging dominant narratives is to identify them and then to take action to challenge them. This initiative is representative of one such attempt; challenging the dominant narrative about who can speak for people with learning disabilities and who has the skills and expertise to be 'involved' in the education of qualifying social workers. This was not just about ensuring the presence of a person with profound and multiple learning disabilities within the teaching but of handing over control. Whilst our work did involve partnership, the role of the academic was to provide more practical support; arranging teaching spaces and materials, introducing the team and participating in some of the exercises. Christian developed and led the teaching with the support of his team.

This was a two day course on working with people with learning disabilities which was offered as an option to students on a qualifying social work programmes. Students could choose two 'electives' to help them develop specialist knowledge in a particular area. The electives were part of a final year module which emphasised life course and whole family approaches to practice (Hughes, 2010; Morris et al., 2008). The teaching had previously been delivered by Nicki. In 2011, building on other work Nicki had undertaken to involve people with learning disabilities in social work education (Mencap, 2010), Christian was commissioned to lead on and deliver the two-day programme.

Inclusive involvement requires positive guidance, support and mentoring and this was particularly important here. Although Christian had begun working in service user involvement some years before and had been involved with the Department of Health in the development of resources for Valuing People Now (DoH, 2009), this was his first experience of delivering social work education in a higher education setting and was a daunting prospect: 'the difference between doing a one-hour workshop and doing the whole module was a big thing' (Matthew, cited in Mencap, 2012). We had several meetings before the teaching was delivered for the first time, initially at Christian's home and then at the University so that Christian could familiarise himself with the surroundings. Nicki provided information about student numbers, level and programme of study and the broader curriculum within which the electives were located. The teaching notes and materials used previously were also provided to Christian and his team as a guide to developing the module. There was no expectation that Christian should use these and it was particularly important to Christian and his team that he had control over the development and delivery of the teaching. Both the original delivery and that by Christian and his team took a workshop approach within which presentations were interspersed by group activities and discussion with students along with the use of audio-visual (AV) material.

One primary difference between the original programme and Christian's teaching was the emphasis on the lived experience. Although the original design had drawn heavily on AV material to provide 'real life' examples of good practice (DoH, 2009), it was not able to capture the lived reality in the same way. Here examples were located in Christian's own life experiences and those of his 'Circle of Support' who have been working alongside Christian since he left school. The circle helps Christian to consider his ambitions and aspirations and to plan his life (For further information on Circles of Support see Burke & Ball, 2015; circlesnetwork.org.uk), various members of Christian's circle came along with him to deliver the teaching. This included Vicki, Matthew as well as others involved in supporting Christian. As well as presentations and discussions materials such as Christian's diaries, photographs and videos were used to illustrate key points, model good practice and promote discussion. Developing and delivering the teaching in this way had a number of benefits. It provided the students with a very explicit example of the importance of the whole family approach and the need to respond flexibly. It also demonstrated the potential benefits of working with a circle of support when working with someone with profound and multiple learning disabilities. The teaching took on a decidedly auto ethnographic approach drawing 'upon the experience of the author/researcher for the purposes of extending sociological understanding' (Sparkes, 2000, p. 21). Christian's team maintained the life course approach developing this through a focus on different 'chapters' in Christian's life including birth, childhood, transition and adulthood. These were illustrated with reference to their biographic experiences and students were able to question directly what professionals did well and what they might have done differently to improve the situation. By exploring Christian's experiences, students were able to consider the impact of social structural issues, the impact of legislation such as the Mental Capacity Act (2005) and the historical development and impact of policy such as educational segregation and personalised and self-directed support. Time was devoted to considering and practising person centred practice and how tools such as PATH[2] planning might be used with people with learning disabilities.

Evaluation—The Student Experience

This case study is based upon the evaluation questionnaires completed by three successive cohorts of students and on reflective interviews which took place between the authors when writing this article.

The teaching was available for 15–20 students in each year. The evaluation form was circulated at the end of the two days teaching. Students were asked about their previous experience of working with people with learning disabilities, their experience of the teaching, assessment of their learning and key learning points and recommendations for the development of the teaching. Finally they were asked to provide feedback on Christian's role in the teaching. This was a new initiative for all of us and we felt it was important to explore how students had experienced being taught by someone who had profound and multiple learning disabilities. Christian and his team especially wanted to know if students felt he was effectively included in the teaching and learning process. As this was a teaching evaluation rather than a research study formal ethical approval was not sought; however the students were informed that their feedback would be used to help Christian develop his work opportunities and may also be used in future publications. The results of these evaluations will be discussed here before moving on to Christian's reflections and those of his team.

Forty students completed the evaluation. Students were not asked to indicate their programme of study (PG or UG), or to provide other demographic data such as gender, age or ethnicity. They were however all asked to indicate whether or not they had previous experience of working with people with learning disabilities and if so, whether or not they had ever worked with someone with profound and multiple learning disabilities. A majority of the students ($n = 30$) had had previous experience of working with people with learning disabilities with a little under half of these having experience with people with profound and multiple learning disabilities.

The types of experience which students had ranged from significant work roles in day and residential settings or personal experience supporting family members to more limited experience on placements whilst at university or interaction through school projects. It is however interesting that most of the students did have some previous experience and it may be that this generated their interest in taking the elective in the first place. However 25% of those who completed the evaluation had no previous experience (Figure 1).

Students were also asked to assess their own learning development as a result of participating in the teaching. Two Likert scales asked students to rate their knowledge of working with people with learning disabilities on a scale of 1–5 (where 1 = 'no knowledge' and 5 = 'significant knowledge') both *before* and *after* the teaching. Across all three deliveries of the module students indicated a growth in their knowledge of between 1.29 and 1.42 points on this scale. For the students who had no previous experience this margin increased, rising 2.25 points from an average of 1.5 to 3.75 on the Likert scale.

Five of the 40 students completing the evaluation indicated no increase in their knowledge all having assessed their knowledge as 'significant' at the outset. However, all of these students indicated things that they had learned from the teaching including tools that

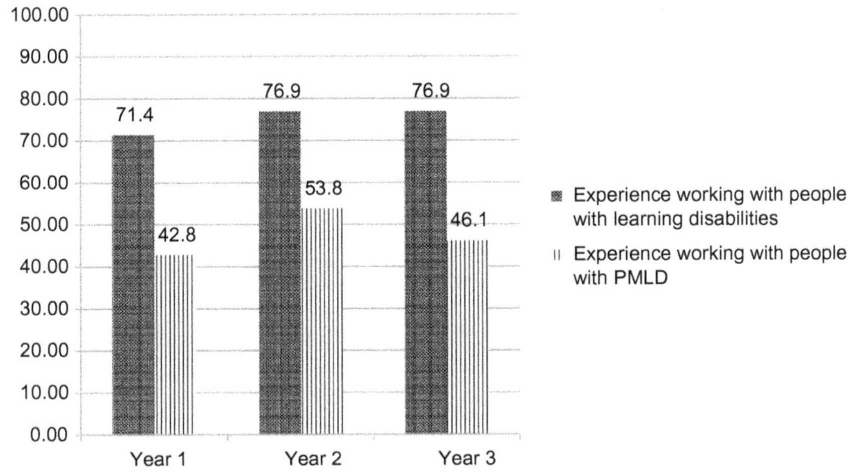

Figure 1. Students previous experience of working with people with learning disabilities.

could be used for person centred planning such as PATH, the importance of challenging of assumptions and how to overcome difficulties in transition.

The evaluation questionnaire invited free text responses to the question 'please identify at least two things that you have learned from the teaching'. The question was purposely phrased in this way, rather than providing a tick box of the different topics covered in the teaching so that we could assess the extent to which the experience itself had informed student learning as well as the content. Responses to this question suggest that both aspects were important with some students mentioning particular elements of the teaching and others referring more broadly to the experience as a whole. Thematic analysis suggests that the most significant topics for students included those related to personalisation and tools for person centred practice as well as the importance of family experiences and the role of communication in working with people with learning disabilities (see Table 1).

Other important but less frequently mentioned learning points included transitions, sources of practical support and wider networks.

Table 1. Key aspects of learning as assessed by the students.

Theme	Description	Number of times mentioned
Person centred planning	This includes specific reference to person-centred planning and also to the tools which may be used to support it such as PATH	17
Circles of support	All references to [co-author's] circle and the way that this approach may help others are included here. This is treated separately to references to more general sources of support and family experiences	8
Personalisation	Here are included all references to personalisation, individual budgets and other forms of self-directed support (i.e. direct payments)	9
Communication	References here included those to different types of communication and the non-verbal communication which took place between [co-author] and his circle	6
Family experiences	This included all references to [co-author] experience and to the importance of understanding wider family experiences and listening to families	7

More significantly, especially for our argument that inclusive involvement is about challenging assumptions and enabling voices to be heard, is the feedback which demonstrates that student learning was highly experiential. It did not just occur through didactic teaching methods in which the lecturer imparted the knowledge to the students. It derived from participatory and observational learning as the following quotes suggest:

> it allowed me to witness new communication methods and it helped me to better understand how non-verbal service users can express themselves
>
> I've never seen such a successful example of personalisation
>
> it enabled me to recognise the importance of communication in terms of verbal, non-verbal and body language
>
> observing Christian communicating with his team was lovely to see
>
> Having Christian there really helped me to imagine the life of somebody with complex needs. I will have lots to think about and consider
>
> talking about someone is very different to actually meeting them.

The learning gained through being part of the process and being able to observe Christian and his support network in practice moved beyond an increase in knowledge and skills; it challenged assumptions and expectations. Within the free text comments, students talked about the importance of having positive expectations, the impact a lack of aspiration can have on a person's life, and the importance of a biographic approach. Others noted the way that the experience had challenged their own assumptions about what a person with learning disabilities might achieve:

> People with learning disabilities are capable of achieving far more than I thought possible
>
> Challenged assumptions about ability to understand information and being able to articulate
>
> it broke down my prejudices that I held by having Christian there
>
> it was great to see Christian there, in fact it was a surprise to me.

One student's comments even reflected a realisation that she and Christian shared common interests noting that she most enjoyed 'seeing and hearing about his love of festivals as that is something that he and I share'.

Bamford argues that working with service users and carers can actually give practitioners a more insightful understanding of 'the *real needs*' of service users rather than their assumed needs' (2015, p. 105 – our emphasis). This is reflected in our evaluation. The student feedback suggests that the teaching not only provided them with additional tools to draw upon in working with people with learning disabilities but that it also challenged some of their assumptions about what type of life was possible for someone with complex needs. However, if we are to argue that inclusive involvement in social work education is a strategy which furthers anti-discriminatory practice then it is also important to consider how this initiative was experienced by Christian and those supporting him.

Evaluation—The Experience of Christian's and his Circle

Christian, along with his circle of support, had identified as part of his PATH that it was important for him to pursue employment opportunities and he had begun to draw upon his personal expertise to work as a self-advocate and to provide training to various health and social care agencies (org ref, 2012). He was therefore ideally placed to be involved in this teaching. He had the skills, experience and support network necessary to deliver the teaching and wanted to develop his skills in this area. It is important however to recognise both the opportunities and challenges which the teaching presented.

Whilst Christian does not communicate verbally if he is not happy or interested in what he is doing then he will communicate this through his actions. In addition, if Christian is stressed or upset with a situation this impacts on his physical and emotional health. When Christian began work his family and friends reported an improvement in his health which resulted in less hospital admissions; this along with his calm demeanour and engagement during the teaching told us that he enjoyed the work that he was doing.

There was also the benefit of being in work, and being able to use the language of 'employment' and being a 'lecturer'. In this way, Christian's involvement not only challenged the attitudes and assumptions of the students but also others who he came into contact with. People with learning disabilities, especially those with more complex needs, are often cast in the role of dependent (Ward, 2011) and employment can be seen as unachievable (Mansell, 2010). However, being employed provides opportunities to occupy valued social roles which in turn present a challenge to the assumptions of others (Mansell, 2010; Ward, 2011). Christian's experience as a lecturer not only influenced the student social workers he came into contact with but also others within his social network. One explicit example of this was during learning disability awareness week when Christian and his family invited their neighbours in for afternoon tea. They used this as an opportunity to talk about Christian's work and many of the neighbours expressed initial surprise hearing about his work as a lecturer. Benbow et al. argue that service user involvement 'carries the potential to subvert attitudes and beliefs that … others hold' (Benbow, Taylor, Mustafa, & Morgan, 2011, p. 632). In this instance Christian and his family directly drew on his experience to educate and challenge assumptions about the lives of people with learning disabilities.

Christian's involvement also had potential impact beyond those students directly involved in the teaching. We noted above that one student identified shared interests that they had in common with Christian whilst others were surprised by his presence. For Christian, it offered him an opportunity to inhabit an environment which is rarely open to those with learning disabilities, to socialise with his peers in an educational environment. It also meant that students and staff within the university also had their assumptions challenged, as Christian moved around the campus and used the campus facilities. Consequently, this work and the other employment opportunities which Christian was engaged in broadened his social circle. In 2015 Christian took a 'gap year' during which he spent time travelling and visiting friends, many of whom he met as he developed his employment opportunities. Here Christian's experience reflects the arguments of Priestley (2003) and Mansell (2010) that inclusion in the socially valued sphere of employment also helps people to develop their broader social networks.

Whilst Christian and his circle experienced a number of positive outcomes from their work at the university, there were also many challenges. Christian had the expertise required for this role because of his life experiences; the teaching was rooted in his autobiography and that of his family and friends. Drawing on this experience and recounting it repeatedly to different groups of people, and being prepared to respond to questions about it, is emotionally draining. Whilst Christian has a very positive package of support now, and a team who know him well and provide excellent support, it has not always been so. For the team having the trust of the academic partner, being able to take control of the teaching and develop and deliver it in ways which were comfortable for them and sensitive of the affective nature of the work was a key consideration informing their willingness to take part.

There were also practical challenges. This teaching was delivered on three separate occasions and on each occasion a different room was allocated. This was something we had no control over and whilst all were accessible some were more conducive to the teaching and more comfortable for Christian and his team, than others were. This in turn had an impact on the experience of students. In spaces where Christian was more comfortable he was more inclined to own the space and move freely around it— sometimes sitting with students at their tables or just circulating—and this was something students commented on as a positive:

> there was much freedom for Christian to move and use the space and communicate when and how he wanted to.

Others have written about the difficulties of negotiating bureaucracies (Beresford, 2013) whilst at the same time ensuring a positive experience and that was also an issue here. Whilst our room booking system allows us to request 'accessible' rooms, this tends to take a narrower, physical view of accessibility.

For the people supporting Christian there were also some practical considerations. For example, on days when Christian was less well decisions had to be made about whether he should attend or whether it would be better for him to remain at home or in his hotel room. Christian did always attend the teaching but there were some occasions when he was experiencing seizures and unable to interact with students as much. This required a delicate balance for Christian's supporters who at these times had to take a lead in delivering the teaching as well as caring for and supporting Christian. For the students seeing Christian when he was less well informed their learning. This was apparent in student feedback which suggested that students found it useful to be with Christian because they had never 'been around someone with such profound learning disabilities' or that they 'found it difficult when Christian has a seizure' having never witnessed one before but that 'it helped me understand how to respond'. However, striking the balance between an opportunity for learning and Christian's welfare and dignity was a delicate one for his circle to manage.

Discussion

Nancy Fraser discusses the importance of recognition, as well as redistribution in considering issues of marginalisation and inclusion. For Fraser, this is about engendering situations which allow for all members of society to interact with each other as peers, to have parity of participation (1997, 2003). In this initiative Christian and his circle of support were able to take on a relatively powerful role, not just engaging with students as 'contributors' alongside academics, but designing and delivering the teaching as a visiting lecturer. This was important in committing to the principles and *practice* of service user involvement. The model adopted here was one of service user control, just as with any other visiting lecturer Christian was provided with a remit for the teaching but within this he was free to develop and deliver the teaching; as such parity of participation in this arena was achieved. The discussion above demonstrates that this was not only important for Christian and his team, but also provided a clear example to the students which challenged their beliefs and assumptions about what could be achieved by people with profound and multiple learning disabilities.

Aiyar (2010) explores participation in governance processes in India and concludes by posing a number of questions, two of which seem particularly important to the discussion here. Firstly are we 'romanticising' participation and secondly whether, in placing such emphasis on it, we are at risk of overburdening our citizens. These are pertinent questions to pose, not in order to undermine the importance of service user and carer involvement and the ongoing development of inclusive involvement but in order to ensure that we are realistic about the possible benefits of involvement for all the stakeholders. Are we romanticising service user involvement? Perhaps a little. We have travelled far but we have not arrived yet; involvement is not always inclusive and in considering who we might recruit to support the education of social workers we need to be prepared to explore and challenge our own prejudices as well as the structural barriers of our institutions. As noted above, there were times when Christian's health needs were apparent within the teaching environment and whilst this added to the students experience and understanding this had to be balanced against Christian's health and welfare. This suggests that we need to think carefully about how we balance the educational benefits of involvement for students with the needs of service users; involvement is important but it should not be at the expense of overburdening those who are in receipt of services.

Bamford (2015) suggests that the benefits of involvement for service users are both short and long term. In the short term, they can lead to enhanced self-respect and improvements in the quality of care 'especially if service users are involved in training practitioners' (2015, p. 100). This would seem to reflect Christian's experience in the short term; he experienced improvements to his well-being and self-confidence through his employment and was also able to broaden his social network. It is difficult to know whether this experience improved the quality of care. This was not an issue for Christian personally but it is hoped that this experience will have improved the quality of care to others with profound and multiple learning disabilities; either through the practise of the students involved or as a result of Christian's broader discussions about his work.

Irvine, Molyneux, and Gillman (2014) suggest that as we develop our understanding of user involvement in social work education we need to focus more on outcomes. Whilst this is not something which we have measured here some of the student feedback suggests that the experience will have longer term outcomes on their practice as indicated by the student who noted:

> this experience had had a profound impact on me on a personal and professional level and I will always remember how it is possible to achieve anything in life when you have people believe in you and show you genuine support.

However as authors, we also believe that there is an important social justice argument for inclusive involvement. We should do it because people have a right to be involved, to have a say in their lives, to have parity of participation— it should not be dependent on the measurement of outcomes.

This experience was a largely positive one; we were successful in furthering our aims of challenging the attitudes and beliefs of student social workers about the potential of people with profound and multiple learning disabilities and Christian had an opportunity to develop his skills in relation to employment and inclusion. However, it is important to note that in the longer term there is a risk that this experience could become a burden to Christian. As we have demonstrated few people with profound and multiple learning disabilities are currently engaged in service user involvement and, as far as we have been able to identify, Christian is the only person with profound and multiple learning disabilities who has been actively involved in designing and delivering teaching to social work students. This presents ongoing challenges both for Christian and his circle and for the social work education community more broadly. For Christian it is his life experiences and opportunities—both positive and negative—which have provided him with the skills, knowledge and support to be able to be involved in this way. His biography, his negative experiences during childhood and the transformations made possible through personalised support, are the basis of his expertise. But becoming 'the' expert involves considerable pressure and more recently he and his circle have identified concerns that involvement on this basis could become a more negative experience; one which requires him to constantly 'relive' some difficult periods in his life and which detracts from the development of different work opportunities. For the academic community difficult questions are posed about how we develop the involvement of those with profound and multiple learning disabilities and provide students with experiences which challenge their assumptions and beliefs about what it possible when so few people with profound and learning disabilities have had the opportunities in their lives to develop the experience and skills which would enable them to be involved in this way. There is, in this sense, a vicious circle of exclusion for people with profound and multiple learning disabilities which can present a barrier to their involvement.

Conclusion

Within the introduction, we suggested that we needed to question our assumptions in order to develop inclusive involvement for people with profound and multiple learning disabilities. Within this article, we have demonstrated that people with learning disabilities, and particularly those with profound and multiple learning disabilities are amongst those who have been identified as 'seldom heard', their voices excluded from involvement. We have argued that a key to challenging this exclusion for people with profound and multiple learning disabilities, and therefore putting an end to the normative violence they experience through having their voices silenced, is to change the attitudes and assumptions of others.

For people with profound and multiple learning disabilities, building inclusive practice means respecting their expertise and knowledge and learning how to hear their voices. In our experience, people with profound and multiple learning disabilities are often seen as unable to communicate a belief which was also reflected in the student evaluations. As social workers we need to consider how our assumptions and expectations might contribute to the silencing of the voices of people with profound and multiple learning disabilities. Social work education has a key role to play here, we cannot rest upon our laurels and assume that we have done all we need to in terms of service user involvement. For people with profound and multiple learning disabilities having access to academia and the right to be involved in the education and training of the professionals who will often have a key role in supporting them in their lives, gives the voices of people with profound and multiple learning disabilities the opportunity to challenge the attitudes and assumptions of those who often occupy positions of power within their lives and shape anti-discriminatory practice. Through this, as Christian has demonstrated, people with profound and multiple learning disabilities are able to actively model what positive communication and person centred planning should look like. However, if we are to make these spaces available then, we also have to question our own beliefs and assumptions about who does and does not have the expertise and knowledge to 'teach' and how (and if) we represent the lives of people with profound and multiple learning disabilities in our broader curriculum.

A key principle of inclusive involvement must be that people are well supported, have access to guidance, support and mentoring and that it is constructed in within the context of a partnership through which the expertise of the person with profound and multiple learning disabilities is respected; they have to be able to control how they are involved and what they choose to share. This requires careful preparation and planning and, as illustrated above, very few people with profound and multiple learning disabilities currently have the opportunities to be involved in this way. We hope that this example will provide some insight into how other such initiatives could be developed.

Notes

1. ASSIA, Social Policy and Practice, PsychInfo, Medline, Embase and HMIC.
2. PATH stands for 'Planning Alternative Tomorrow with Hope' and is a style of person centred planning which has been found to be particularly valuable with people with learning disabilities. It begins by identifying people's hopes and ambitions and then works backwards to identify the key stages which need to be addressed in order to achieve the ambition (Further information can be found at http://www.parent2parentqld.org.au/planning/path.php).

References

Abbott, S., & McConkey, R. (2006). The barriers to social inclusion as perceived by people with learning disabilities. *Journal of Learning Disabilities, 10*, 275–287.

Aiyar, Y. (2010). Invited spaces, invited participation: Effects of greater participation on accountability in service delivery. *India Review, 9*, 204–229.

Arnstein, S. (1969). A ladder of citizen participation. *Journal of the American Institute of Planners, 35*, 216–224.

Baldwin, C. (2013). *Narrative social work: Theory and application*. Bristol: Policy Press.

Bamford, T. (2015). *A contemporary history of social work: Learning from the past*. Bristol: Policy Press.

Benbow, S. M., Taylor, L., Mustafa, N., & Morgan, K. (2011). Design, delivery and evaluation of teaching by service users and carers. *Educational Gerontology, 37*, 621–633.

Beresford, P. (2007). User involvement, research and health inequalities: Developing new directions. *Health and Social Care in the Community, 15*, 306–312.

Beresford, P. (2013). *Beyond the usual suspects: Towards inclusive user involvement*. London: Shaping Our Lives.

Bollard, M., Lahiff, J., & Parkes, N. (2012). Involving people with learning disabilities in nurse education: Towards an inclusive approach. *Nurse Education Today, 32*, 173–177. doi: 10.1016/j.nedt.2011.10.002

Boxall, K. (2011). Research ethics committees and the benefits of involving people with profound and multiple learning disabilities in research. *British Journal of Learning Disabilities, 39*, 173–180.

Burke, C., & Ball, K. (2015). *A guide to circles of support*. London: Foundation for People with Learning Disabilities. Retrieved from http://Learningdisabilities.org.uk

Cairney, J., Chettle, K., Clark, M., Davis, A., Gosling, J., Harvey, R., ... Russell, L. (2006). Editorial. *Social Work Education, 25*, 315–318.

Carr, S. (2004). *Has service user participation made a difference to social care services?* (Position Paper No. 3). Bristol: Policy Press, Social Care Institute for Excellence.

Clement, T., & Bigby, C. (2009). Breaking out of a distinct social space: Reflections on supporting community participation for people with severe and profound learning disability. *Journal of Applied Research in Learning Disability, 22*, 264–275.

Commission for Social Care Inspection, Mental Health Act Commission, & Healthcare Commission. (2009). *Commissioning services and support for people with learning disabilities and complex needs: National report of joint review*. London: Author.

Cowden, S., & Singh, G. (2014). A critical analysis of service user struggles. In C. Cocker & T. Hafford Letchfield (Eds.), *Rethinking anti-discriminatory & anti-oppressive theories for social work practice* (pp. 93–107). Basingstoke: Palgrave MacMillan.

Department of Health. (2001). *Cmnd 5086 valuing people, a new strategy for learning disability for the 21st century*. London: Author.

Department of Health. (2002). *Requirements of social work training*. London: Author.

Department of Health. (2009). *Valuing people now resource pack*. London: Author.

Fawcett, B., Fillingham, J., River, D., et al. (in press). *Service user and carer involvement in health and social care: A retrospective and prospective analysis*. London: Palgrave.

Fraser, N. (1997). *Justice interuptus: Crticial reflections on the post-socialist condition*. London: Routledge.

Fraser, N. (2003). Social justice in an age of identity politics: Redistribution, recognition and participation. In N. Fraser & A. Honneth (Eds.), *Redistribution or recognition* (pp. 7–109). London: Verso.

General Social Care Council. (2005). *Post qualifying framework for social work education and training*. London: Author.

Green, L., Featherstone, B., & Butler, J. (2014). Power and social work. In C. Cocker & T. Hafford Letchfield (Eds.), *Rethinking anti-discriminatory & anti-oppressive theories for social work practice* (pp. 31–44). Basingstoke: Palgrave MacMillan.

Gilbert, T. (2004). Involving people with learning disabilities in research: Issues and possibilities. *Health and Social Care in the Community, 12*, 298–308.

Health and Care Professions Council. (2009). *Service user and carer standard and guidance* (SET 3.17). Retrieved from http://www.hcpc-uk.org/assets/documents/1000295EStandardsofeducationandtraining-fromSeptember2009.pdf

Hernandez, L., Robson, P., & Sampson, A. (2010). Towards integrated participation: Involving seldom heard users of social care services. *British Journal of Social Work, 40*, 714–736.

HM Government. (2009). *Valuing people now: A new three year strategy for people with learning disabilities, making it happen for everyone*. London: DH Publications.

House of Commons Health Committee. (2007). *Patient and public involvement and the NHS*. London: The Stationery Office.

Hughes, N. (2010). Models and approaches in family-focused policy and practice. *Social Policy and Society, 9*, 545–555.

International Federation of Social Workers. (2004). *Ethics in social work: Statement of principles, international federation of social workers*. Retrieved July 8, 2014, from http://ifsw.org/policies/statement-of-ethical-principles/

Irvine, J., Molyneux, J., & Gillman, M. (2014). Providing a link with the real world: Learning from the student experience of service user and carer involvement in social work education. *Social Work Education, 34*, 138–150.

Lawton, A. (2009). *Personalisation and learning disabilities: A review of evidence on advocacy and its practice for people with learning disabilities and high support needs*. London: Social Care Institute for Excellence.

Maestri-Banks, A. (2013). Learning disability, education and empowerment: Learning from individuals who live with a learning disability. *Health and Social Care Education, 2*, 21–24.

Mansell, J. (2010). *Raising our sights: Services for people with profound intellectual and multiple disabilities*. Kent: Tizard Centre. Retrieved July 8, 2016, from https://kar.kent.ac.uk/24356/1/DH_2010_Raising_our_sights.pdf

McClimens, A., & Allmark, P. (2011). A problem with inclusion in learning disability research. *Nursing Ethics, 18*, 633–639. doi:10.1177/0969733011404588

McClimens, A., Lewis, R., & Brewster, J. (2012). Dr. Tulp attends the soft machine: Patient simulators, user involvement and intellectual disability. *Journal of Intellectual Disabilities, 16*, 173–182. doi:10.1177/1744629512451213

McLaughlin, H. (2009). What's in a name: 'Client', 'patient', 'customer', 'consumer', 'expert by experience', 'service user' – What's next? *British Journal of Social Work, 39*, 1101–1117.

McLaughlin, H. (2010). Keeping service user involvement in research honest. *British Journal of Social Work, 40*, 1591–1608.

Mencap. (2004). *PMLD network – Partnership board survey 2004*. London: Author.

Mencap. (2010). *Good practice in involving families in your workforce development: The what, why and how*. London: Author.

Mencap. (2012, May/June). Quietly confident. *Viewpoint*, Issue 128, 20–21.

Mental Capacity Act. (2005). London: HMSO.

Morris, K., Hughes, N., Clarke, H., Tew, J., Mason, P., Galvani, S., … Burford, G. (2008). *Think family: A literature review of whole family approaches*. London: Cabinet Office.

Pendred, B., & Chettle, K. (2006). What being a trainer means to me. *Social Work Education, 25*, 415–417.

Priestley, M. (2003). *Disability a life course approach*. Oxford: Blackwell Publishing.

Public Health England. (2014). *People with learning disabilities in England 2013*. Retrieved January 20, 2016, from http://www.improvinghealthandlives.org.uk/securefiles/151009_1537//People%20with%20learning%20disabilities%20in%20England%202013.pdf

PMLD Network. (n.d.). *About profound and multiple learning disabilities*. Retrieved January 20, 2016, from http://pmldnetwork.org/

Scior, K., & Werner, S. (2015). *Changing attitudes to learning disability: A review of the evidence*. Retrieved January 20, 2016, from https://www.mencap.org.uk/sites/default/files/documents/Attitudes_Changing_Report.pdf

Sparkes, A. C. (2000). Autoethnography and narratives of self: Reflections on criteria in action. *Sociology of Sport Journal, 17*, 21–43.

Tew, J., Gell, C., & Foster, S. (2004). *Learning from experience: Involving service users and carers in mental health education and training: A good practice guide*. Nottingham: Higher Education Academy/NIMHE/Trent Workforce Development Confederation.

The College of Social Work. (2014, June). *Endorsement by the college of social work of qualifying social work programmes: An information and guidance booklet for universities and colleges version 5.0*. London.

Tuffrey-Wijne, I., & Butler, G. (2010). Co-researching with people with learning disabilities: An experience of involvement in qualitative data analysis. *Health Expectations, 13*, 174–184.

Ward, N. (2015). Reciprocity and mutuality: People with learning disabilities as carers. In M. Barnes, T. Brannelly, L. Ward, & N. Ward (Eds.), *Ethics of care: Critical advances in international perspective* (pp. 165–178). Bristol: Policy Press.

Ward, N. J. (2009). Social exclusion, social identity and social work: Analysing social exclusion from a material discursive perspective. *Social Work Education, 28*, 237–252.

Ward, N. J. (2011). Care ethics and carers with learning disabilities: A challenge to dependence and paternalism. *Ethics and Social Welfare, 5*(2), 168–180.

Zaviršek, D., & Videmšek, P. (2009). Service users involvement in research and teaching: Is there a place for it in Eastern European social work. *ljetopis Socijalnog Rada, 16*, 207–222.

The benefits of prisoner participation in interdisciplinary learning

Ben Raikes and Rachel Balen

ABSTRACT

This paper considers the provision of an inter-disciplinary workshop day held for Social Work, Police and Nursing students at a UK university. The focus of the day was to give the students an insight into the reality of being a mother in prison, and the impact that having a mother in prison has upon children. A key feature of the day was the involvement of a group of imprisoned mothers from an open prison, who shared their experiences and engaged with students in small groups. The workshop allowed the stereotypes that the prisoners and student professionals held in relation to one another to be challenged. The planning, aims, process and outcomes of the day are considered along with feedback from those taking part. Students reported increased awareness of the stigma faced by this often overlooked vulnerable group of service users, an increased recognition of the needs of children with mothers in prison and an appreciation of the power of interdisciplinary working to deliver a good service. The imprisoned mothers welcomed the chance to educate the students about the issues faced by themselves and their children, and they found the experience of participating to be positive and empowering.

Introduction

Involving service users in the teaching of Social Work courses is now established as an essential aspect of any programme offered (Warren, 2007). However, serving prisoners rarely have a chance to directly express their views and to describe their lived experience to the professionals based *outside* the prison whose decisions and judgements can have a profound impact upon their lives (Crewe & Bennett, 2012). It is important to note that within prisons, there is a commitment to gathering feedback from prisoners regarding aspects of how the prison is run and what improvements can be made. In their 2011 report on service user involvement in the criminal justice system, CLINKS, which supports voluntary organisations that work with offenders and their families, noted that 84% of prisons have prison-wide consultations (Chapman Gibbs, Hayes, & Thomson, 2011, p. 4).

Those serving prison sentences are at the extreme end of the continuum of 'involuntary' service users (Trotter, 2006). They do engage with professionals for the purposes of preparing reports but all too often these reports focus on a particular issue, and there is no time to dwell on the impact of being imprisoned as an issue in itself. This reflects what some have argued is a tendency for Social Workers to only see service users in 'instrumental terms and as a means to end', for example only considering their ability to parent (Featherstone, White, & Morris, 2014, p. 13). The danger of this approach is that service users can cease to be viewed as beings in their own right, with their own needs, which can have a dehumanising effect. The views of prisoners are sometimes gathered by researchers, but in reality, the possibilities of them participating in research are very limited (Charles, Rid, Davies, & Draper, 2016). If prisoners do have the chance to participate in research, they are dependent upon researchers to accurately portray their perspectives in the publications produced, and they have little control over what is written.

Prisons are by definition closed worlds, and often professionals have little knowledge of the issues faced by prisoners and their families. In the absence of knowledge, the danger is that professionals will rely on stereotypes, which in turn might cause them to decide that prisoners and their families are undeserving of their time and resources, especially in the current economic climate where both are scarce. Therefore, the inter-disciplinary event aimed to create the opportunity for the imprisoned mothers attending to speak directly to the student professionals about the particular issues they faced, articulating and personalising their experiences in their own words. It has been recognised that hearing from service users 'in the flesh' generally has a much more lasting impact on students than other forms of teaching (Irvine, Molyneux, & Gillman, 2015, p. 144).

Why focus on imprisoned mothers and their children?

Women prisoners form only 6% of the overall prison population in the UK (Prison Reform Trust, 2015). As a minority group in a prison population that is overwhelmingly male, it is easy for the needs and views of female prisoners to be marginalised. It is estimated that 65% of women in prison are mothers with dependent children (Carlen & Worrall, 2004), which equates to approximately 17,200 children in the UK experiencing the imprisonment of their mother each year (Wilks-Wiffen, 2011). Our focus on imprisoned mothers was also driven by the additional disadvantage faced by children whose mothers are in prison compared to those children who have a father in prison. Whereas 90% of children whose fathers are in prison live with their mothers (Caddle & Crisp, 1997), only a mere 9% of those with a mother in prison are cared for by their fathers (Corston, 2007). The rest experience a disruptive change in living arrangements, with an estimated 25% being cared for by a grandmother (Corston, 2007), 15% looked after by another female relative and the remaining 51% residing with foster carers or in a children's home (Prison Advice & Care Trust [PACT], 2011), organised by Social Workers. This means that there is a high likelihood that children with imprisoned mothers will often be moved away from support systems such as friends and school just at the time when they need them the most. For this reason, the negative impacts for children are generally much worse when their mother is imprisoned compared to those with an imprisoned father (Burgess & Flynn, 2013; Murray & Farrington, 2008). It is also recognised that children with parents in prison have an increased likelihood of experiencing mental health problems (Jones et al., 2013). This may in part be due to the lack of understanding and empathy that children and young people in this situation experience if they are brave enough to talk to others, including some professionals. It has been likened to a bereavement, but one that does not attract the same amount of sympathy as if a parent had actually died (Robertson, 2007). This has been referred to as a *disenfranchised* form of grief in which *social support for the mourner may be less than sufficient* (Worden, 2009, p. 63). Therefore, another key aim of the workshop was to enable the student professionals attending to gain an understanding of these issues to enable them to practise more sensitively with families where a mother has been imprisoned.

Goffman defined stigma as *an attribute that is deeply discrediting* that serves to diminish those it attaches to *from a whole and usual person to a tainted discounted one* (Goffman, 1963, p. 3). Stigma is attached to all prisoners to some extent (LeBel, 2012) and this stigma is transferred on to family members too. However, due to the small number of female prisoners, the stigma associated with being a mother in prison is likely to be greater. Criminologists have recognised for some time that female offenders can be judged twice when they come before the criminal courts. Firstly, for the crime they have committed and then a second time for engaging in behaviour that breaks the stereotype of how women are expected to behave (Heidensohn, 1985). (I experienced this first hand when I was a student Probation Officer in the early 1990's, in the Crown Court with a female offender who I had written a report for regarding an offence of violence. The male judge opened his comments by observing that the defendant had engaged in *most unladylike behaviour*). It has been reported that foster carers looking after children whose mothers and fathers are in prison are more likely to agree to contact between the children and their fathers than with their mothers. Their rationale is that if a mother has been sent to prison, she must have committed a *very* serious offence, whereas fathers being imprisoned is seen as more commonplace and acceptable (Moyes, 1997).

Children with parents in prison have been referred to as 'invisible' (O'Keeffe, 2013; Smith et al., 2007) as their needs are often overlooked by agencies that could assist them. This is partly due to the fact that often they do not want to identify themselves as having a family member in prison due to the fear of being judged. Therefore, the interdisciplinary workshop that we held aimed makes the needs and lived experience of imprisoned mothers and their children more visible to the students who participated. It was also an attempt to reduce the stigma faced by these service users. The planning, aims, process and outcomes of this workshop day, held for Social Work, Nursing and Police students, are discussed below.

Inter-disciplinary learning and service user involvement in teaching

Inter-disciplinary learning (IDL) has been defined as

> when two or more professions learn with, from and about each other to improve collaboration and the quality of care (www.caipe.org.uk/about-us/defining-ipe/)

It is recognised that it has many benefits which include

> improved joint working practices not only between professions and organisations but also with service users and carers, thus improving care and quality of life. (Balen, Rhodes, & Ward, 2010, p. 417)

The importance of the role of IDL in improving collaboration between and within health and social care teams is well documented, for example in relation to modifying negative attitudes and perceptions, and being a solution for trust and communication between professions (Dickinson & Carpenter, 2005).

IDL has been found to result in better 'cooperation, coordination and sharing' (Mccallin, 2001, p. 419) which in turn assists workers to cope with problems that exceed the capacity of only one profession. Some of the advantages of interdisciplinary activity within the teaching environment are that different areas of the curriculum can be linked; common learning outcomes can be shared; 'silo working' can be minimised whilst staff themselves model interdisciplinary working; and the involvement of service users can be maximised. It is recognised that service user inclusion in teaching activities greatly benefits learners. For example Balen et al. (2010) discuss how a 'user narrative'-based interdisciplinary workshop day that involved hearing users' own stories can provide meaningful learning experiences for students as illustrated by feedback given by a student who took part: *It is important to hear from those who use services. You can never get this understanding from reading books* (Balen et al., 2010, p. 7).

The workshop on the subject of imprisoned mothers and their children was congruent with the strategy of the University Social Work department that aims to enhance student learning through making service user and carer involvement central to as many of our teaching and learning activities as possible. For example, the Social Work BSc and MSc students currently undertake a module entitled 'Working with Service Users and Carers' in which the majority of the sessions are facilitated by service users and carers.

Our 'Imprisoned Mothers' workshop day was attended by over 90 students from 6 professional groups – Social Work, Health Visiting, Mental Health Nursing, Children's Nursing, School Nursing and the Police. Nine imprisoned mothers participated, who were released on temporary licence for the day to attend. These professional groups were chosen on the basis of their relevance to practice in relation to children and families affected by imprisonment and the total number of participants was governed, as is often the case within educational settings, by the number and size of available rooms as much as by the availability of workshop facilitators.

Planning – Teaching staff

The workshop was planned over several months. It was crucial that the planning group had representation from all the academic disciplines that taught the students who would be participating, in order to ensure that there was a commitment to the workshop from each course. It was agreed that the student places on the workshop would be allocated equally between the different disciplines. All of the students who participated were in their final year of study, meaning that they had been out on their practice placements, with the result that they could consider what they learned in the workshop in the light of their experience to date.

We were very fortunate to have very strong links with an open women's prison that is situated about 50 miles from the university. The links had developed as a result of myself and a colleague conducting an evaluation of a facility within the prison that allowed children to stay overnight with their mothers. In the course of liasing in relation to the evaluation, we could discuss other opportunities for collaboration. The governor who was in charge of family services was very keen to make the workshop happen when I suggested it to her. Therefore, we did not encounter the problems in accessing service users that have been highlighted as a potential obstacle (McKeown, Malihi-Shoja, & Downe, 2010). Due to her other commitments, it was hard for her to attend our planning meetings. However, I kept her informed by email and sought her views on any important decisions that needed to be made.

Preparing the imprisoned mothers

From the outset, we knew that it was very important to provide many opportunities for the imprisoned mothers who participated to prepare. Preparation has been identified as key to the success of training events that involve service users (Scammell, Heaslip, & Crowley, 2016). Therefore, a number of colleagues on the planning group went to the prison on two occasions. On the first occasion to explain what we were doing and to invite imprisoned mothers to participate. In terms of breaking down stereotypes, this process started at the first meeting at the prison in which one of the participants was a Police Officer. He used humour to build rapport with the imprisoned mothers who came to the meeting, acknowledging that many of the mothers might regard him with a great deal of suspicion. Likewise, representatives from Social Work such as myself recognised that for many of the prisoner participants, their engagement with Social Workers may not have been positive. This naming of what could have been the 'elephant in the room' served to break down barriers and build trust. We were very mindful that in a prison environment there could be the potential for subtle coercion that might push some of the women into attending against their will. Therefore, when we had our initial meeting with prisoners, we emphatically stressed that participation was entirely voluntary, with the option to withdraw at any time. Twelve women came forward expressing an interest in participating. We knew that this number was likely to drop before the actual workshop, and as predicted the number dropped to nine women attending on the day of the workshop.

After discussions with the imprisoned mothers, it was agreed that there would be an introduction to the reality of prison life through the 'Prison Me? No Way!' format in the morning, followed by workshops in which groups of prisoners would meet with groups of students in the afternoon in a workshop facilitated by members of staff who both had knowledge of the issues and experience of facilitating workshops. The Prison Me? No Way! Trust (http://www.pmnw.co.uk) was founded by a group of Prison Officers in 1993 who wanted to bring alive the lived reality of being in prison for school children, to put them off a life of crime. Many of the women were familiar with getting messages across about their experience of prison and the criminal justice system using this format in school settings. It involves a Prison Officer asking the women in turn hard-hitting questions about the journey from arrest to imprisonment. It can be excruciating to watch as for example one of the prisoners becomes tearful about the guilt she has in relation to not being present for her children, or another discussing the indignity of not being able to shower or change underwear whilst detained for a number of days in a Police station. When I first witnessed this method of evoking responses from the prisoners, I was concerned it was exploitative. However, having spoken to the women who participated, they have always reassured me that it is cathartic for them and that they gained the satisfaction of knowing they have engaged an audience to understand more about how it is to be an imprisoned mother.

We visited the prison on another occasion two weeks later to allow the women a chance to rehearse what they would share with students in the workshops. Many of the prisoners who were going to participate had prepared scripts which were rich in material to share. The idea was that they would share their thoughts and then give students the chance to ask questions. They also assured us that they would feel comfortable to refuse to answer any questions that they did not feel comfortable with. We offered to go up to the prison on a third occasion but the imprisoned mothers told us they would be able to support one another to prepare and engage the support of staff where necessary.

The format for the workshop

The planning group thought carefully about the content of the workshop to come up with a structure that was stimulating, enjoyable and informative. It was important to have many opportunities for the students to engage with the prisoners, but also for students from different disciplines to work together. Brown and Young (2008) suggest that there are three ways that service users can be involved in teaching: facilitated dialogue; conversations about personal histories; and acting as co-facilitators of workshops. We incorporated elements of all three of these formats.

The prisoner officer who brought the women was keen that they sat amongst the audience so that nobody knew who the prisoners were until they introduced themselves. This worked because the students were from different disciplines who did not know one another and were mainly female, and the prisoners were wearing their own clothes and not prison uniform. Therefore, at the start of the workshop, the prisoners introduced themselves one by one, standing up and giving their name and offence. Surprised looks on the faces of the students were evident when they realised they were sitting next to a prisoner convicted of murder or drug dealing. It was a very powerful way of making the point that anybody could end up in prison, and that you cannot tell by looking at a person that they are a prisoner. After revealing themselves, the prisoners answered questions posed to them by the Prison Officer who facilitated Prison Me? No Way! Examples of the questions were: *how did you feel when you were arrested in front of your children?* or *what was going through your mind when the judge sentenced you to 15 years?* Inevitably, the answers evoked a tearful and emotional response, but you could see that every student participant was listening intently and taking it all in.

After 'Prison Me? No Way!', students were put in mixed discipline groups with two prisoners in each group, to undertake a multiple choice quiz in relation to issues relating to imprisoned mothers and their children. The quiz was facilitated by a PhD student and a Research Fellow. The purpose of the quiz was to establish what the students knew about these issues. In many cases, the prisoners had held back from helping the students answer the questions, thereby revealing the limits of their knowledge. However, although the subject matter was serious, the quiz was conducted in a light-hearted way, and generated energy and laughter as the planning group had intended. After the quiz, there were three speakers: the Director of Partners of Prisoners Support Service (www.partnersofprisoners.co.uk) which provides support to prisoners and their families and manages prison visitor centres in the north of England; The Director of the Together Women's Trust (www.togetherwomen.org) which provides projects to support female offenders and the Prison Governor in charge of family work. There was a chance for students and anyone else to ask questions.

We then allowed plenty of time for lunch, and put on the best spread that the budget would allow. Fair payment for service users who contribute to teaching has rightly been identified as very important (Anghel & Ramon, 2009). We were mindful that providing lunch was the only way we could show our appreciation for the women who attended as they were not allowed to accept gifts (with permission from the Prison Officer we gave the prisoners all the leftover food to eat on their way back to the prison). Throughout lunch time, I was very pleased to note that at all times the prisoners were engaged in talking informally to groups of students, providing the opportunity for pre-conceptions on both sides to be challenged.

After lunch, we held the workshops. We had 10 students and 3 prisoners in each workshop, which we held twice during the afternoon. I had the privilege of facilitating one of the workshops. We had agreed that there would be a minimum of three imprisoned mothers in each workshop, so that they could support and bounce ideas off one another. Each workshop had a mixture of student Police Officers, Social Workers and Nurses within it. There were ground-rules for the workshops that confirmed that the imprisoned mothers could choose not to answer any questions they were not comfortable with, and to leave the workshop at any time. The other ground-rule was that there were to be no interruptions or disrespectful comments. McKeown et al. (2010) have noted that one hazard of involving service users is that they can feel excluded by the use of professional jargon. During our workshops, the power dynamics in relation to jargon were turned on their head as it was the students who needed to seek clarification from the prisoners regarding frequently used terms such as Release on Temporary Licence (ROTL).

In the workshop, I facilitated there were some very frank, but at all times respectful, exchanges. A critique that is made in relation to service user involvement is that the voices of service users who have negative experiences of services can be absent (Irvine et al., 2015). This was not the case in our workshops. For example, one of the Police Officers and one of the prisoners discussed the issue of when Police Officers have to undertake dawn raids of houses. The imprisoned mother described how her teenage son was still traumatised by the Police smashing down her front door in the early hours of the morning, which he experienced as being akin to a burglary. The Police Officer acknowledged the impact upon children of these raids. However, he explained that while the Police tried to avoid dawn raids wherever possible when children and young people were around, there were occasions, for example if they were trying to find drugs or firearms, when they had no other option. He also confirmed that in accordance with the UK Human Rights Act (1998), any intrusion on the rights of citizens to privacy and private life had to be agreed by a magistrate when a warrant was obtained to confirm that the proposed manner in which the warrant was executed was both *necessary and proportionate.* An equally candid discussion occurred between an imprisoned mother who had a negative experience of Social Services and a Social Work student. The prisoner considered that she had not been listened to or valued in the course of an assessment. The Social Work student listened carefully to what she said, and did not seek to minimise how she had felt about that assessment. She did point out that there were times when the only option for protecting a child was to remove the child. During the course of the workshop discussions, it appeared that understanding between the professionals and imprisoned mothers was promoted through respectful communication and listening to one another's points of view.

We ended the day with a plenary session where all participants fed back on what they had learned and gained from the day which will be reflected in the feedback detailed below.

Evaluation: participant feedback

Evidence suggests that students react positively to interprofessional activities when they can clearly see their relevance to practice (Pirrie, Hamilton, & Wilson, 1999). This certainly seems to be borne out by the feedback comments from the students who took part in this workshop. We were interested in their experience of participating in an interdisciplinary learning event, their acquisition of knowledge and in the development of their practice skills. Therefore, student participants were asked to complete an evaluation form that focused on what they had learned from spending the day with students from other professional groups, what they had learned about the experiences of imprisoned mothers and their families and what they felt they would take away from the day into their practice. Evaluation forms were returned to us by virtually all the 90 participants and their responses can be grouped into 3 key themes:

- Challenging stereotypes, awareness of stigma and changed views
- Recognition of the needs of the children of prisoners
- Appreciation of the power of interdisciplinary working to deliver a good service

Challenging stereotypes/changing views

These were reflected in comments offered by students from all the professional groups involved in the day. Some focused on the service users:

> A changed view of people in prison and offenders (Children's Nurse)
>
> Not to stereotype. The impact on mothers and children (Social Worker)
>
> Not to stigmatize (people) who are sent to prison (Mental Health Nurse)
>
> More humility needs to be used in certain situations (Police trainee)

Others reflected on previously held views about other agencies and professionals:

> A changed view of the prison service (Health Visitor)

One social work student not only noted her changed views on her evaluation sheet, but sought out one of the workshop facilitators at the end of the day to emphasise how much her experience of the day had changed her outlook:

> I will research about women in prison and I am actually now thinking of working down those lines. My thinking has changed and I am more open and able to relate to them (prisoners)

Recognition of the needs of the children of prisoners

> The importance of supporting children and families to work through emotional issues that are created when a parent is incarcerated. The value of providing support to family members who have taken over the caring role in the absence of a parent. Importance of having a network of support services when released. (Social Worker)
>
> It has highlighted for me the lack of accountability and lines of communication which represent the very vulnerable population of children of imprisoned mothers. Huge safeguarding implications (Health Visitor)

> I will always consider the impact on children (Police trainee)
>
> That it is not just prisoners that are affected when someone goes to prison.
>
> It has a knock on effect and punishes the children and their families (Social Worker)

Appreciation of the power of interdisciplinary working to deliver a good service

> Good to see that there are other agencies out there to work with (Police student)
>
> I will clarify practice relating to how info is shared about mothers who go to Prison (Health Visitor)
>
> Learned how important multidisciplinary communication and teamwork is (Children's Nurse)
>
> Liaise with other agencies, forge contact – exchange information (Police student)

Another Police student had been inspired by the workshop to call in on all agencies who might be working with children of prisoners to have a cup of tea and to make himself known to them.

Interestingly, several of the mental health nurses commented on how they would transfer their learning into work with other groups of service users:

> To take children into consideration when parents are being sectioned, visiting hospital etc.
>
> As a mental health nurse, the same principles apply when we go into service users' homes and section patients. Planning and liaising with service providers to enable appropriate support for children is paramount.

The women prisoners who took part in the workshop offered us their own positive insights into their experience of the day. One commented: *I enjoyed taking part and giving the students an insight into prison life*. They were also able to make suggestions to inform the planning of future events. The quiz answers had revealed the levels of student knowledge/ignorance in relation women in prison: *clearly students knew little about this subject, but I wasn't surprised*. However, other feedback comments from the women revealed that the inter-professional workshop discussions had brought benefits not only for the students, but for the prisoners themselves:

> It gave students the chance to ask personal questions ... e.g. the Police understood the impact of not having a wash. Only way you would get personal questions answered was from the people who were there. I was surprised how open I was.
>
> Being a prisoner and having spent so long in prison ... You don't know how much work you have done (on yourself) until you are tested.

The prisoner's suggestions for future workshops centred on having more time for this personal contact: *More time for talking with students in small groups*.

Discussion and conclusion

It is clear from the feedback that the workshop had fulfilled its objectives of raising awareness, reducing stereotyping and stigma, and encouraging the students from different disciplines to work more closely together. Students were honest in relation to the previously held stereotypes they had regarding prisoners and the Prison service. Meeting prisoners and prison staff in person had the desired effect of humanising both groups. The result was that students were less likely to judge prisoners and more likely to engage with their prison service colleagues. I was particularly struck with the student Police Officer's comment that more '*humility*' needs to be shown, which means being humble and not believing you are better than other people. Again this implies that his thinking changed as a direct result of attending the event. Terry (2012) considers that involving service users has the potential to develop emotional intelligence, provided the recipients have some emotional intelligence to begin with to allow them to engage with the service users meaningfully. I consider the comments from that trainee Police Officer demonstrate how that occurred.

Likewise, it was very encouraging to hear the student Social Worker's comment about how they would practice differently as a result of the day, in which they recognised the importance of assisting families to work through the emotional impact of having a parent incarcerated. Again this evidences the emotional impact of hearing the accounts of the imprisoned mothers directly and the changes created in terms of aspirations for future practice as a result. Another student Social Worker commented that she was now more open and felt much more comfortable relating to prisoners as a result of attending the workshop. Again this very honest feedback suggests that prior to meeting the prisoners she was perhaps wary of engaging them, no doubt by negative and sensational portrayals of prisoners in the media. Clearly, this will have a direct impact upon her practice when she is required to meet prisoners in the course of her work. However, it also indicates that many professionals will be relating to prisoners during the course of their work informed not by a real experience of prisoners, but by absorbing negative cultural stereotypes about them. This clearly will impact on the quality of the professional relationships that can be created.

It was also very positive to see through the feedback the extent to which students had taken on key points about the needs of imprisoned mothers and their families. For example, they recognised the ripple effects upon the whole family when a mother is imprisoned. They also picked up on the potential safeguarding issues, and also the degree to which children with a parent in prison, especially an imprisoned mother, are particularly vulnerable. This knowledge galvanised them to consider how support networks could be developed for families in this position, and also brought home to them the importance of multi-agency working to achieve this. It was also very encouraging to hear the Mental Health Nursing students start to transfer the knowledge they gained to the work they undertake with sectioned parents.

An increase in confidence and a sense of purpose are recognised as one of the benefits for service users who participate in teaching events (Anghel & Ramon, 2009; Brown & Young, 2008). This was borne out by the feedback we received from the imprisoned mothers who participated. This confidence arose from the fact that the prisoners were aware that they were able to deliver something unique to the student professionals in terms of sharing their personal experience and perspectives, which provided an insight the students could not gain from any other source. A prisoner reflected that only the prisoners present were able to answer the personal questions posed by the students. Another prisoner clearly found the experience of taking part was a chance to take stock of her progress during her sentence. It confirmed to her what she had achieved while in prison and she '*surprised*' herself in terms of how open she was. This recognition of how her self-confidence had grown during her sentence was possible through being '*tested*' during the course of the workshop. This would suggest the workshop produced increased self-esteem and confidence for the prisoners. We were concerned that the workshops might have been too raw and demanding for the prisoners. However, their ability to articulate their experiences during them so well and their feedback that they would have valued more one to one time with the students, convinced us that the workshops provided the right format for small group discussions.

We were fortunate to have such a close pre-existing working relationship with a prison which we could build on to make this workshop a reality. However, I imagine that there are a number of universities that have similar well established relationships with prisons that could potentially allow a similar workshop to be delivered. My literature review did not identify any other universities which had engaged in a similar workshop so I am left wondering whether it was a unique event.

Acknowledgements

The author would like to thank Rachel Balen for having the idea for this workshop in the first place, and for having such a clear vision about how it would be planned and delivered. I would also like to thank other colleagues who were involved in the planning of and delivery of it: Dr. Kelly Lockwood, Dr. Christine Rhodes, Kath Padgett and Ruth Neville from the University of Huddersfield School of Human and Health Sciences; Inspector Kevin Robinson and P.C. Robert Winslade from West Yorkshire Police; Carol Burke MBE, now retired, but who was at that time Head of Family Services Governor at Askham Grange prison, and Graham Holgate, the Prison Officer who so skilfully facilitated the Prison Me? No Way! part of the workshop. In addition to this, I would like to thank the imprisoned mothers who kindly gave their time to courageously participate and for sharing their experiences so frankly.

Disclosure statement

No potential conflict of interest was reported by the authors.

ORCID

Ben Raikes http://orcid.org/0000-0001-5853-8522

References

Anghel, R., & Ramon, S. (2009). Implicarea beneficiarilor de servicii sociale si a sustinatorilor lor in pregatirea profesionala a asistentilor sociali: Un studiu de caz britanic [Service users and carers' involvement in social work education: Lessons from an English case study]. *European Journal of Social Work, 12*, 185–199.

Balen, R., Rhodes, C., & Ward, L. (2010). The power of stories: Using narrative for interdisciplinary learning in health and social care. *Social Work Education: The International Journal, 29*, 416–426.

Burgess, A., & Flynn, C. (2013). Supporting imprisoned mothers and their children: A call for evidence. *Probation Journal, 60*, 73–81.

Brown, K., & Young, N. (2008). Building capacity for service user and carer involvement in social work education. *Social Work Education, 27*, 84–96.

Caddle, D., & Crisp, D. (1997). *Imprisoned women and mothers*. London: Home Office.

CAIPE. (2002). *Defining IPE*. Retrieved January 23, 2016, from http://www.caipe.org.uk/about-us/defining-ipe/

Carlen, P., & Worrall, A. (2004). *Analysing women's imprisonment*. Cullompton: Willan.

Chapman Gibbs, P., Hayes, C., & Thomson, M. (2011). *Best practice in service user involvement in prisons and probation trusts'*. London: Clinks.
Charles, A., Rid, A., Davies, H., & Draper, H. (2016). Prisoners as research participants: Current practice and attitudes in the UK. *Journal of Medical Ethics, 42*, 246–252.
Corston, B. J. (2007). *A review of women with particular vulnerabilities in the criminal justice system*. London: Home Office.
Crewe, B., & Bennett, J. (2012). *The prisoner*. London: Routeledge.
Dickinson, C., & Carpenter, J. (2005). "Contact is not enough": An inter-group perspective on stereotypes and stereotype change in interprofessional education. In H. Colver, M. Helme, & I. Jones (Eds.), *The theory-practice relationship in interprofessional education* (pp. 23–30). London: Higher Education Academy: Health Sciences and Practice.
Featherstone, B., White, S., & Morris, K. (2014). *Re-imagining child protection: Towards humane social work with families*. Bristol: Policy Press.
Goffman, E. (1963). *Stigma: Notes on the management of spoiled identity*. Englewood Cliffs, NJ: Prentice Hall.
Heidensohn, F. (1985). *Women and crime*. London: Macmillan Press.
Irvine, J., Molyneux, J., & Gillman, M. (2015). 'Providing a link with the real world': Learning from the student experience of service user and carer involvement in social work education. *Social Work Education, 34*, 138–150.
Jones, A., Gallagher, B., Manby, M., Robertson, O., Schutzwohl, M., Berman, A. H., … Christmann, K. (2013). *Children of prisoners: Interventions and mitigations to strengthen mental health*. Huddersfield: University of Huddersfield.
LeBel, T. P. (2012). Invisible stripes? Formerly incarcerated persons' perceptions of stigma. *Deviant Behavior, 33*, 89–107.
Mccallin, A. (2001). Interdisciplinary practice – A matter of teamwork: An integrated literature review. *Journal of Clinical Nursing, 10*, 419–428.
McKeown, M., Malihi-Shoja, L., & Downe, S. (2010). *Service user and carer involvement in education for health and social care*. Oxford: Wiley-Blackwell.
Moyes, J. (1997, 18th July). Double stigma for women in jail. The Independent.
Murray, J., & Farrington, D. (2008). The effects of parental imprisonment on children. *Crime and Justice, 37*, 133–206.
O'Keeffe, H. (2013). The invisible child: Perspectives of head teachers about the role of primary schools in working with the children of male prisoners. *The Prison Service Journal, 209*, 24–28.
Pirrie, A., Hamilton, S., & Wilson, V. (1999). Multidisciplinary education: Some issues and concerns. *Educational Research, 41*, 301–314.
Prison Advice and Care Trust. (2011). *Protecting the welfare of children when a parent is imprisoned*. London: Author.
Prison Reform Trust. (2015). *Bromley briefings prison fact file Autumn 2015*. London: Author.
Robertson, O. (2007). *The impact of parental imprisonment on children*. Geneva: Quaker United Nations Office.
Scammell, J., Heaslip, V., & Crowley, E. (2016). Service user involvement in preregistration general nurse education: A systematic review. *Journal of Clinical Nursing, 25*, 53–69.
Smith, R., Grimshaw, R., Romeo, R., & Knapp, M. (2007). *Poverty and disadvantage among prisoners' families*. York: Joseph Rowntree Foundation.
Terry, J. (2012). Service user involvement in pre-registration mental health nurse education classroom settings: A review of the literature. *Journal of Psychiatric and Mental Health Nursing, 19*, 816–829.
Trotter, C. (2006). *Working with involuntary clients: A guide to practice*. London: Sage.
Warren, J. (2007). *Service user and carer participation in social work*. Exeter: Learning Matters.
Wilks-Wiffen, S. (2011). *Voice of a child*. London: Howard League for Penal Reform.
Worden, J. (2009). *Grief counselling and grief therapy: A handbook for the mental health practitioner* (4th ed.). New York: Springer.

Gaining by giving? Peer research into service user and carer perceptions of inclusivity in Higher Education

Joy M. Rooney, Peter F. Unwin and Nina Osborne

ABSTRACT
Service users and carers (SUAC) have made significant contributions to professional training in social work courses in Higher Education (HE) over the past decade in the UK. Such participation has been championed by government, academics and SUAC groups from a range of theoretical and political perspectives. Most research into the effectiveness of SUAC involvement at HE has come from the perspectives of academics and very little SUAC-led research exists. This qualitative peer research was led by two members of the University of Worcester's SUAC group. Findings were that SUAC perceived their involvement brought benefits to students, staff, the University and the local community. Significant personal benefits such as finding a new support network, increased self-development and greater confidence to manage their own care were identified in ways that suggested that the benefits that can flow from SUAC involvement at HE are perhaps more far-reaching than previously recognised. Barriers to inclusion were less than previously reported in the literature and the humanising effects of SUAC involvement are presented as a partial antidote to an increasingly marketised HE culture.

Introduction

For more than a decade, the University of Worcester, England, has included service users and carers (SUAC) in the recruitment and education of its students, in its quality processes and in its research endeavours. In England, the use of SUAC in academic settings is encouraged by both legislation and policy, particularly given recent concern about standards in practice (e.g. Francis, 2013). SUAC involvement in qualifying social work training has been mandatory since 2002 (Department of Health, 2002) and SUAC involvement within policy was first identified in The National Health Service and Community Care Act (1990) wherein a model of consumerism was promoted in an emerging patient- led NHS. Part of New Labour's marketisation and modernisation agenda for the NHS was designed to enable more choice for SUAC with a focus on including them in the delivery and service design of their own care (Department of Health, 2006). Similar policies of modernisation and marketisation have also come to dominate HE (Higher Education) in England (Jary,

2014). This consumerist agenda can be critiqued as an anti-professional neoliberal stance which views health and social care services as businesses in which the customer is king (Harris, 2003). Glasby and Beresford (2006) promote SUAC involvement, specifically in the research arena, as a necessary antidote to the elitist hierarchy that has characterised western academic research. Such a view positions SUAC knowledge as a different kind of knowledge, rather than an inferior type of knowledge, to that held by senior academics and professionals.

This paper reports the results of research led by the University of Worcester's SUAC group, 'IMPACT', into perceptions regarding the SUAC role both within the University and in regard to the wider community. SUAC perceptions regarding any associated achievements, benefits or barriers to inclusion were also explored. The IMPACT group has been involved in teaching and learning, recruitment and selection, quality assurance and research since 2008 and had 21 members at the time of the research project. Apart from one BME group member, all other participants are white British. The IMPACT group is made up of a variety of people who use services relating to physical disability (n. 6), mental health services (n. 2), substance abuse (n. 2), domestic violence (n. 1) chronic illness (n. 1) or are carers (n. 8) or care leavers (n. 1). The research team comprised two IMPACT members and an academic, the IMPACT members taking the lead in all aspects of fieldwork, analysis and write-up with the academic member being involved in the research analysis and write-up.

Literature review

SUAC involvement might be usefully analysed via Arnstein's (1969) Ladder of Citizen Participation (Figure 1):

This seminal model portrays a hierarchical construct of participation, placing 'Manipulation' on the bottom rung, along with 'Therapy', which are together classified as representing forms of non-participation in that they are seen as dishonest and patronising. The next rungs on the ladder—'Informing', 'Consultation' and 'Placation' are grouped together as 'Tokenism' in that a decision has probably already been made by the organisation in question and citizens are being given information rather than choice, being asked questions about a decision already made or being falsely reassured that there is nothing to worry about. The top three rungs on the ladder—'Partnership', 'Delegated Authority' and 'Citizen Control' are grouped together as 'Citizen Power'—and are seen to apply when decisions and planning matters are joint affairs, when citizens genuinely have at least some delegated authority to make a decision. Citizen Control indicates a form of participation whereby citizens design, plan and carry executive responsibility for an organisation or part of an organisation. Arnstein's model was developed from the field of urban planning but can be adapted to the situation of SUAC involvement in HE.

There is some reported SUAC-led research (e.g. Barber, Beresford, Boote, Cooper, & Faulkner, 2011; Brett et al., 2014; Faulkner, 2010; Gillard, Simons, Turner, Lucock, & Edwards, 2012; Gillard & Stacey, 2005; Hutchinson & Lovell, 2013; Patterson, Trite, & Weaver, 2014; Wallcraft, Fleischmann, & Schofield, 2012), which particularly relates to the health-oriented patient and public involvement (PPI) literature. With regard to the effect of SUAC involvement in research, Brett et al. (2014) systematically reviewed 66 studies of PPI involvement and demonstrated that, despite a relatively weak evidence base (due partly to the nature of SUAC involvement not always being made clear), health and social work

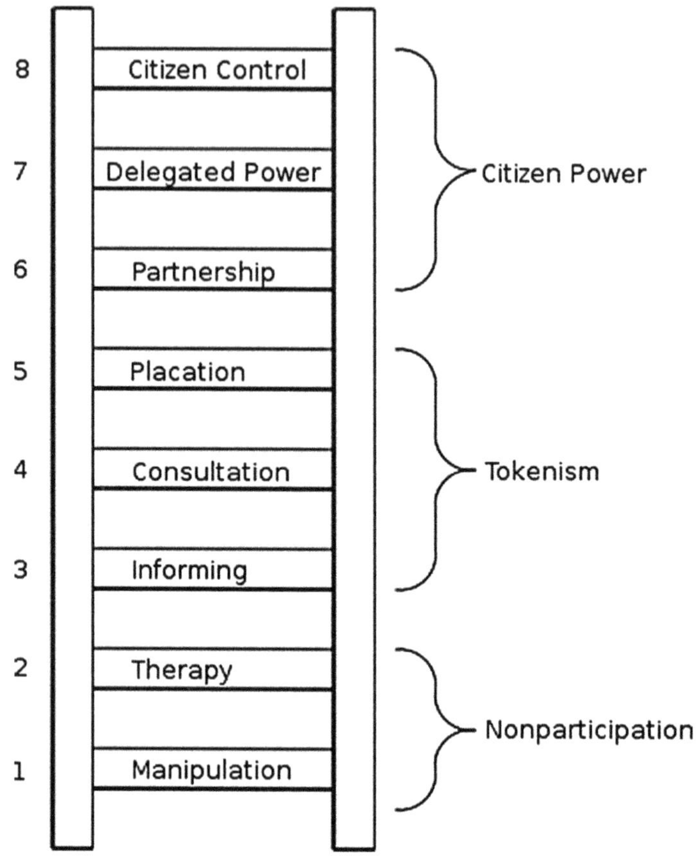

Figure 1. Eight rungs on a Ladder of Citizen Participation (Arnstein, 1969).

research has benefitted from PPI in the enhancement of the quality of research and in having better assured its appropriateness and relevance. This was particularly found to be the case when SUAC involvement was towards the top rungs of Arnstein's (1969) ladder, namely when SUAC were involved from design through to analysis and dissemination, rather than in sporadic or tokenistic ways.

McKeown et al. (2012) included three SUAC researchers in focus group research into why people elected to participate in the University of Central Lancashire SUAC group 'Comensus'. Their key findings suggested that SUAC participants used 'activist' concepts in making sense of their social relations. SUAC wished for social change, not personal gain, became more self-aware and felt valued, worked in a democratic way and benefitted from comradeship and sociability with other Comensus members. SUAC participants also became involved in a wider set of issues than their initial initiative and also wrote and led their own modules on the practice of involvement (McKeown et al., 2012).

In respect of SUAC involvement in health and social work in the UK, there has been little systematic progress made in evidencing its nature and its outcomes (McCutcheon & Gormley, 2014; Wallcraft et al., 2012). Despite some government initiatives (e.g. Department of Health, 2002) to further develop initiatives between SUAC, academics and practice, Rhodes (2012) concluded a literature review by stating that much more research is necessary to determine the effect of service users in transformative learning and care delivery. Towle et al. (2010) reviewed active patient involvement in the education of health professionals internationally and found a wide range of activity but no evidence suggesting any change in the behaviour of learners as a result of exposure to SUAC as part of their education.

Barriers to SUAC participation in health and social care education

Barriers are widely reported to still exist regarding the meaningful inclusion of SUAC in professional education across health and social care (Basset, Campbell, & Anderson, 2006; Lathlean et al., 2006 & Speed, Griffiths, Horne, & Keeley, 2012). Basset et al. (2006, pp. 395–400) identified 10 barriers to SU participation in mental health education and training. These were:

- hierarchies that exclude,
- stigma and discrimination—not a service user-friendly atmosphere,
- validation and accreditation processes,
- academic jargon and 'put-downs',
- clever people/clever excuses,
- knowledge as king and topics/levels,
- individual and not team approach,
- gaining access in the first place,
- bureaucratic payment systems,
- lack of support for trainers/educators.

Lathlean et al. (2006, p. 425) cited four barriers to SUAC involvement in health care education:

- the perception of service user involvement as being threatening to staff and their sense of professional autonomy,
- the stress of involvement may damage users' health,
- service users themselves may be reluctant or lack interest with factors such as age, gender, cultural background, diagnosis, previous health care experiences, personality characteristics and educational background playing a part,
- service users are not adequately remunerated for their contributions.

Speed et al. (2012), from a sample of 38 SUAC groups across the North West of England, determined the potential barriers to SUAC involvement in nurse education as:

- not knowing the context of the group,
- lack of preparation of the group,
- not being supported, not being allowed to be real,
- not receiving feedback,
- not being paid appropriately.

As suggested by these above barriers, the involvement of SUAC in HE is not straightforward, rather it is a complex undertaking full of issues around power/hierarchies/rights/language/stigma/remuneration and logistics. The methodology outlined below of using SUAC researchers to seek SUAC views in this project was designed to minimise some of these hierarchical/language and power barriers in the belief that fuller and franker data might result.

Methodology

The present research project came about as the result of an IMPACT subgroup which promotes and carries out research. Members suggested that a focus on the motivations for involvement seemed to be an area lacking in research which could possibly be used to add to knowledge as well as inform future recruitment/retention strategies. After an initial group discussion, two IMPACT members volunteered to take the lead in research design and implementation, working in partnership with the academic facilitator of IMPACT on subsequent analysis, write-up and dissemination of findings.

The method chosen by the two IMPACT researchers was one of conducting semi-structured interviews by Skype telephoning, a method previously used by the researchers and one which could produce rich data, as well as offering IMPACT members choice over when the interviews took place. Recordings were subsequently anonymised and transcribed. Core questions, designed by SUAC researchers, revolved around exploring whether there were any perceived benefits or disadvantages to students, the Institute of Health and Society, the University and the wider community from SUAC involvement. Questions were concerned with whether any personal achievements and benefits were perceived as flowing from their involvement within the fields of teaching and learning/recruitment, quality assurance and research. Additionally, a question was asked about any perceived barriers to fuller involvement with IMPACT and whether there were any views about whether IMPACT involvement brought any benefits to other community groups of which the participant might also be a member.

Ethical approval was granted by the Ethics Committee of the Institute of Society and Health at the University of Worcester. Invitations to participate and the associated consent forms were sent by e-mail to individuals on the database of the IMPACT group (n. 21). The two SUAC researchers, also members of IMPACT, were not included in the research sample. Each IMPACT member who expressed interest in the research was then telephoned and invited to return their consent form if they wished to participate. Fifteen semi-structured interviews with 11 female and four male respondents were subsequently carried out by Skype telephoning, this response level constituting 79% of the IMPACT membership eligible for interview. Reasons for those who did not participate included ill health or ill health in those they cared for, and lack of available time.

Recordings of the interviews were subsequently anonymised and transcribed. Both SUAC researchers independently analysed the interviews using thematic analysis and then met with their academic colleague to discuss and agree their findings.

Key findings

The research found that SUAC perceived that their involvement in HE brought benefits to students, to the Institute of Health and Society, to the University and to the wider community. Additionally, there was significant evidence of contributions made and personal achievements and benefits received by being members of IMPACT. Barriers preventing greater involvement were identified and suggestions for improving SUAC involvement were also made. The six key themes that emerged were those of:

(1) Perceived direct benefits to the students in the Institute of Health and Society through SUAC involvement in learning, selection and teaching.
(2) Perceived corporate benefits to the University.
(3) Perceived benefits of 'the two-way street' whereby group members brought experience and insight to the University and took new knowledge and insights back to their organisations.
(4) Perceived value of contributions made to students and staff across the Institute of Health and Society that may translate into practice.
(5) Perceived achievements and benefits to SUAC.
(6) Perceived barriers to SUAC involvement including accessibility, organisational and personal barriers.

These themes are presented in detail below:

Perceived direct benefits to the students in the Institute of Health and Society through SUAC involvement in learning, selection and teaching

The direct benefits of SUAC activities were mentioned 20 times by 15 respondents and fell into the following three categories—student learning, the teaching of students and student/staff selection:

With regard to student learning, students' confidence was perceived as having been built up through direct contact with the SUAC experience (4), either by direct testimony received or by SUAC having interacted with the same students over the duration of a course. Students were perceived as having been enabled to learn what impacts people's lives across a wide range of diverse groups and situations (3) and the quality of student readiness for practice was seen as having improved. SUAC respondents also believed that they provided a safe learning and research resource for students (2).

With regard to teaching, students were perceived as having benefitted from exposure to the reality of SUAC emotion in the 'safety' of the classroom (2); theory was related more to practice in the SUAC teaching sessions (1); a rounder, more holistic learning experience for students was offered (1) and there was opportunity to question SUAC within a classroom environment (1) without fear of sanction.

With regard to student selection, there were perceived impacts on the quality of students recommended for admission across social work and related courses (2) and a different perspective to the selection processes was provided, emphasising assessment of soft skills and value base (3) from the SUAC perspective.

Commentary—The above findings suggest that SUAC believe that they bring distinctive and valued aspects to student learning, teaching and student selection, perspectives that have not been detailed in the literature.

Perceived corporate benefits to the University

The corporate benefits of IMPACT as an organisation were recognised in 19 instances by 15 respondents and comments encompassed the following themes:

- IMPACT brings a humanising perspective to a world of academia that is increasingly preoccupied with targets and league tables (8).
- IMPACT was perceived as a 'hub' for the dissemination SUAC involvement across the University (2).
- Helping to meet course requirements for accreditation (4).
- Enhanced reputation for inclusion (2).
- Ticks boxes and gets 'brownie points' (2).
- Increases opportunities to access funding for courses/research (1).

Commentary—It is interesting to note respondents' views that staff also benefit from being reminded of the human side to their teaching and learning activities, which can all too easily be marginalised in a performance-managed culture. Respondents clearly demonstrated their awareness of the University's need to be able to demonstrate sufficient levels of SUAC engagement to gain accreditation and to pass audits/inspections but these comments were interpreted as being realistic rather than cynical and there was no suggestion that involvement was perceived as either mercenary or tokenistic.

Perceived benefits of 'the two-way street' whereby group members brought experience and insight to the University and took new knowledge and insights back to their organisations

Respondents mentioned that they carried out paid work in social care settings (2). Other respondents mentioned organisations or community initiatives with which they were involved (8). These were mainly voluntary organisations plus one member was an SUAC representative on The College of Social Work (TCSW) Board (The English Coalition Government had established TCSW in 2012 to champion and promote best practice across social work, including the involvement of SUAC. The College was in place at the time of this research but was unexpectedly shut down by government in 2015, some of its functions transferring to the British Association of Social Workers (BASW), others to the private sector and others being lost).

From the above responses, it can be seen that the type and level of contributions to the widening community are very varied, but in all cases members felt that IMPACT both provided benefits to, and benefitted from, their various other involvement and employment roles. Responses included:

> I take increased awareness and ideas about how to do service user and carer involvement into my job role

> … two-way general benefit through self-broadening

> I'm more open to different ways of working

> …. work experience enhances IMPACT role play, learning from diverse membership of IMPACT can be applied in work situations

> …. definitely a two-way flow- able to suggest speakers, think of different ways of working, more thoughtful about the kind of services needed and understanding of how things could be streamlined.

Commentary—The above responses demonstrate a two-way flow of learning and awareness facilitated by IMPACT members which helps the University to both deliver courses more effectively and to discharge its expressed strategies of inclusivity and widening participation. The sharing of insights, information and skills with those organisations with which IMPACT members are also involved was mentioned by a majority of respondents as an important spin-off from participation.

Perceived value of contributions made to students and staff across the Institute of Health and Society

Specific areas of experience that SUAC respondents believed they offered included:

- Helping staff learn/gain breadth of understanding about SUAC issues, leading to them valuing SUAC colleagues more (2).
- Presenting a strong and credible SUAC voice that offered real-time, contemporary information on issues such as the effects of social policy and legislation (2).
- Modelling advocacy in acting as a proxy for SU lacking capacity (1) and speaking as a member of ethnic minority (1).
- Improvement of course materials and policies through listening to the views and experiences of SUAC and acting on these perspectives in activities such as involving SUAC in the design and audit of curriculum (4).

Commentary—Respondents valued the richness of their diverse backgrounds and experiences and seemed very aware of how important these grass-roots perspectives were for both staff and students.

Perceived achievements and benefits to SUAC

Fourteen respondents identified having made positive personal achievements, between them giving 38 examples of what they felt they achieve:

Sense of achievement/purpose (19)

The greatest response was that of feeling valued (5), followed by making a difference/contributing (3), the knowledge that they were helping/useful (2) and finding the experience itself rewarding (2) were also significant positives mentioned by respondents. Other notions were those of self-satisfaction, still working to benefit others, using skills and professional expertise, promoting disabled people as equals, seeing people you have helped to select go on to become professionals, being recognised by students for their contributions, finding students' regard for SUAC involvement a 'breath of fresh air' and being given a new lease of life:

> With my involvement with IMPACT, I felt treated very much like an equal and somebody with something to offer, and so that's been very positive

> Well I feel that I've come in with a fresh approach to how I perceive how I would like to be treated as a patient

> You are valued as a carer … and there are things for you to do which are meaningful, that does give me a really good sense of value.

Access to training/learning (9)

A diverse set of issues were recognised in this area regarding the broadening of understanding/increasing one's own knowledge (2). Some other areas mentioned were keeping up to date in health and social care, being encouraged to take further training, being enabled to rekindle research skills and having access to University facilities/learning.

Enjoyment/increased emotional well-being (11)

Responses in this area included regained confidence (3), interesting/enjoyable work (2), helped me come out of myself, personal development, treated with respect/as equals, sense of belonging, changed attitude about work opportunities and finding the IMPACT work enjoyable/having a good laugh—'Oh gosh, yes. It's amazing, yeah. It's actually given me a lot more confidence, definitely. It's helped me to come out of myself a little bit more'.

People also felt that being a member of IMPACT gave them a voice, made them better at building relationships and helped them develop a more positive outlook on their personal situation:

> Yeah, so personal development, because I have sort of developed as a person, and the way I speak and I'm more focused on trying to get the outcomes to when I first started. So it's obviously been appealing to me as well as to the students and the academics that I've worked with.

Social networking/group support (6)

In this group, 20 separate references were made to the emotional and supportive benefits of involvement including the opportunity to work with interesting/varied people (3), social networking/group support (2) and help in overcoming risks of isolation/deskilling.

Fifteen responses cited practical benefits stemming from involvement which included being part of a community, knowing what is going on at the University and having contact with others about lived experience. Other responses included being paid (2) and one person had achieved a job beyond the University which they partly attributed to confidence gained by way of IMPACT activities. People also appreciated being able to update or gain new knowledge, learning reflective and resilience techniques, doing something properly in a supported setting and being able to work for the local good in terms of influencing the next generation of health and social care professionals. An overarching benefit of doing something stimulating is highlighted in the following quotes:

> It stops the brain cells, I suppose, from vegetating completely in retirement. Because it is stimulating and makes me think. I'm interested. It gives me another tack to think about and to explore

> Actually being a part of the University, I never would have thought I'd be working alongside the University. That's absolutely amazing. So yeah, I absolutely love it.

Commentary—This section is emphatic in its acknowledgement of the achievements and benefits perceived by individuals through participation in IMPACT. The identification of new social support networks, peoples' increased levels of self-awareness, confidence and emotional resilience suggest that there are overall long-term benefits to participation for SUAC.

Perceived barriers to SUAC involvement including accessibility, organisational and personal barriers

The four themes that emerged in this area were those of Accessibility, Organisational barriers, Personal barriers and Time constraints

Accessibility barriers

Accessibility barriers were perceived by respondents (12) as comprising:

- Inappropriate/repetitive work times such as early starts or late finishes that are challenging for those needing or arranging care (2).

This matter has been raised by the IMPACT facilitator with colleagues and is being addressed by working with staff to increase awareness about appropriate timings, rooming and the need for appropriate breaks in long sessions.

- Expectation that members are competent with technology.

Training is offered to IMPACT members in the use of technology and alternative communication methods are also being used which respect individual SUAC circumstances and abilities.

- Poor communication regarding meeting details.

A set format for communications and a 'catch all' plan has been developed for last-minute instructions. Dedicated administrative support for IMPACT has been successfully lobbied for by IMPACT members and the IMPACT facilitator.

- Excessive distances to travel (3).

It has been accepted that it is not reasonable to ask IMPACT members to travel significant distances for short sessions. Wherever possible, extra activities are planned that are designed to account for at least a half-day input.

- Mileage being 'mean' at 25p a mile (2).

Travel is paid for all IMPACT activities but this rate set is a corporate rate which it has not, as yet, proved possible to change.

- Formatting of e-documents for screen reader/individual needs.

The particular needs of IMPACT members are being addressed incrementally by the University's IT specialists, many of these needs being similar to those of students with impairments.

- Arrangements and costs of support workers and scribes.

A strategy has been developed for organising such support, making use of services previously only made available to students. All additional support worker costs incurred by partaking in IMPACT activities are paid from the IMPACT budget, which has been increased accordingly. A system has been brought into play with the help of the new administrative support that better guarantees equality of opportunity and participation of all IMPACT members in all activities.

- University perceived as an elite establishment 'not for people like me':

Community facilities are now offered as an option for initial meetings with potential IMPACT members to lessen any stigma that might be attached to University premises for people who have never been to a University.

Organisational barriers (10)

The major one was seen as:

- Not enough members/diversity within membership.

Prior to this study, recruitment to IMPACT had largely been by word of mouth. This strategy tended to attract similar members to the existing members, the vast majority of whom were white British, wider recruitment drives are now in place, supported by an information pack and a user-friendly application form, designed by IMPACT members. Members from a wider range of ethnic backgrounds have been recruited as a result of this new approach.

- Lack of awareness of what is happening in IMPACT.

A communication strategy has been developed which includes periodic updates on all work streams. The work streams of Recruitment and Selection/Quality Assurance/Learning and Teaching and Research meet three times per year, now supplemented by a twice-yearly meeting of the whole group. An online newsletter is also in the process of development.

- Limited utilisation of some members/systems for work allocation not clear/short notice of work allocation.

A clear strategy is now in place that avoids any perceptions of favouritism in respect of letting IMPACT members know about work opportunities. This appears to be working well. Staff have been asked to give reasonable time frames when requesting IMPACT involvement although some requests for IMPACT involvement inevitably come with short notice requirements.

- Rate of remuneration not having increased.

The rate of pay has now been increased from £2.50 p.h. to £12.50 p.h. The rate for teaching/leading seminars has remained static at £18.00 in line with wider University policy regarding visiting lecturer rates.

Personal barriers (10)

- Personal health/stamina (5).

Flexibility is built into work delivery plans and it is accepted that some SUAC will need to 'step back' from time to time. A cooperative culture has developed within the group and members will sometimes ask each other to substitute in regard to a commitment they are unable to fulfil due to personal circumstances.

- Lack of care cover/child care (2).

While IMPACT cannot facilitate the actual child care, any additional costs incurred by way of IMPACT duties are now covered by its budget.

- Lack of skills or knowledge (2).

Training sessions regarding activities such as Research and Recruitment/Selection are run on an annual or biannual basis and a system of individual appraisal is being developed to better ensure that all IMPACT members work to their potential.

- Need for a regular income.

Engagement of IMPACT members is dependent on demand, which fluctuates from semester to semester; hence, it is not possible to assure a regular level of income from IMPACT duties.

Time constraints (10)

- Busy lifestyle/family life (5), work/study commitments (2) and carer responsibilities (3).

It is inevitable that the everyday caring and coping demands on SUAC will limit their availability for IMPACT. Such pressures are accommodated within IMPACT's systems, including payments to cover caring responsibilities. Clear communication to enable advanced planning is taking place with improved awareness of replacement carer/child-care payments.

Commentary—Although the above comments indicate the presence of real and ongoing barriers for respondents continuing their involvement with IMPACT, these are being addressed within IMPACT and the University as discussed above. The presentation of such candid comments might be seen as partly due to the research having been led by peer researchers. The wider resonance of these issues with previous research in this area will be further discussed below.

Discussion

This current study, led by two SUAC researchers, has produced some noteworthy findings, particularly around the themes regarding perceived achievements and benefits to SUAC participants in HE. These add to those achievements and benefits of wider SUAC participation reported elsewhere (e.g. Barber et al., 2011; Brett et al., 2014; Faulkner, 2010; Gillard & Stacey, 2005; Gillard et al., 2012; Hutchinson & Lovell, 2013; Patterson et al., 2014; Wallcraft et al., 2012). Other findings of this study, such as those that perceive considerable benefits to the education of students, corroborate other non-SUAC-led research findings about such benefits (e.g. Anghel & Ramon, 2009; Chambers & Hickey, 2012).

Brett et al. (2014) found that research benefitted from SUAC involvement when that involvement was systemic from conceptualisation through to dissemination. The present study can be viewed as according with this model and is also valuable in respect of its clarity regarding the actual parts played by SUAC in the overall research. Brett et al. (2014) criticised much previous literature due to its lack of specificity about the SUAC role. Involvement in IMPACT can be seen to be largely perceived by SUAC respondents as fitting with Arnstein's (1969) 'Partners' rung, which is within the subgrouping of 'Citizen Control', although the two higher rungs in this sub-category—'Delegated Power' and 'Citizen Control' do not seem to be reflected in the findings. Indeed, in respect of co-production as applied to SUAC involvement in HE, more delegated power and citizen control might not equate as being 'top of the ladder'. For example, in social work student recruitment and in the assessment of role plays and biographical, reflective pieces, SUAC already have delegated authority but any marking is always negotiated with an academic partner. This joint knowledge is seen as the best knowledge and there were no respondents asking for more power and control in this research, rather they wished for closer and more transparent partnerships.

Glasby and Beresford (2006) view that SUAC knowledge should be seen as of equal value to academic knowledge appeared to be reflected in SUAC perceptions of the value they bring to staff and students in HE. The perception that this knowledge, combined with personal growth and development, is also carried back to benefit their own organisations is a new research finding, warranting further enquiry. Positive partnership working between staff and SUAC is demonstrated in this study, as is the lack of stigma and discrimination associated with SUAC involvement that has been widely reported in previous publications (Basset et al., 2006; Lathlean et al., 2006; Speed et al., 2012). Basset et al. (2006) listed 10 types of barriers to participation and only two, namely the gaining of access in the first place and SUAC groups at HE perhaps operating on an individual rather than a team basis, can be seen to feature in the present study's findings. Lathlean et al. (2006) identified barriers to SUAC involvement to comprise staff seeing such involvement as threatening, SUAC finding involvement damaging to their health, SUAC being reluctant to engage and remuneration being inadequate. There was some evidence of reluctance to engage found in the present study, largely to do with feelings that universities were not for 'people like me' although steps have since been taken to allay such stigma with potential new recruits, such as offering first meetings outside of University premises. The issue of inadequate remuneration did feature in the present study and steps have again been taken since the study to remedy some of these concerns, although others, such as mileage rates, have remained unchanged. Speed et al. (2012), with specific reference to nurse education, had found that SUAC were often unprepared and unsupported by staff in regard to the context of their involvement, that no feedback was received and that remuneration was again inadequate. These issues, apart from that of remuneration, were absent from the present study.

Nevertheless, the research project also acted as a 'Health Check' for IMPACT after eight years of operation and, despite its many positive findings, the perceived barriers to participation were of particular concern, leading to some of the changes in practice discussed above. It is perhaps encouraging that these barriers were largely perceived by SUAC respondents as barriers that could be overcome in a spirit of partnership, suggesting that some of Glasby and Beresford's (2006) aspirations for a lessening in hierarchical practices within HE are actually happening. The responses regarding barriers were candid and might have been so as a result of SUAC peers having conducted the field research. As suggested by Barber et al. (2011), peer researchers might be viewed as theoretically more likely to bring out candid responses in fieldwork. While this study cannot claim generalisability, the extent and depth of disclosure as well as the level of constructive criticism about changes needed in IMPACT, can be hypothesised to have been less likely to have flowed from a more hierarchical form of research, such as that led by academics.

Conclusions

The overall achievements and benefits perceived by SUAC participants in this study are considerable. SUAC respondents reported being given a sense of purpose, access to training/learning, personal development/increased emotional well-being, practical and material benefits, social networking and peer support. Such findings are similar, although more far-ranging, to those reported by Towle and Godolphin (2015).

The rich and candid findings that have emerged from this peer-led research study are distinctive in their depiction of SUAC themselves benefiting significantly from their own involvement in HE. 'Gaining by Giving' is the overarching and novel theme which stands out from the key findings, a theme which represents an important role for universities in the ever-marketised world of HE. The SUAC members of the IMPACT group perceive that they benefit greatly in terms of personal development and well-being, while the University of Worcester receive the input of the widening community to give added value across a wide range of functions. This added value was perceived as relating to the selection of students, teaching, learning, staff knowledge and awareness, curriculum development, feedback, research and corporate compliance with national policies and requirements. However, in line with the findings of Towle et al. (2010) and Rhodes et al. (2014), no hard evidence emerged in this study regarding SUAC involvement having brought about transformative change in the learning or practice behaviour of students, which is the main aim of SUAC involvement within HE. Further research, co-produced between academics and SUAC, into the effects on subsequent practice in social work and associated fields is needed to ascertain whether SUAC learning is translated into practice.

Universities in England operate on business models whereby league tables and performance indicators can make them lose sight of one of their core purposes, namely being part of, and educating, a community. Widening participation and including non-traditional members is an aim often to be found in the corporate-speak of universities' prospectuses and strategic plans. The University of Worcester's IMPACT Group has convinced its own members that inclusivity and widening participation are realities rather than aspirations. This is not to forget also that the educational experiences of staff and students were perceived as being well-served via their exposure to the diverse and varied experiences of IMPACT members, experiences that will hopefully be translated into practice.

References

Anghel, R., & Ramon, S. (2009). Service users and carers' involvement in social work education: Lessons from an English case study. *European Journal of Social Work, 12*, 185–199. doi:10.1080/13691450802567416

Arnstein, S. (1969). A ladder of citizen participation. *Journal of the American Planning Association, 35*, 216–224. doi:10.1080/01944366908977225

Barber, R., Beresford, P., Boote, J., Cooper, C., & Faulkner, A. (2011). Evaluating the impact of service user involvement on research: A prospective case study. *International Journal of Consumer Studies, 35*, 609–615. doi:10.1111/j.1470-6431.2011.01017.x

Basset, T., Campbell, P., & Anderson, J. (2006). Service user/survivor involvement in mental health training and education: Overcoming the barriers. *Social Work Education, 25*, 393–402. doi:10.1080/02615470600593675

Brett, J., Staniszewska, S., Mockford, C., Herron-Marx, S., Hughes, J., Tysall, C., & Suleman, R. (2014). Mapping the impact of patient and public involvement on health and social care research: A systematic review. *Health Expectations, 17*, 637–650. doi:10.1111/j.1369-7625.2012.00795.x

Chambers, M., & Hickey, G. (2012). *Service user involvement in the design and delivery of education and training programmes leading to registration with the health professions council.* Retrieved from http://www.hpc-uk.org/assets/documents/10003A08serviceuserinvolvementinthedesignanddeliveryofapprovedprogrammes.pdf

Department of Health. (2002). *Requirements for social work training.* Retrieved from http://webarchive.nationalarchives.gov.uk/20050831173515/, http://www.dh.gov.uk/PublicationsAndStatistics/Publications/PublicationsPolicyAndGuidance/PublicationsPolicyAndGuidanceArticle/fs/en?CONTENT_ID=4007803&chk=Cg4OdW

Department of Health. (2006). *Our health, our care, our say: A new direction for community services.* CM6737. Retrieved from http://www.official-documents.gov.uk/document/cm67/6737/6737.pdf

Faulkner, A. (2010). *Changing our worlds: Examples of user controlled research in action.* Eastleigh: INVOLVE.

Francis, R. (2013). *Report of the Mid Staffordshire NHS Foundation Trust Public Inquiry.* Retrieved from https://www.gov.uk/government/publications/report-of-the-mid-staffordshire-nhs-foundation-trust-public-inquiry

Gillard, S., Simons, L., Turner, K., Lucock, M., & Edwards, C. (2012). Patient and public involvement in the coproduction of knowledge: Reflection on the analysis of qualitative data in a mental health study. *Qualitative Health Research, 22*, 1126–1137. doi:10.1177/1049732312448541

Gillard, S., & Stacey, E. (2005). All talk: Experiencing user-led research. *A Life in the Day, 9*, 27–30. doi:10.1108/13666282200500017

Glasby, J., & Beresford, P. (2006). Who knows best? Evidence-based practice and the service user contribution. *Critical Social Policy, 26*, 268–284. doi:10.1177/0261018306059775

Harris, J. (2003). *The Social work business*. London: Routledge.

Hutchinson, A., & Lovell, A. (2013). Participatory action research: Moving beyond the mental health 'service user' identity. *Journal of Psychiatric and Mental Health Nursing, 20*, 641–649. doi:10.1111/jpm.12001

Jary, D. (2014). The marketisation of UK higher education. *Journal of Widening Participation and Lifelong Learning*, 16, 71–77. doi:10.5456/WPLL.16.3.71

Lathlean, J., Burgess, A., Coldham, T., Gibson, C., Herbert, L., Levett-Jones, T., … Tee, S. (2006). Experiences of service user and carer participation in health care education. *Nurse Education Today, 26*, 732–737. doi:10.1016/j.nedt.2006.07.017

McCutcheon, K., & Gormley, K. (2014). Service-user involvement in nurse education: Partnership or tokenism? *British Journal of Nursing, 23*, 1196–1199. doi:10.12968/bjon.2014.23.22.1196

McKeown, M., Malihi-Shoja, L., Hogarth, R., Jones, F., Holt, K., Sullivan, … CIT. (2012). The value of involvement from the perspective of service users and carers engaged in practitioner education: Not just a cash nexus. *Nurse Education Today, 32*, 178–184. doi:10.1016/j.nedt.2011.07.012

The National Health Service and Community Care Act. (1990). Retrieved from http://www.legislation.gov.uk/ukpga/1990/19/section/46

Patterson, S., Trite, J., & Weaver, T. (2014). Activity and view of service users involved in mental health research: UK survey. *British Journal of Psychology, 205*, 68–75. doi:10.1192/bjp.bp.113.128637

Rhodes, C. (2012). User involvement in health and social care education: A concept analysis. *Nurse Education Today, 32*, 185–189. doi:10.1016/j.nedt.2011.11.012

Rhodes, C., Hardy, J., Padgett, K., Symons, J., Tate, J., & Thornton, S. (2014). The health and well-being of service user and carer educators: A narrative enquiry into the impact of involvement in healthcare education. *International Journal of Practice-based Learning in Health and Social Care, 2*, 51–68. doi:10.11120/pblh.2013.00025

Speed, S., Griffiths, J., Horne, M., & Keeley, P. (2012). Pitfalls, perils and payments: Service user, carers and teaching staff perceptions of the barriers to involvement in nursing education. *Nurse Education Today, 32*, 829–834. doi:10.1016/j.nedt.2012.04.013

Towle, A., Bainbridge, L., Godolphin, W., Katz, A., Kline, C., Lown, B., & Thistlewaite, J. (2010). Active patient involvement in the education of health professionals. *Medical Education, 44*, 64–74. doi:10.1111/j.1365-2923.2009.03530.x

Towle, A., & Godolphin, W. (2015). Patients as teachers: Promoting their authentic and autonomous voices. *The Clinical Teacher, 12*, 149–154. doi:10.1111/tct.12400

Wallcraft, J., Fleischmann, P., & Schofield, P. (2012). *The involvement of users and carers in social work education: A practice benchmarking study*. London: Social Care Institute for Excellence. Retrieved from http://www.scie.org.uk/publications/reports/report54.pdf

Being a service user and a social work academic: balancing expert identities

Joanna Fox

ABSTRACT

I am a service user and academic working in a university social work department. My hybrid identity allows me to draw on different types of knowledge in all aspects of my work, including: academic, practice and experiential wisdom. Service user involvement is mandated across social work education but the scope and breadth of different kinds of participation is developed in diverse ways across university contexts. This article affirms the value of service user involvement in health and social care education, exploring its positive impact on students. When lecturers share personal experience of using services alongside practice and academic wisdom in the course of teaching, sometimes the value of experiential knowledge is doubted and its influence dismissed. I examine the importance of experiential wisdom in social work education, specifically when it is embedded in an academic role in a university social work department, and consider how it can be respected and valued. The parallel experiences of involving peer support workers in mental health services, who use their knowledge of recovery to mentor other service users, are then briefly examined, together with reflection of the concerns across mental health with professionals sharing their experiential wisdom with the people that they support.

Introduction

Service users are increasingly becoming involved in all aspects of UK health and social care professionals' pre-qualifying training (Anghel & Ramon, 2009; Rush, 2008) and often in their continuing professional development (Webber & Robinson, 2012), with social work having adopted this requirement for their participation in qualifying courses since 2002 (Levin, 2004). The professional regulator of UK social work education, formerly the General Social Care Council (Levin, 2004) and now the Health and Care Professions Council (HCPC, 2009); mandates the involvement of people who use services and their carers in all aspects of pre-qualifying training including: programme development, admissions processes, assessment practices, teaching and learning, and programme management. The increased participation of service users in health and social care education demands their recognition as experts-by-experience. This inevitably changes the perception of their role from passive recipients of services to active citizens (Barnes & Bowl, 2001); however many questions remain unresolved about the nature of a service user's authority and expertise as they contribute their knowledge from experience to developing and delivering education.

Although it is a requirement that service users and carers contribute to social work education (HCPC, 2009; Levin, 2004), in many university contexts, there is a division between the status to the different kinds of knowledge possessed by service users and lecturers respectively: experiential, practice and academic wisdom. I am a social work lecturer, a service user, a social work researcher and an activist; a hybrid identity central to all aspects of my work. In the classroom, I share many of my own experiences of mental ill-health with students to enable them to understand this lived reality and to underline the need for mental health services to support recovery. In my capacity as a service user, alongside that of being a social work academic, I am able to reflect on experiences of oppression, discrimination and stigmatisation which are central to my identity as a mental health service user, and am able to convey multiple perspectives derived from experience, academia and practice.

My experience as a person who both uses mental health services and teaches social work leads me to disclose personal experience, and mix discussion of what occupies the personal and the professional realms. I encourage students to consider how services may be perceived by the user as oppressive when practitioners consider them to be supportive and effective in managing risk. For example, when I relate that, as both a prospective mother and an identified mental health service user, I was provided with an enhanced provision from maternity services (Fox, 2012, 2016) I reflect on how I felt I had to be a compliant patient as I was subject to professionals' authority and yet wanted to be a self-advocate who challenged deficits-focused practice. Yet should we as social worker lecturers share experience or should we focus on 'scientific' and theoretically based academic and practice wisdom?

This consideration is underpinned by an implicit belief in how we value the different kinds of wisdom derived from experience, practice and education, and how we utilise these different perspectives in the professional arena. It leads to questions about the nature of expertise, authority, and wisdom. In this article the value of user involvement is underlined in health and social care education by highlighting the impact of experiential knowledge on student learning, with consideration of the diverse ways in which they contribute to education programmes. This leads to discussion of the potential role of the service user lecturer in social work academia, and reflection on the nature of their wisdom and experience. The article concludes with consideration of the best ways to embed real learning from expertise-by-experience in social work education.

Background

As previously stated, service users' contribution to health and social care programmes can enable students to relate to their clients as experts-by-experience (Anghel & Ramon, 2009) leading them to apply the strengths approach in their practice (Fukai, Goscha, & Rapp, 2012). Gregor and Smith (2009, p. 24) note that social work students may 'embark on their social work training with a strong conviction that they want to "help" people in distress and it may therefore be more difficult for them to reconcile the fact that service users are indeed capable individuals who may not always require "help"'. Service user involvement in education has the potential to rebalance and redefine power relationships (Fox, 2015) even when social workers traditionally hold the power; as indeed with additional training as Approved Mental Health Professionals social workers may invoke the law in specific circumstances to compel people experiencing mental ill health to be detained in hospital (Golightley, 2014).

Similarly, there is now growing evidence of the positive influence of service user involvement in the adjoining field of nursing education (Rush, 2008), with it now becoming an integral part of health care training (The Willis Commission, 2012). Rush (2008), in an early study in nursing training, highlights how nursing students experienced a sense of transformational learning (Mezirow, 2000) as they participated in a module developed in partnership between educationalists and service recipients. This allowed the power and authority between the different stakeholders to be redefined: the students sought to make sense of the service user's story by engaging in dialogue with the service user and learning about their experiences. This demanded a reversal of the traditional roles with the service user becoming the helper and the students the helped. This approach, which emphasised a change in power differentials influenced the emotions of the student as their assumptions about people with mental health needs were changed. This led them to resolve to change future practice, thus reflecting a process of transformational learning.

There is a strong evidence base of the positive impact of service users' contribution to the training of social work students (Allain et al., 2006; Anghel & Ramon, 2009; Gregor & Smith, 2009). Although many small scale qualitative studies have been undertaken in which the value of user involvement in education has been confirmed, a limitation of current research is its focus on evaluation of the process of service user involvement with little consideration of its impact on outcomes (Webber & Robinson, 2012).

Arnstein's (1969) Ladder of Involvement was the first model that sought to quantify and understand the nature of service users' involvement in decision-making processes. This has been widely used in community development work to evaluate the nature of power and influence that service users hold; similarly it can be used in education. Building on Arnstein's (1969) Ladder of Involvement, Tew, Gell, and Foster (2004) proposed five stages of service user involvement that can be applied to professional training:

Level 1: No involvement
Level 2: Limited involvement
Level 3: Growing involvement
Level 4: Collaboration
Level 5: Partnership

Additionally Webber and Robinson (2012) evaluated service user involvement in the training of post qualifying social work students and developed four levels of involvement: consultation, partnership, political and user control. This model reflects the stages developed by Tew et al. (2004), building on Arnstein's (1969) work. However, the latter two stages of political involvement and user control emphasise the importance of utilising a democratic model of involvement that is underpinned by equality between service users and other partners. Webber and Robinson (2012, p. 1268) highlight the political aspects of service user involvement which 'model radical social work … by building a community of service users and carers and by seeking to contribute to wider political change'.

Despite strategic mandates which drive the participation agenda forward (HCPC, 2009; Levin, 2004; The Willis Commission, 2012), as teaching programmes are developed, power and control tends to become concentrated in the hands of educationalists rather than in those of service users; although educators may choose, from a position of authority, to share some of their power with service users. Some lecturers confine user involvement to that of wheeling out the service user to tell their story (Gregor & Smith, 2009); this reduces user knowledge merely to the service user identity and undermines the potential ways in which experts-by-experience can contribute to professional development. This aligns in part to Arnstein's (1969) notion of 'tokenism'; and merely reinforces the idea of service users as passive recipients of services rather than active citizens who are experts-by-experience (Barnes & Bowl, 2001).Despite this, when all stakeholders collaborate to build effective involvement, service users can begin to share power. Allain et al. (2006, p. 412) note that as experts-by-experience contributed in more creative and innovative ways to the development of the social work programme at Middlesex University they began to feel they had 'reached rung six (partnership) where we are just beginning to negotiate a more effective participatory role'.

Sometimes lecturers, from a position of power, are anxious about the negative impact of involvement on service users' well-being; despite service users often demanding their increased participation in ever more creative and innovative ways. Duffy, Das, and Davidson (2013) discuss how students and staff perceived service users' involvement in role plays which were used in a social work module to assess students' readiness for direct practice. Concerns were expressed about using *real* service users in the role play scenario as it was believed that they could be negatively impacted by insensitive questioning from inexperienced students. Does this coincide with a professional's duty of care to protect service users from harm? Or does it concord with risk averse practice? Social role valorisation (Wolfensberger, 1972), an early concept developed during transition from institutionalised care to independent living in the community, reinforces the need for professionals to support service users to develop positive social identities that can be respected by the wider community. Ion, Cowan, and Lindsay (2010) note how this concept can help us to understand the respect and authority that service users can gain when they make a useful contribution to training mental health professionals.

Despite this, it is noted that the attainment of a 'positive' identity, which is central to the notion of social role valorisation (Wolfensberger, 1972), is framed by the constructions of the community – i.e. a valued role is socially constructed by the normative framework. Moreover, the recognition that is acceded to expertise-by-experience in social work education is also socially constructed and framed by those who have the power; this means that expertise-by-experience and its value and acceptability in social work education is defined by the dominant social work discourse. This begs the question: is the place of expertise-by-experience in social work education transient or is it perceived as a permanent and powerful aspect of social work education?

Coulter, Campbell, Duffy, and Reilly (2013), drawing on Freire's (1970) work, emphasised the notion of education as a liberating, anti-oppressive, political endeavour, in their context in a university setting in Northern Ireland. Their study, based in a community which had experienced the political conflict of the 'Troubles', evaluated the students' responses as lecturers brought the 'victims' and 'perpetrators' of political violence into the classroom. This process enabled the social work students to reflect on the possible challenges of working with people who had both experienced and perpetuated political violence. Focusing on sharing diverse and challenging perspectives of conflict underlines the premise that user involvement in education can be a form of political expression (Freire, 1970; Webber & Robinson, 2012) as indeed the students own political perspectives were challenged and confronted. In support of this, McLaughlin (2009, cited in Duffy & Hayes, 2012) reminds us of the anti-oppressive nature of social work and its underpinning tradition of sharing power by working in partnership with those who receive services or who have experienced violence and oppression, reinforcing its political nature. More widely, the discourse of expertise-by-experience (Fox, 2015), which highlights the capacity and skills of people who receive services, goes some way to challenging the prevailing belief in professional hegemony by underlining the value of experiential wisdom – emphasising the political nature of user expert knowledge.

This article has explored the nature of user involvement in education as a catalyst for transformative learning (Rush, 2008); as an anti-oppressive and liberating process (Coulter et al., 2013); and as a potentially political action (Webber & Robinson, 2012). In the next section, I reflect on my hybrid identity as a lecturer who uses services and consider whether this is seen as an authoritative and effective way to convey the reality of experience.

Discussion

Social workers are encouraged to be reflective practitioners who critically consider the connections between their personal and professional ethics and how these influence their behaviour (Beckett & Maynard, 2013). When lecturers have lived experience of using services, which is central to their teaching, it is unclear on what basis their authority is founded and how their wisdom is valued by both lecturers and students in academia. My authority as an academic in the classroom is derived from my professional knowledge, yet it is the story of my lived experiences that most inspires my students. In order to resolve this conundrum, it is necessary to explore how academic and experiential wisdom interact and to consider what happens when the lines between professional and personal knowledge are blurred, and more widely how user involvement can be most effectively embedded in social work education.

Intersectionality, developed by Crenshaw (1989), provides a framework for understanding how the different identities that people possess can compound their sense of oppression. Crenshaw (1989) reflected on the multiple experiences of oppression of African-American women in USA arguing that this was not related merely to their gender or their ethnicity, but was rather located in the intersectionality of both identities. The multi-dimensional experiences of exclusion experienced by women of colour were derived from being a part of a society that was patriarchal and which comprised a white majority, locating power in the hands of white men who failed to understand and relate to the needs of women of colour. As a lecturer, I possess the authority from my status as an academic located in a university institution which expounds academic and scientific knowledge intersecting with the powerlessness and stigma of being a service user in a discriminatory society. How do students relate to this authority that intersects with experiences of powerlessness and discrimination?

Gregor and Smith (2009) noted that when a service user comes into a classroom and becomes the lecturer, it can be difficult for the lecturer labelled as the service user to maintain a sense of authority, they may instead be labelled as 'that person who has done really well to get to where they are'. Gregor and Smith (2009, p. 27) consider that the 'service user identity can be confusing for all parties, for they are neither a fulltime service user, nor social worker, nor full-time lecturer. This either/or/neither/nor' can be projected on to the student group who may also become confused as to what role the service user is fulfilling'. They however highlight that because one in six people experience mental ill-health at one point in their lives, there may inevitably be a blurring of boundaries between who is the service user and who is the potential professional; despite this they contend that it is often easier for students to 'other' service users by putting them into pigeon holes. Ion et al. (2010, p. 7) reflect that students may hold 'damaging stereotypes' about people with mental health issues and that 'by introducing students to service users in the role of lecturer, we go some way to challenging these unhelpful and corrosive portrayals of, most often, very ordinary people who are struggling to cope with extraordinary experiences and circumstances'.

Simons et al. (2007) advocate that the best way for service user knowledge and authority to be embedded in a university context is for the creation of a service user academic post to support the participation agenda. They built on a model developed in an Australian university that sought to develop the specific role of service user academic (Happell, Pinikahana, & Roper, 2003) However, some failures with this model in the English context were highlighted by Simons et al. (2007) during implementation; they noted that the service user academic didn't have the normal employment support such as an academic induction and she failed to undertake normal academic roles (like marking) as part of her normal day-to-day duties. This was designed to enable her to focus her time on developing service user involvement but her role was inevitably perceived as endowing her with less authority and influence.

Webber and Robinson (2012, p. 1264) argue that meaningful involvement 'ideally requires embedding service users and carers in university social work departments as lecturers'. They however highlight that such a role concords with the model of consultation, as presented earlier, rather than that of political or user control. They argue that this framework is focused on consulting a limited number of people rather than genuinely empowering service users or fostering a movement of control to them – although acknowledging that different service user academics will utilise such a role in different ways depending on their strengths and skills. Furthermore, Beresford and Branfield (2012) note that current models of service user involvement draw on the consumerist model of involvement rather than the democratic model. The former is based on the idea of market forces in public services, whereas the latter emphasises the importance of citizenship, equal opportunities and the development of a rights- and responsibility-based society (Beresford, 2002).

Furthermore a consideration of the changes in health and social care discourse shows that it is a *collective* movement that challenges established power, rather than the actions of *individual* experts. For example, physically disabled people, as a collective group rather than as individual experts, redefined established knowledge as they developed the social model of disability (Finkelstein, 1990; Oliver, 1983, 1990; Shakespeare, 2006). This radical movement led to a reinterpretation of the way physical barriers which prevented disabled people's access to and participation in society were understood. This action by disabled people began to define the role of service users not just as service recipients but as citizens living beyond the label of their impairment (Shakespeare, 2006). Similarly, the collective power of the mental health service user movement led to user involvement in service review and development (Rose, 2001).

This above discussion highlights wider concerns about the nature of effective user involvement in social work education and the concomitant value placed on individualised expert experience compared to that of collective knowledge. Harrison (2002), in an early paper on representation of users in service development and service review, questions the status of the individual service user as an effective representative. Harrison (2002, p. 29) notes that service users who speak on behalf of their peers can be perceived as professional users, 'not typical users'. He considers that it is very difficult for service users to represent their group's views unless accountability processes are transparent; where this does happen, their credibility as service consultants is increased, and thereby their credibility with other professionals. Without an established network, a representative cannot take a mandate from their peers, they are not accountable to the group, and cannot be said to represent the group (Barnes, 1997). This analysis directly challenges the premise that embedding a lecturer with lived experience in a university department is a sustainable model for implementing user involvement in social work education.

Furthermore, Stickley (2006) radically questions the reality of service user involvement in mental health services by asking if the participation agenda is tokenistic, conforming to empty rhetoric. He argues that if service users sit on committees and become too professionalised then they can no longer challenge the dominant mental health discourse which has disempowered and disabled service users throughout many years. Stickley (2006, p. 576) contends that 'The very system employed by those within positions of power to apparently promote more democratic change, that is, service user involvement in the existing powerful psychiatric system, is the very structure that will continue to retain overall control'. He argues for the necessity to confront the hegemonic authorities to enable service users to challenge the oppression of mental health services.

This analysis highlights that the very processes of involvement impact on what we consider are effective ways to convey authentic and tangible expertise-by-experience to health and social care students. However, the questions remain: does my role as a service user and lecturer suggest an innovation that has potential to transform education and focus it on user expertise, or does it rather suggest a concession to the user involvement agenda? And even more widely; is a singular model of user representation credible or should a collective model of representation be developed in university social work departments? This allows us to return to the original question: how and when should lecturers who use services share experiential wisdom in teaching and what is the nature of their expertise and authority?

Contention about the knowledge that a professional lecturer should share when teaching social work students parallels much debate in mental health care as we consider the role of Peer Support Workers (PSWs) in supporting recovery. PSWs are employed to use their experiences of recovery to mentor other service users and are beginning to gain a greater presence in mental health care (Ockwell, 2012; Repper & Carter, 2010) as their authority is becoming more recognised. The debate about the role of PSWs in mental health care can help us to locate current arguments about the role of the service user lecturer in social work education for there are many parallel issues.

When service users contribute to education, they can help students to understand the need to work from a strengths perspective (Fukai et al., 2012) and to work in a way which promotes hope and optimism – in a context which is akin to the contribution that PSWs can make to the service users they mentor (Ockwell, 2012). Health and social care lecturers often question the ability of service users to maintain appropriate professional boundaries between themselves and students; this is similarly highlighted by practitioners as they consider the role of PSWs working with service users and in using their own experiences to support recovery (Repper & Carter, 2010). Duffy et al. (2013) wanted to protect the mental well-being of service users as they considered whether they should take part in role play scenarios; such concerns are similarly held by health professionals as they consider the needs of PSWs (Repper & Carter, 2010), highlighting the need to ensure they didn't take on too many shifts particularly during waking nights.

In a wider debate, concerns expressed about social work educators incorporating experiential wisdom alongside practice and academic wisdom in teaching is paralleled in debates in practice. How do we locate the place of trained professionals, such as social workers, CPNs and psychiatrists, who also use services, and want to use experiential wisdom to support their practice? Indeed, all such debates relate to occupational and professional status and what is the best way to deliver best practice care and support in education, practice and research. As a service user lecturer, I share many of the experiences similarly played out in mental health services, these are based on the stigmatisation of mental ill health and the accompanying suspicion that it is better to remain silent about these experiences and confine them to the personal realms.

Conclusion

This article has described the evidence base that underpins the usefulness of service user involvement in health and social care education, and considered the diversity of the ways in which service users contribute to different programmes. I have considered the potential ways in which the authority and influence of service users can be secured in social work education by embedding them in academic roles in universities, and highlighting the challenges to this more widely, by asking if a singular model of user representation is even credible or whether it should be replaced by a collective model of involvement, I have concluded by drawing parallels between the experiences of PSWs in mental health services and service user lecturers in social work education.

Many studies have indicated that students themselves value listening to service users' experiences in education (Anghel & Ramon, 2009) and note how it can lead to transformative learning (Rush, 2008). Students themselves affirm experiential wisdom is important in changing practice, therefore we must seek to increase the opportunities they have to learn from authentic experience. This will enable us to ensure that education is based on parity of influence between different stakeholders (Tew et al., 2004), and not on a foundation that allows lecturers to confine the service user perspective to them 'telling their story' (Gregor & Smith, 2009) – which often points to tokenism rather than partnership working (Arnstein, 1969).

As I teach students about social work, I mix professional language and underpinning theory with personal experience. I remind students of the importance of understanding experience through authentic reflection and underline the impact of their power on service users' lives (Fox, 2012, 2016). I am therefore able to make experiences of service receipt real and tangible to students. However, more widely the diagnosis of mental ill health continues to be stigmatised and the professional utilisation of experiential experiences in education and in practice is still under-explored and under-valued; despite the mandate that service users and carers should be involved in all aspects of health and social care education. It is important to ensure that lecturers who acquire knowledge through experiential wisdom experience similar levels of authority and power as those who acquire expertise through their education and practice.

References

Allain, L., Cosis Brown, H., Danso, C., Dillon, J., Finnegan, P., Gadhoke, S., ... Whittaker, F. (2006). User and carer involvement in social work education – A university case study: Manipulation or citizen control? *Social Work Education, 25*, 403–413. doi:10.1080/02615470600593790

Anghel, R., & Ramon, S. (2009). Service users and carers' involvement in social work education: Lessons from an English case study. *European Journal of Social Work, 12*, 185–199. doi:10.1080/13691450802567416

Arnstein, S. (1969). A ladder of citizen participation. *Journal of the American Institute of planners, 35*, 216–224.

Barnes, M., & Bowl, R. (2001). *Taking over the asylum: Empowerment and mental health.* New York, NY: Palgrave.

Barnes, M. (1997). *Care, communities and citizens.* Harlow: Addison Wesley Longman.

Beckett, C., & Maynard, A. (2013). *Values and ethics in social work.* London: Sage. ISBN 9781446203200.

Beresford, P. (2002). User involvement in research and evaluation: Liberation or regulation? *Social Policy and Society, 1*, 95–105.

Beresford, P., & Branfield, F. (2012). Building solidarity, ensuring diversity: Lessons from service users and disabled people's movements. In M. Barnes & P. Cotterell (Eds.), *Critical perspectives on user involvement* (pp. 33–45). Bristol: Policy Press.

Coulter, S., Campbell, J., Duffy, J., & Reilly, I. (2013). Enabling social work students to deal with the consequences of political conflict: Engaging with victim/survivor service users and a 'Pedagogy of Discomfort'. *Social Work Education, 32*, 439–452. doi:10.1080/02615479.2012.668180

Crenshaw, K. (1989). Demarginalizing the intersection of race and sex: A black feminist critique of antidiscrimination doctrine, feminist theory and antiracist politics. *University of Chicago Legal Forum (PhilPapers), 140*, 139–167.

Duffy, J., Das, C., & Davidson, G. (2013). Service user and carer involvement in role-plays to assess readiness for practice. *Social Work Education, 32*, 39–54. doi:10.1080/02615479.2011.639066

Duffy, J., & Hayes, D. (2012). Social work students learn about social work values from service users and carers. *Ethics and Social Welfare, 6*, 368–385. doi:10.1080/17496535.2012.654497

Finkelstein, V. (1990, March 22). Conductive education: A tale of two cities. *Therapy Weekly*, pp. 6–7.

Fox, J. (2012). Best practice in maternity and mental health services: A service user perspective. *Schizophrenia Bulletin, 38*, 651–656.

Fox, J. (2015). The contribution of experiential wisdom to the development of the mental health professional discourse. *Schizophrenia Bulletin.* doi:10.1093/schbul/sbv082

Fox, J. (2016). A personal reflection on working with parents with mental ill-health: Obstacles and opportunities for delivering best practice. In M. Diggins (Ed.), *Parental mental health and child welfare work* (pp. 25–29). Hove: Pavilion Publishing and Media.

Freire, P. (1970). *Pedagogy of the oppressed.* New York, NY: Seabury.

Fukai, S., Goscha, R. J., & Rapp, C. A. (2012). Strengths model case management fidelity scores and client outcomes. *Psychiatric Services, 63*, 708–710.

Golightley, M. (2014). *Social work and mental health.* Exeter: Learning matters.

Gregor, C., & Smith, H. (2009). "I'm not a performing monkey": Reflections on the emotional experience of developing a collaborative training initiative between service users and lecturers. *Journal of Social Work Practice, 23*, 21–34. doi:10.1080/02650530902723290

Happell, B., Pinikahana, J., & Roper, C. (2003). Changing attitudes: The role of a consumer academic in the education of postgraduate psychiatric nursing students. *Archives of Psychiatric Nursing, XVII*, 67–76.

Harrison, M. (2002, September 28–30). Perils of engagement. *Mental Health Today.*

Health and Care Professions Council. (2009). *Standards of education and training.* London: Author. Retrieved from http://www.hcpc-uk.org/assets/documents/1000295EStandardsofeducationandtraining-fromSeptember2009.pdf

Ion, R., Cowan, S., & Lindsay, R. (2010). Working with people who have been there: The meaningful involvement of mental health service users in curriculum design and delivery. *The Journal of Mental Health Training, Education and Practice, 5*, 4–10.

Levin, E. (2004). *Involving service users and carers in social work education. Resource guide No 2.* London: Social Care Institute for Excellence. Retrieved from http://www.scie.org.uk/publications/guides/guide04/

McLaughlin, H. (2009). What's in a name: "Client", "Patient", "Customer", "Consumer", "Expert by Experience", "Service User" What's next? *British Journal of Social Work, 39*, 1101–1117.

Mezirow, J. (2000). Learning to think like an adult: Core concepts of transformation theory. In J. Mezirow & Associates (Eds.), *Learning as transformation: Critical perspectives on a theory in progress* (pp. 3–33). San Francisco, CA: Jossey-Bass.

Ockwell, C. (2012). Challenges and triumphs: Developing an inpatient peer support project. *The Journal of Mental Health Training, Education, and Practice*, 7, 94–100. doi 10.1108/17556221211236501

Oliver, M. (1983). *Social work with disabled people.* London: Macmillan, British Association of Social Workers.

Oliver, M. (1990). *The politics of disablement.* Basingstoke: Macmillan.

Repper, J., & Carter, T. (2010). *Using personal experience to support others with similar difficulties:A review of the literature on mental health in peer support services.* Nottingham: University of Nottingham/Together. Retrieved from http://www.together-uk.org/wp-content/uploads/downloads/2011/11/usingpersexperience.pdf

Rose, D. (2001). *Users' voices: the perspectives of mental health service users on community and hospital care.* London: The Sainsbury Centre for Mental Health.

Rush, B. (2008). Mental health service user involvement in nurse education: A catalyst for transformative learning. *Journal of Mental Health, 17*, 531–542. doi:10.1080/09638230802053383

Shakespeare, T. (2006). *Disability rights and wrongs.* Abingdon: Routledge.

Simons, L., Tee, S., Lathlean, J., Burgess, A., Herbert, L., & Gibson, C. (2007). A socially inclusive approach to user participation in higher education. *Journal of Advanced Nursing, 58*, 246–255.

Stickley, T. (2006). Should service user involvement be consigned to history? A critical realist perspective. *Journal of Psychiatric and Mental Health Nursing, 13*, 570–577.

Tew, J., Gell, G., & Foster, S. (2004). *Learning from experience: Involving service users and carers in mental health, education and training. A good practice guide.* MHHE (Mental health in higher education), NHS (National Institute for Mental Health in England), Trent NHS Workforce Development Confederation.

Webber, M., & Robinson, K. (2012). The meaningful involvement of service users and carers in advanced-level post-qualifying social work education: A qualitative study. *British Journal of Social Work, 42*, 1256–1274.

Wolfensberger, W. (1972). *The principle of normalization in human services.* Toronto: NIMR.

The Willis Commission. (2012). *Quality with compassion: The future of nursing education. Report of the Willis Commission on nursing education.* London: Royal College of Nursing. Retrieved from www.rcn.org.uk/williscommission

Role-played interviews with service users in preparation for social work practice: exploring students' and service users' experience of co-produced workshops

Sara Hitchin

ABSTRACT
Within a *Theory and Practice of Social Work* module, prior to embarking on practice placements, social work students practised professional communication skills with people who had used social work services. They undertook role-played interviews with service users about real issues, which had led individuals to seek assistance in the past. Using principles of co-production, the workshop was developed in partnership with members of the University's social work service users and carers' group. Care was taken to safeguard service users' well-being, as well as developing an effective learning opportunity. Drawing on evaluations by students and feedback from service users, this paper discusses the process of planning and delivering the workshops, as well as perceived outcomes for both groups. Findings indicate that students valued the opportunity to engage with service users, gaining key learning about their own practice skills. Service users described a boost to self-esteem through contributing to students' learning. The workshop provides an example of how service user involvement in social work education has evolved from a primary focus on sharing personal testimonies to active participation in student skill development. It underlines the importance of investment in service user involvement to achieve an appropriate context for such projects to develop.

Introduction

This paper explores how a service users and carers' involvement group in one Scottish University, arrived at a point whereby six members felt confident enough in their role as student educators to allow students to practise professional communication skills with them. This involved using role-play around experiences that led them to seek social work support in the past. The paper argues that this type of engagement with students is significantly more demanding of service users than traditional forms of involvement, such as sharing personal stories, but that, with appropriate preparation and support, such an experience can be beneficial to both students' learning and service users' self-esteem and personal development.

Through exploration of the planning and delivery of the workshop and drawing on evaluation by both students and service users, the paper highlights the evolution of service user and carer involvement, and will argue that this is only possible when there is investment by academic staff and group members in such work.

Whilst people who have experience of using social work services are referred to here as 'service users', this paper acknowledges that this and alternative terms in current usage fail to accurately reflect the relationship between social workers and the people we work with (McLaughlin, 2009). It is, therefore, avoided where possible but, in the absence of a preferred alternative term, used on a number of occasions.

Background to the workshop

The Framework for Social Work Education in Scotland (Scottish Executive, 2003) sets out the requirements and standards for social work education in the Scottish context. This includes service user and carer involvement, which is seen as integral to the development, re-approval and delivery of the BA (Hons) and MSc/PG diploma programmes delivered by eight Scottish Universities. Service user and carer participation was initially supported by an annual Scottish Government grant of £5000 per University for the first five years of the new degree in Scotland (2005–2010).

The Unity service user and carers' group was established in 2005 with some founder members still currently involved. A model of partnership with local services proved effective, with agency staff supporting the involvement of their members to attend monthly meetings, deliver teaching workshops, etc. and becoming members of the group themselves. A range of local services were represented—five different mental health agencies, a self-advocacy service for people with a learning disability, people with a physical disability and parents of children who were receiving support from a voluntary agency. All members were white Scottish adults. Whilst the group recognized that it lacked diversity amongst its membership, in terms of representation of young people, people from minority ethnic groups and those from seldom-heard groups, this proved difficult to address and, whilst this cannot be explored in depth here, work on this issue is ongoing.

It soon became apparent that direct work with students was most members' main interest and that this was taking place, primarily within agency groups. For example, service users and staff from one mental health service developed and delivered a workshop on experiencing symptoms of mental ill health. Whilst this input appeared to be effective for student learning, it meant that not all group members were having regular opportunities to work with students. This was potentially divisive and early signs of a competitive dynamic began to emerge. In 2009, opportunities to work together on the production of a DVD for teaching purposes and developing a new workshop entitled 'The ideal social worker' opened the doors to a more inclusive approach to involvement. Networking opportunities arose; members got to know each other and each other's agencies better and sharing lunch following monthly meetings encouraged social contact. Relationships between members of the group, including with academic staff appeared to be strengthened and celebrations of successes such as the launch of the DVD galvanized the group as a vibrant, committed and enthusiastic body with a clear sense of group identity, shared role and purpose.

An underpinning philosophy of the group emerged as it became clear that, for the group to work well, everyone involved should feel that they were getting something out of it;

benefits should be reciprocal. Ager, Dow, and Gee (2005) report a similar process whereby group values were forged and this is in line with guidance set out by Levin (2004). Whilst the language of co-production was not being used at the time, the operation of the group was consistent with core principles of co-production: *Reciprocity, Equality, Accessibility* and to a lesser extent, *Diversity* (Social Care Institute for Excellence [SCIE], 2013). Co-production is a process, which involves working in partnership by sharing power with people who use services or are carers (SCIE, 2013). The staff involved in working with Unity attempted to promote a partnership approach so that members were welcomed, their ideas were listened to and valued and they had a central role in decision-making around the work of the group.

Scottish Government funding enabled the group to take on projects such as the development of the DVD, printing of newsletters as well as the core business of reimbursing travel expenses and providing catering for meetings. As a group, members decided that payment for teaching contributions was unnecessary. Whilst this is an ethically uncomfortable position, which cannot be fully explored here, it became apparent that the established level of service user and carer involvement could not possibly be sustained if a going rate was paid for contributions, primarily because workshops involved several members at a time (up to 15). As a compromise position, members received gift cards on an annual basis as a token thank you. Feedback from members indicated that they valued their involvement in teaching students on a personal level, gaining confidence and increasing self-esteem. This group consolidation set the firm foundation on which it was possible to develop the role-played interview workshop.

Government funding came to an end in 2011 leading to uncertainty about the viability of properly supported service user and carer participation. At this University, one student cohort recognized the risks that lack of ring-fenced funding posed to the work of the group and, valuing their involvement, organized a sponsored event in order to raise funds.

The use of role-play

Role-play is a recognized method of teaching social work skills (Hargreaves & Hadlow, 1997; Skilton, 2011; Wilson & Kelly, 2010) and forms a central element of the *Theory and Practice of Social Work* module. This takes place in the semester preceding the first assessed practice placement (Year two of the four-year honours degree and year one of the MSc/PG diploma). The module is taught over eight days with a large group lecture and small group work format in the mornings and two practice skills groups, each working with one tutor in the afternoons. Opportunities to develop core communication and engagement skills before embarking on placements are crucial if University staff are to be confident of students' readiness to work effectively with service users (Moss et al., 2007; Scottish Executive, 2003; Skilton, 2011). Indeed, such readiness is assessed, on this module, through a video recorded role-played interview along with an accompanying written assignment. The module must be passed before students can proceed to their first practice learning opportunity.

Although, undoubtedly a valuable tool for skills practice, role-play between students has limitations. Some struggle to get beyond the unreality of the scenarios they are asked to submerge themselves into, both in the roles of service user and social worker. Wilson and Kelly (2010) found that students identified role-play as a strength of preparation for practice teaching whilst also identifying the artificial nature of role-play as a weakness.

Naylor and Finger (as cited in Faherty, 1983) suggest a framework for analysing the effectiveness of role-play in terms of *Internal, External* and *Interactive* consistency. They highlight the difficulties, which can arise with *Internal Consistency* when a student in service user role introduces new and contradictory information, for example. Similarly, *External Inconsistency* can arise when the student in social worker role lacks accurate information about law, policy or procedure. Issues relating to *Interactive consistency* can occur when existing role relationships e.g. being friends, impact on the reality of the role-play. This is apparent when students give overly positive feedback to each other. The opportunity to practise skills with people who have experience of using social work services seems to offer significant advantages, therefore, in terms of increasing both *Internal* and *Interactive Consistency*. Issues of *External Consistency* can be addressed by giving students time to research a scenario prior to undertaking the role-play or, as in this case, by setting learning objectives which focus on establishing a rapport and gaining an understanding of the person's concerns rather than planning any form of intervention.

Practicing skills with service users who are focused on student learning, in a safe, classroom environment appears to offer more in-depth learning and preparation for practice than student-to-student role-play alone. Moss et al. (2007) report that a higher degree of realism was achieved in skills laboratories when service users and carers were role-playing an agreed set of scenarios. Duffy, Das, and Davidson (2013) give an account of service users undertaking assessed role-plays with students where relevant scenarios rather than real experiences were used. Ethical concerns are highlighted around service user involvement in role-play and the use of real-life experience, some of which are addressed in the following section of this paper.

Developing the workshop

Unity members were invited to take part in a workshop, which involved using role-play with students in order for them to practise professional communication and engagement skills. A planning meeting was arranged in order for service users and carers' group members to plan the workshop with two academics, both experienced social workers, one of whom was the module coordinator as well as being convener of the Unity group. Members opted into the session and came along on the understanding that they were under no obligation to take part in the workshop but would be able to gain a better understanding of what would be involved before deciding whether to take part and contribute to its design. Informed choice and opportunities to influence how the workshop would operate were fundamental in terms of co-production (SCIE, 2013).

Some members described themselves as familiar with role-play, whilst for others it was entirely new. Everyone was given an introduction to the use of role-play in student skill development followed by an opportunity to practise role-play with a staff member and to discuss how the session would be structured.

A central concern of group members was whether or not to draw on real experiences from their past or to use fictional scenarios. Following group discussion, everyone opted to draw on an experience that had led to them seeking assistance from social work services. Members gave the rationale that it would be easier for them to draw on their own experiences and, therefore, more authentic for students. Members expressed concerns about having insufficient understanding of specific experiences to be able to elaborate accurately on fictitious scenarios. Such concerns are consistent with Naylor and Finger's consideration of *Internal Consistency* (as cited in Faherty, 1983).

Each member was supported to develop a brief written scenario as referral information to be given to students before undertaking the role-played interview. Scenarios were selected on the basis that they warranted an initial meeting, rather than being part of an ongoing situation and did not include overly complex information or that which might result in a child or adult protection response. This was intended to enable students to focus on using their interpersonal skills to engage with the individual, establish a rapport and begin to undertake an initial assessment rather than worrying about how they should respond to an urgent, high risk situation. Hargreaves and Hadlow (1997) highlight the importance of setting clearly defined learning objectives for role-play in order to avoid distraction by the many interesting issues that are likely to arise.

A further important criterion for scenario development was that Unity members were comfortable revisiting aspects of their life that had been difficult for them. This was particularly important as the students would be learning the basics of interview skills and, as inexperienced practitioners, may not always handle the encounters with complete sensitivity. Skilton (2011) highlights the potential emotional impact of crossing the boundary between role-playing and acting out one's own issues, whilst Duffy et al. (2013) raise concerns around the possibility that participation in role-play might expose service users to risk of distress and harm. With such concerns in mind, respecting members' choice to draw on their own experiences and careful preparation with opportunities to debrief were crucial.

The value of the planning meeting was particularly apparent as one member, Lorna, identified an issue, undertook a practice role-play with a staff member and realized that the situation she had chosen was still too painful for her to explore in this way. She considered withdrawing from the workshop at this point but was able to identify another, less painful, issue to use for the role-play. Lorna decided to remain involved and has subsequently taken part in the workshops for two years with plans to be involved next time round. How Unity members manage the emotional impact of taking part will be discussed later.

In the first year of the role-play workshops, six members took part; five of them were users of mental health services, one also being a carer. One person had a learning disability and participated with the support of a worker from the self-advocacy group of which he was a member. Five of the same people took part in the second year, one person being unwell at the time but indicating a desire to be involved next time. The group comprised of three men and three women, all within the 50–65 years age range.

It was apparent from the planning stage that this was different from other teaching sessions that members had taken part in. Those who volunteered were experienced members of the group, had been involved for several years, had good relationships with staff and with each other and had grown in confidence throughout their time with the group. They were used to taking part in sessions, which involved giving their personal testimonies, talking to small groups of students about their experiences and facilitating workshop exercises. In the second year, a newer group member opted to come to the planning session but later decided not to take part in the role-play workshop, although they did take part in other teaching input. This is, perhaps, a further indication of the different level of engagement required of service user volunteers in this workshop.

Benefits to service users through involvement in social work education have been identified in a number of studies and these include having a valued role, increased skills and confidence (Brown & Young, 2008), finding the experience enjoyable (Moss et al., 2007), being valued, helping others and coming together as equals (Scheyett & Kim, 2004). Rhodes et al. (2014) reported similar benefits to service user and carer educators involved in health care education. It became apparent that participation in the role-played interview workshop asked service users to step back from an *expert* role, where they shared their views on what makes a good social worker, for example. Rather, through undertaking role-play with students, they were being asked to return to a former situation where they needed help and experienced relative powerlessness. Some situations would inevitably involve a strong emotional component (Hargreaves & Hadlow, 1997). Given that documented benefits to service users, primarily relate to more traditional forms of engagement with students, it is important to be mindful that taking part in the role-play aspect of the workshop is inherently different and benefits to service user participants cannot be assumed. Therefore, both in terms of ethical partnership and the principle of reciprocity, it was important that members emerged from the sessions without experiencing a negative impact on themselves, at the very least, and hopefully experiencing benefits from their involvement. This highlights the importance of members being able to de-role from that of *service user seeking help* and resume the role of *expert with experience of using services and in educating students* by giving feedback to students and entering into discussion around issues arising from the role-play.

Service user members were, in fact, given limited guidance on how to give feedback, although they were encouraged to consider non-verbal communication and to focus on how the interaction made them feel. They were given an explanation of the purpose of the exercise and the module's role in preparing students for their first assessed practice placements. The process of giving feedback in a balanced and supportive way was also discussed. On the basis of this paper's findings, future planning sessions will pay greater attention to the process of giving feedback to students. Skilton (2011) found that training workshops for service users and carers were successful in increasing confidence including around giving feedback, whilst 91% of students in their study reported finding the feedback helpful.

The workshops

In the first year, the opportunity for students to undertake role-played interviews with Unity members was offered as an option for students who would otherwise be undertaking role-played interview skills practice with each other. Following overwhelmingly positive feedback from participants, an additional workshop was offered so that more students could take part in year one and the workshop was built into the programme in such a way that all students undertaking the *Theory & Practice* module would experience this opportunity over the course of two, two-hour workshops in future. Workshop sessions were structured so that students were allocated to triads. This allowed them to practise professional communication skills using role-play scenarios in the main class, enabling them to alternately take on the role of service user, social worker and observer. Hargreaves and Hadlow (1997) highlight the valuable learning available to students through undertaking all three roles. One tutor worked with this group of around 30 students with two Practice Educators. Their role was to facilitate the use of scenarios, observe role play and give feedback to students on the skills demonstrated.

In a second classroom, the module coordinator met with Unity members prior to the session in order to go over the workshop aims and format and to ensure that all members were feeling confident and happy to proceed. The room was set out so that each Unity member had a space with three chairs beside them. Student triads were invited to come to the room in groups allowing for one triad to work with one Unity member at a time. On arrival, the students, from each triad, were given brief scenarios. These acted as referral information and allowed the student and service user to go straight into the role-played interview. For example:

> You are meeting Michael for the first time and are visiting him at home. He has contacted the social work office, where you are on placement, with concerns about his housing support which is funded by social work.
>
> You are meeting Oliver for the first time and are visiting him at home. Oliver has a learning disability and lives with his father. He has been upset by young people in the area shouting names at him and throwing stones and would like some support in relation to this. (NB, Oliver is being supported to take part in the workshop today by Joe who will not be participating in the role play)

Triads were directed to the relevant service user, where those not undertaking the role of social worker took on the role of observers. After a 10-minute role-play, student observers, Unity member and in some cases the tutor, gave feedback to the student in social worker role. Triads then moved around the room so that each student in the triad undertook the role of social worker with a different service user. Once all the students had undertaken the role of social worker and received feedback, students returned to the main teaching room and another group of students joined the service users.

The tutor role involved monitoring and offering support to both Unity members and students as well as facilitating the session. Ensuring that all the students had the opportunity to work with service users necessitated maintaining tight timescales. This had implications for both student and service user experience of the workshop, as student triads often entered into lengthy discussions with service users after undertaking the role-play. This time enabled service users to come out of *service user seeking help* role and resume the role of *expert* by giving feedback to the student and sharing experiences. Whilst this was valuable in itself, time constraints meant that groups had to move on in order for others to have the opportunity to take part. Getting this balance right was important in order for service users to experience their involvement as beneficial, as well as for students to recognize the ways in which people had been able to move on with their lives and use their experiences to contribute to student learning (Brown & Young, 2008; Scheyett & Kim, 2004).

Following the sessions, the module coordinator spent time with service user group members to debrief. This is an important element of engagement, which enables both staff and service users to reflect on and learn from the experience and to ensure that individuals are feeling supported and haven't been unsettled by taking part (Duffy, 2006).

Evaluation

Evaluation was undertaken in line with the British Sociological Association Statement of Ethical Practice (British Sociological Association, 2002). Arrangements were discussed and approved by a member of the School of Applied Social Science's ethics committee.

Following the workshops, students were asked to complete anonymous evaluation forms. As these were not expected to be used for publication at the time, retrospective consent was sought with students being invited to opt out if they had any objections to their anonymous feedback being used. No objections were made.

Evaluation by Unity Members took place through verbal and written feedback as well as anonymous evaluation forms immediately after the workshops. A focus group also took place several months after the second workshop. Each participant signed a consent form, agreeing to participation and to their anonymous comments being used in publication.

Student evaluation

> I really enjoyed it. I felt that the interview with the Unity member felt almost like I was in practice as it was their real problems which allowed me to feel empathy. (Student quote, 2015)

In 2014, the workshop was optional for students ($n = 47$) so both those who participated and those who chose not to take part were invited to give feedback. In 2015, the workshop involved all students, with two sessions scheduled into the module timetable ($n = 45$).

The students who chose not to participate but returned evaluation forms in 2014 ($n = 21$) gave a number of reasons for their decision, the majority of these relating to lack of confidence and feeling that it was too soon to put underdeveloped skills into practice. There is learning from this in terms of the timing of workshops with service users, to ensure that students have the opportunity to practise skills together before hand. Several students commented that they regretted not taking part and recognized the value of the workshop.

In both student cohorts, the majority of students indicated some apprehension before undertaking the role-played interviews. In response to a question on the 2015 evaluation form: *How did you feel before taking part in the workshop?*, 78% of students indicated that they had been feeling nervous, worried or anxious ($n = 28$), yet comments suggest that the experience was, in fact, positive. For example,

> Role-play is not as terrifying as everyone thinks; I can do this!

In response to the question: *How did you find the experience?*, 100% of students who took part in the workshops and returned evaluation forms, in both cohorts, gave positive responses ($n = 22$ in 2014 and $n = 36$ in 2015). One hundred per cent also indicated that they thought future students would benefit from undertaking the workshop.

In both student cohorts, 100% indicated that they had learned something but there was wide variation in what they had learned, for example: 'The importance of listening', 'Not to dive in too quickly to "fix" things', 'To be more empathetic', 'How to deal with silence', 'To stay calm and really listen to what they say'. Whilst these different areas of learning cannot be explored in depth here, reasons for such variation might relate to a number of factors. Firstly, the nature and extent of feedback they received varied widely as they were receiving feedback from different students, different service users and some also had feedback from a tutor. One member's feed back to students was supplemented by additional contributions from his support worker.

A second potential explanation for the different areas of learning relates to variation in the role-play experience itself. At one point, the tutor supported a service user to refocus on role-play rather than engaging in a conversation with the students, for example. This might relate to the Unity member being drawn to the more comfortable role of *expert* as discussed earlier.

Given the range of responses from students, however, variation in what they learned may relate to individual learning needs. Skilton (2011), for example, found that some students engaging in role-play had little experience of working with service users. It is likely that this will also have been the case in this workshop. As they practised the skills of professional communication and engagement, feedback was given on students' abilities to maintain attentive non-verbal communication, to make the individual feel comfortable, to engage in a conversation about difficult issues, to structure the interview and a myriad of other factors which contribute to effective communication in a social work context. On this basis, there appeared to be particular value in the individually tailored learning experience that the workshop offered to students.

In drawing a comparison between undertaking role-play with service users rather than with other students, feedback from both student cohorts was overwhelmingly in favour of role-play with service users (86% in 2014, 97% in 2015). Student quotes indicated: 'It felt much more realistic', 'It was much easier to do', 'It felt much more natural', 'Feedback was much more helpful'. Some students also used the evaluation form as a mechanism for expressing their appreciation of Unity members' involvement (*n* = 8 in 2014, *n* = 21 in 2015): 'Thanks Unity- really helpful to our learning', 'It's wonderful that Unity give up their own time to help students', 'Loved it- great experience. Can't wait to go on placement now'.

Service user evaluation

Feedback was overwhelmingly positive, with members indicating that participation in the workshops had been a positive experience for them and that they wanted to take part again. Several Unity members focused on the importance of their role in working to produce the best possible social workers. Lorna, for example, wrote about students giving her hope for the future as they had 'treated her as a person not as an illness'. Louise wrote about working with the students so that they can become the best social workers they can be and another member wrote about the value of the workshop in tackling stigma around mental ill health.

Members indicated that participating in the planning sessions had been helpful in terms of preparation for what would happen on the day. One member stated on their evaluation form: 'They [the planning meetings] were extremely useful and made me feel empowered in being able to help and educate student social workers. Everyone has a say, the meetings are relaxed and informal and everything said is confidential'.

Service users also advised that they felt the students appreciated their involvement, they felt valued, it had increased their confidence and self esteem, they felt empowered and had enjoyed taking part. This feedback is in line with the findings of other service user involvement work (Brown & Young, 2008; Moss et al., 2007). This is, arguably the crux of effective service user and carer involvement. The sense of well-being that members gain through taking part underlines the importance of reciprocity in service user involvement in social work education. Without this, fewer people would continue to be involved, to give up their time for meetings, programme committees and direct work with students. This seems especially likely within a context where there is no ring-fenced funding to pay people for their involvement. The camaraderie of the group, trusting relationships that have developed and the recognition that members have something important to offer social work education all contribute to the momentum of the group.

The perceived benefits to service user members should not, however, be taken for granted. Lorna talked about how she managed the emotional impact of taking part. She recognized that revisiting such painful times in her life might leave her feeling down after the session so made sure she had something nice planned for afterwards. Others referred to their own nerves about taking part. Michael also talked about having chosen an issue that he knew would not be too painful for him.

It was apparent that Unity members had assumed a nurturing role with students—giving thought to whether their stories might be distressing, so leaving out aspects that they thought would be too upsetting. They also found themselves trying to put students at ease at the start of the role-plays. Whilst realizing that this should have been the role of the student social worker, all recognized the importance of creating a positive learning environment (Hargreaves & Hadlow, 1997; Moss et al., 2007).

Unity members identified areas for development amongst the students relating to use of jargon, lack of confidence, issues with non-verbal communication and not remembering referral details such as their name or the fact that they were visiting the service user at home rather than meeting in the office. The clear focus on learning, sensitivity, insight, honesty and tact that Unity members used in giving feedback to students was impressive. They were also aware of a difference between the students across the two years; finding that they were more confident, more able to talk about issues such as confidentiality and generally seemed better prepared in the second year. This highlights the importance of preparation for students planning to engage in such a learning opportunity. In the second year, the first workshop took place two days later in the eight-day module, so students had received more taught input as well as opportunities to practise communication and engagement skills through role-play with each other before working with Unity. As a result, they appear to have been able to make better use of the learning opportunity in the second year.

Members recognized that their own level of experience and confidence in the staff member and in each other helped them to undertake the role-play task, which, most felt they would not have been able to take on at an earlier stage. Michael commented that, 'Group members have the self esteem and confidence to do the role-play now'. Louise stated: 'I just feel that as the group is growing, I'm growing as well'.

Members also expressed confidence that their work was beneficial in developing student practice. Jack commented: 'I enjoyed it greatly – it gives me a sense of actually being listened to. It put the things that happen in life to great use that benefitted – I hope – the students who will be able to help change things in other people's lives for their good, so indirectly I have helped those people get their lives together'.

Conclusion and implication for future practice

The workshop provides an example of how service user and carer involvement in social work education has evolved from a primary focus on sharing personal stories to active participation in student skill development (MacSporran, 2015; Sadd, 2011; Taylor & Le Riche, 2006). Whilst, there is, undoubtedly, value in the former, commitment to service user involvement can support the emergence of a culture in which service users can grow in confidence and develop their ability to engage in more challenging learning opportunities to the benefit of student learning and development. There are a number of other examples of such innovations including service user involvement in skills laboratories (Moss et al.,

2007), in assessed role-plays with students (Duffy et al., 2013; Skilton, 2011) and as mentors for social work students on observational practice placements (MacSporran, 2015).

Whilst opportunities for innovative service user and carer involvement in social work education are evident, this paper also considers the potential risks to service users if such work is not carefully planned and supported. Key factors in supporting the role-played interview workshop have emerged as:

- A well-established service users and carers' involvement group in which members' contributions are valued, staff are able to contribute both time and enthusiasm and principles of co-production underpin practice.
- Members are supported to recognize the demands and potential impact on themselves of this type of teaching contribution and choose whether or not to be involved.
- Priority is given to planning and preparation, support through delivery and debriefing time over a cup of tea.

A key finding of this paper is the importance of service users being able to resume the role of student educator following role-play with students, in order for them to experience benefits from their involvement. Sufficient time for this must be incorporated into the workshop as well as planning sessions including detailed guidance and discussion around how to give feedback.

The full impact of the loss of direct government funding for service user and carer involvement in Scotland is perhaps still to be felt, as groups run out of funds. Further investment in service user involvement will be necessary in order to achieve and maintain an appropriate context for projects such as the role-played interview workshop to develop and to avoid tokenistic or exploitative involvement (Ager et al., 2005; Brown & Young, 2008; Levin, 2004; Sadd, 2011). This paper calls for recognition of the important contribution to social work education made by people who have experience of using social work services. It also aims to highlight the scope for innovation and development in service user involvement when appropriately supported.

Confidentiality

Individual service users are referred to using pseudonyms in order to preserve anonymity.

Acknowledgements

Grateful thanks to members of the service users and carers' group: Unity, at the University of Stirling. Without their enthusiasm and commitment to helping social work students become the best they can be, the workshop would not have been developed.

References

Ager, W., Dow, J., & Gee, M. (2005). Grassroots networks: A model for promoting the influence of service users and carers in social work education. *Social Work Education, 24*, 467–476.

British Sociological Association. (2002). *Statement of ethical practice for the British Sociological Association*. Retrieved June 29, 2016, from http://www.britsoc.co.uk/media/27107/StatementofEthicalPractice.pdf?1467195794130

Brown, K., & Young, N. (2008). Building capacity for service user and carer involvement in social work education. *Social Work Education, 27*, 84–96.

Duffy, J. (2006). *Participating and learning. Citizenship involvement in social work education in the Northern Ireland context: A good practice guide.* London: Social Care Institute for Excellence [online]. Retrieved February 3, 2016, from www.scie.org.uk/publications/misc/citizeninvolvement.asp

Duffy, J., Das, C., & Davidson, G. (2013). Service user and carer involvement in role-plays to assess readiness for practice. *Social Work Education, 32*, 39–54.

Faherty, V. E. (1983). Simulation & gaming in social work education: A projection. *Journal of Social Work Education, 19*, 111–118.

Hargreaves, R., & Hadlow, J. (1997). Role-play in social work education: Process and framework for a constructive and focused approach. *Social Work Education, 16*, 61–73.

Levin, E. (2004). *Involving service users and carers in social work education.* London: SCIE [online]. Retrieved February 3, 2016, http://www.scie.org.uk/publications/guides/guide04/files/guide04.pdf

MacSporran, J. (2015). A mentor's PATH: Evaluating how service users can be involved as mentors for social work students on observational practice placements. *Social Work & Social Sciences Review, 17*, 46–60.

McLaughlin, H. (2009). What's in a name: 'Client', 'Expert by Experience', 'Service User' – What's next? *British Journal of Social Work, 39*, 1101–1117.

Moss, B. R., Dunkerly, M., Price, B., Sullivan, W., Reynolds, M., & Yates, B. (2007). Skills laboratories and the new social work degree: One small step towards best practice? Service users' and carers' perspectives *Social Work Education, 26*, 708–722.

Rhodes, C., Hardy, J., Padgett, K., Symons, J., Tate, J., & Thornton, S. (2014). The health and well-being of service user and carer educators: A narrative enquiry into the impact of involvement in healthcare education. *International Journal of Practice Based Learning in Health and Social Care, 2*, 51–68.

Sadd, J. (2011). *'We are more than our story': Service user and carer participation in social work education.* London: Social Care Institute for Excellence [online]. Retrieved January 4, 2016, http://www.scie.org.uk/publications/reports/report42.asp

Scheyett, A., & Kim, M. (2004). "Can We Talk?": Using facilitated dialogue to positively change student attitudes towards persons with mental illness. *Journal of Teaching in Social Work, 24*, 39–54.

Scottish Executive. (2003). *The framework for social work education in Scotland.* Edinburgh: Author.

Skilton, C. J. (2011). Involving experts by experience in assessing students' readiness to practice: The value of experiential learning in student reflection and preparation for practice. *Social Work Education, 30*, 299–311.

Social Care Institute for Excellence. (2013). *Co-production in social care: What it is and how to do it.* London: Author [Online]. Retrieved January 15, 2016, http://www.ndti.org.uk/uploads/files/Coproduction_Guide51Fin.pdf

Taylor, I., & Le Riche, P. (2006). What do we know about partnership with service users and carers in social work education and how robust is the evidence base? *Health and Social Care in the Community, 14*, 418–425.

Wilson, G., & Kelly, B. (2010). Evaluating the effectiveness of social work education: Preparing students for practice learning. *British Journal of Social Work, 40*, 2431–2449.

Learning from service users' involvement: a research about changing stigmatizing attitudes in social work students

Elena Cabiati and Maria Luisa Raineri

ABSTRACT
Stigmatizing attitudes can create barriers to forming partnership with service users and to developing people's empowerment. So, social work education must help students overcome their stigmatizing attitudes. A useful strategy for bringing about changes is service users' and carers' involvement in social work education, providing students with direct exposure to stigmatized people in roles that emphasize their humanity and strengths, rather than their deficits. The present study assessed the impact of a one-day meeting with service users and carers members of self-help and mutual-aid groups on freshman social work students. Students completed an adapted version of Attitudes to Mental Illness Questionnaire before and after the meeting, and answered several qualitative questions. Data comparisons suggest that after face-to-face contact with service users and carers, social work students showed reduced stigmatizing attitudes. Implications for further research and social work education are discussed.

Social work and stigmatizing attitudes

Stigma is particularly important in social work because most if not all people social workers work with will be subject to some form of stigmatization. 'Simply being a client of a social worker is often enough to attract stigma' (Thompson & Thompson, 2008, p. 216). Furthermore, social work has an important tradition and role in supporting vulnerable populations and in fighting discrimination and stigma (Banks, 2008; Barnes, 2006; Burke & Parker, 2007; Cree, 2013; Dominelli, 2002, 2008; Fook, 2012; Thompson, 2006). Nevertheless, social workers often share the negative view of social problems that is so widespread among general population. Stigmatizing attitudes are not only present in society at large but also in helping professions, including psychiatry, psychology and social work (Nordt, Rössler, & Lauber, 2006; Scheyett & Kim, 2004; Trevithick, 2005). Promoting users' empowerment and partnership is pivotal to social work practice, but stigmatizing attitudes can create barriers to forming partnership and to empowering people. Therefore, it is vital that social work education helps students to overcome their stigmatizing attitudes (Zellmann, Madden, &

Aguiniga, 2014) as means to develop a 'critical understanding of how socio-structural inadequacies, discrimination, oppression, and social, political and economic injustices impact human functioning and development at all levels, including the global' (Sewpaul & Jones, 2005, p. 220).

Various ways to decrease stigmatizing attitudes in general population (e.g. Corrigan & Penn, 2015; Galletly & Burton, 2011; Heijnders & Van Der Meij, 2006; Lebel, 2008; Weiss, Ramakrishna, & Somma, 2006) and among professionals (e.g. Galletly & Burton, 2011) are described in literature. As direct contacts and personal relationships with those stigmatized seem particularly useful to reduce stigma (Corrigan & Penn, 2015; Covarrubias & Han, 2011) an important strategy for bringing about changes in professionals' perceptions of stigmatized people has been to involve the latter in education and training, providing students and practitioners with direct exposure to stigmatized people in roles that emphasize their humanity and strengths, rather than their deficits (Scheyett & Kim, 2004; Shor & Sykes, 2002).

Service users' and caregivers' involvement in social work education

Diffusion

In the last three decades, in the UK, service users' and carers' involvement in social work has become firmly embedded in important aspects of social work education (Branfield, 2009; Edwards, 2003; Taylor, Braye, & Cheng, 2009). In recent years, service users' involvement in university programmes has been started in other European countries—as Denmark, Germany, Norway, Sweden, in Northern Ireland (Agnew & Duffy, 2010), Croatia (Skokandić & Urbanc, 2009) and in Eastern European countries (Zavirsek & Videmsek, 2009). As far as we know, in the Italian social work education system, only two experiences can be found that were carried out by the Catholic University of Milan and by the University of Eastern Piedmont (Allegri, 2015), respectively.

Rationale

The involvement of service users and carers in social work education is thought of as promoting the more collaborative ways of working that contemporary social work theory and practice emphasize (Waterson & Morris, 2005), and as providing a balanced education capable of building a good professional practice in students, especially when service users are involved right from the beginning (Baldwin & Sadd, 2006; Tyler, 2006; Waterson & Morris, 2005). The central idea is that social workers must regard service users and carers as partners in dealing with their life difficulties. So, social workers should not regard them merely as recipients of interventions, but as people from whom to learn, both in professional practice and education.

Service users' everyday experiences are fundamental to equipping would-be social workers with key elements of knowledge and expertise and to improving services (Anghel & Ramon, 2009; Beresford, 2000). The exposition to service user perspectives also aims to help social work students, and freshmen especially, relate theory and practice (Cooper & Spencer-Dawe, 2006; Irvine, Molyneux, & Gillman, 2015).

Power sharing

In order to achieve an effective participation and to avoid the risks of a tokenistic approach, general issues about how users' role could be presented and how programmes could be adjusted to promote effective changes in social work practice should be addressed (Askheim, 2012).

There is the risk that users could be seen as 'case studies' instead of partners, increasing the emphasis on the distance between 'us' (professionals) and 'them' (the users) (Beresford & Croft, 2008; Wilson & Beresford, 2000). Conversely, only if service users and carers feel respected for what they can offer, they are more able to share their perspectives (Anghel & Ramon, 2009, p. 187). When groups or organizations of users are involved, they are in a better position to effectively challenging conventional images of service users (Beresford & Boxall, 2012).

Involvement domains and methods

Service users and carers have collaborated with social work courses in different ways: as personal testimonies, educators, co-teachers, recruiters of students (Askheim, 2012). They have contributed by telling their stories and real-life experiences, as well as by producing written materials (Reynolds & Read, 1999) and videos (Smith, 2013). Gee, Ager, and Haddow (2009) analysed what learning students had gained after spending 24 h with service users and family carers. Quinney and Fowler (2013) described a participatory initiative carried out through online discussion groups run by users and carers.

Judkins and Lahurd (1999) underlined the importance of involving service users and carers in curriculum development and design, and not only as personal testimonies—they should be regarded as partners in developing educational programmes (Molyneux & Irvine, 2004). To this purpose, they may take part to a wide range of tasks, as students' selection, development of teaching approaches and materials, programme planning, teaching and learning activities, feedback and assessment, quality monitoring and evaluation (Health & Care Professions Council, 2014).

Though, service users and carers have been actively involved in assessing the readiness of freshmen students in social work for their first period of practice learning (Duffy, Das, & Davidson, 2013) and in assessing students' achievement both in practice learning and in institution-based learning (Gee et al., 2009), more compelling evidence about the effectiveness of service users in such roles is needed (Skoura-Kirk et al., 2013). According to Gregor and Smith (2009), prior to involving 'service users as educators', their potential role and contribution, as well as their training needs, should be considered.

Recruitment and training

Involving service users and carers can mean working with individuals or working with groups and networks of service users and carers, with voluntary organizations (Health & Care Professions Council, 2014), with community organizations (Gupta & Blewett, 2008), with local activity centres (Askheim, 2012). This outreach work always takes time and requires careful preparation. It is essential to explain the initiative to the different individuals or organizations targeted, and to learn what they may offer, whom else they are involved with and what their engagement conditions are (Levin, 2004).

Service users and carers may need support and training, particularly when they take part in student selection processes or assessment tasks (Brown & Young, 2008). Help with reading, understanding and/or producing written may be necessary too (Gupta & Blewett, 2008).

Preliminary meetings among service users and carers enable them 'to present the views of the group, rather than just their own experiences, which can be emotionally difficult for them and dismissed as unrepresentative by those receiving the training' (Baldwin & Sadd, 2006; Gupta & Blewett, 2008, p. 468; Irvine et al., 2015).

Outcome

Most authors argue that service users' and carers' involvement in social work education is extremely valuable to all parties (Brown & Young, 2008; Morgan & Jones, 2009; Irvine et al., 2015).

Irvine et al. (2015) show that many students come to realize how keeping the service users' perspectives at the core of practice is paramount in order to actualize social work values. Thanks to service users' and carers' testimonies, awareness of the importance of human experience within the social and health service system has grown (McCusker, MacIntyre, Stewart, & Jackson, 2012). A student quoted by Smith (2013) said that he had learnt by service users the importance of being aware of how social workers' behaviour and attitude impact upon them.

Students acknowledged the importance of interacting with service users and carers away from their usual environments and roles (Benbow, Taylor, Mustafa, & Morgan, 2011). The 'us-and-them' distinction between the parties dwindled (Askheim, 2012). Significantly for the purposes of the present article, it has been shown that the stigma associated with certain service user groups, particularly in relation to mental health, decreases. This occurs to varying degrees, depending on students' previous experience (Smith, 2013). One of the most important results of the project carried out in Northern Ireland by Coulter, Campbell, Duffy, and Reilly (2013) was showing how this kind of initiatives appeared to increase students' awareness and capacity in a divided society. After talking with victims of violence and discrimination, students appeared more equipped to meet the requirements of such a society (Judkins & Lahurd, 1999).

Furthermore, learning by and with service users and carers develops communication skills (Skilton, 2011) and emphasizes the value of listening (Branfield, 2009).

There are indications that service users involved in social work education improve their confidence and self-esteem, arising from a sense of making meaningful contribution (Benbow et al., 2011; McCusker et al., 2012). The significant literature review by Robinson and Webber (2013) underlined that little effort has been made to ascertain if the participation of service users in social work education actually improves outcomes for students. After analysing 29 international studies, they showed that none of them addressed the effects on social work practices and only two measured change in social students' attitudes or in their perception of service users and carers.

The study presented in this article attempts to fill a small part of this gap by investigating the effects of a meeting between freshman students in social work and service users and carers in terms of reduction of stigma.

A full-day meeting: students and EBE together

Setting

In Italy there aren't specific policies to promote service users' involvement in social work education programmes, and not even in social services planning and delivery.

Nevertheless, service users' and carers' participation is closely linked to the social work approach taught at the Catholic University in Milan, i.e. Relation Social Work. Relational Social Work (Folgheraiter, 2004, 2007, 2015; Folgheraiter & Raineri, 2012) stems from relational sociology (Donati, 2010) and focuses on relationships as the basis for change. The central idea in Relational Social Work is that change emerges from a reciprocal aid, both among people in difficult circumstances, family members, friends, neighbours and between that network and the social worker. The practitioner helps the network to develop reflexivity and improve it in enhancing welfare, and—in turn—the network helps the practitioner to better understand how s/he can help it (Folgheraiter & Raineri, 2012).

In Relational Social Work, service users are considered as 'experts by experience' (McLaughlin, 2009; Preston-Shoot, 2007; Saleebey, 1996), because they have experience of using care services, and especially because they are experts about their lives, and about their difficulties.

Coherently with the Relational paradigm, the involvement of service users or ex-service users and carers as teachers is an important part of social work education programme at the Catholic University. During the 3 years of bachelor's degree and even in the 2 years of master's degree, the students take part in various activities realized with the contribution of carers and services users. First-year students work together with service users and carers in the activity described below. During the following training years there are two workshops each of 30 h, where service users and carers with different life problems are invited to share their experience with the students, and to discuss with them how social work interventions could be improved. In the third year of bachelor's degree and in the second year of master's degree, groups of service users and carers, students and other stakeholders work in partnership to develop small community social work projects. Service users and carers take part in the annual social work students' congress in which conventional practice placements and off the beaten track placements (Doel, 2009) are presented. Finally, service users and carers are involved in almost all lessons, workshops and other events opened to external professionals too (students supervisors, social and health practitioners, etc.).

The meetings

The present study looked at a learning experience that is part of a Social Work Orientation Workshop (Cabiati, 2016) addressed to freshman students and aimed at providing them with an opportunity to know a life story and change their views of social problems and service users. For 8 years, this annual 'Social Work Orientation Workshop' has been a component of professionalizing modules about Social Work Skills, Values, Approaches and Contexts.

Every academic year, the University organizes a full-day meeting between students and 'Experts by experience' (EBE), who are service user members of self-help and mutual aid groups). The programme of the day is divided in two parts: in the morning, each student talks individually with a service user for two hours. It is not a professional interview but a simple conversation aimed at knowing each other and exchanging life experiences. After the lunch time, shared together in the university canteen, all the participants (students and service users) meet together in 5 groups with about 15 EBEs and 15 students, to express thoughts and feelings about the experience. Every group was facilitated by one of EBEs.

The EBEs who participate in the meetings can be experts in various different problems that can change every academic year depending on the self-help/mutual-aid groups in which EBEs took part. In the year when the present research was carried out (2014), the students met EBEs with experience in the following problems: mental health; drugs addiction; alcohol addiction; unemployment; disability; difficult partner divorce; parents of children in child protection; gambling addiction.

EBE recruitment

EBEs were recruited through self-help and mutual-aid groups organizations, the so-called 'umbrella' organizations that gather a number of self-help and mutual-aid groups for the same type of problem, or many groups with different targets.

Firstly, the initiative was presented to some key persons who were group facilitators and who had already contacts with the teachers of social work course. Then, the University sent a letter to each self-help and mutual-aid group, inviting all those who were interested in participating and suggesting to extend the invitation to other potentially interested groups. The only necessary condition to participate was to be member of a self-help and mutual-aid group for a year at least.

In 2014, a total of 80 self-selected members of mutual-aid groups took part in the full-day meeting. This number can be seen as a significant success, since—according Levin (2004)—the number of individuals actively involved in social work education initiatives usually ranges from 4 to 20, with an average of 8–10.

According to Relational Social Work, service users and carers are 'experts by experience' because they are experts in their lives, in coping one or more life problems, in taking care of a relative or a friend, in managing the relationship with services and practitioners. The recruitment through self-help and mutual-aid groups' organizations was chosen taking into account both the range of benefits arising from working in groups (highlighted above) and particularly what happens in this kind of groups. Self-help and mutual-aid groups produce strengths-driven processes promoting psychological insight and social skills (Steinberg, 2010). Self-help and mutual-aid groups imply an ongoing reflection on personal experiences, starting from the others', in a peer-to-peer logic. In this way, individuals can develop narrations and points of view enhanced by the other members' perspectives. When someone participates in a self-help and mutual-aid group for a period of time, s/he will not only elaborate his/her experience individually but s/he will also enrich it with the coping experiences of the other members. When motivated people who have lived similar experiences talk and listen to each other, they can develop a higher standing life knowledge that expresses the shared experience and is less contingent on individual circumstances. In a self-help and mutual-aid group, the knowledge of individual members upgrades, just because it becomes shared knowledge (Raineri, 2011).Thus, the student who meets an EBE listens to his/her life story, but in the dialogue between them the experiences of other people expert in coping with a particular difficulty also emerge. In this way, the student does not listen only to the individual voice of an expert but listens to his/her experience revisited in the light of experiences of others.

Due to all these reasons, the experience in self-help and mutual-aid groups was considered as an excellent basis of competence for the EBEs involved in social work education. In fact, thanks to their participation in those groups, the EBEs are experts in sharing and communicating their life experience. This expertise needs an adequate amount of time—at least one year—to be elaborated. So, the EBEs were required to participate to a self-help and mutual-aid group for at least a year before taking part in the meeting.

Other minor issues about the EBEs participation were discussed with the key persons who were group facilitators and with the course's teachers.

Research method

The research hypothesis was that face-to-face contact with people coping with life difficulties would produce educational effects in the students, particularly by reducing the level of prejudice towards service users who are experiencing life problems. The research aimed at exploring how this educational experience affected participants and at finding out, by means of a survey, if students' attitudes showed any change.

Students were administered an adapted version of the 'Attitudes to Mental Illness Questionnaire' (AMIQ—Cunningham, Sobell, & Chow, 1993; Luty, Fakuda, Umoh, & Gallagher, 2006), previously translated into Italian, both in the two weeks preceding the meeting (pre-test) and in the two weeks following it (post-test). The second administration included some additional qualitative questions.

The 5-item AMIQ has good psychometric properties and can be used in most situations (Luty et al., 2006). Respondents read short vignettes describing an imaginary service user and answer five questions for each vignette. Respondents are asked to rate how likely some consequent events are to occur on a 5-point Likert scale (from −2 = most likely, to + 2 = most unlikely). The scores for the five questions are then added up, giving a total score that can range between −10 and +10. Low scores indicate negative attitudes.

The data collected by means of the questionnaire were analysed through a statistical programme to look for differences between pre- and post- results. Differences were calculated by subtracting each student's pre-test score from his/her post-test score.

The full-day meeting was part of the common academic activity, so all freshman students were expected to attend it. Prior to the meeting, students were told that they would take part to an initiative aimed at gaining a better understanding of the life and difficulties of people who turn to social services.

Through an email the survey was sent to the students by an external researcher. The online questionnaire came with a note giving assurance about anonymity and explaining that the research intended to gather information about some opinions and attitudes of the students. Students have never known the survey and its aims before. Responding to the questionnaire was discretionary and the teachers didn't participate in the research project. Students responded online anonymously. Each student was asked to insert an alphanumeric code that would allow us to make the pre-/post-comparison. Non-obligatory participation, anonymity and lack of awareness of the specific AMIQ aims were a way to limit the influence by role expectations.

The study was conducted with the freshman students of the Catholic University (Milan, Italy) in 2014. A total of 100 students participated. Most of them (90%) were female and

Italian. The mean age was 20 years. 45% of them came from technical college and 55% from high schools.

Findings

The hypothesis of the present research, i.e. that after face-to-face contact with EBEs students' attitudes towards service users would improve, was supported by the findings of pre-test/post-test analyses. The data obtained through the first and second administration of the AMIQ are shown in Table 1.

Post-test mean scores differ from pre-test mean scores for all the vignettes, with the only exception of the disability vignette. The mean AMIQ scores improved from −0.45 prior to the meeting with EBEs to +0.25 after that meeting, with a mean difference of +0.70.

Through a second analysis, participants were divided into percentiles on the basis of their total score at the pre-test. Three groups were identified: with a high, medium and low level of prejudice. It is apparent that the increase in mean scores is due to improvement by students with lower scores (i.e. students in the sample who initially had a high level of prejudice).

As Table 2 shows, change scores for this group of students are up to 2.71 for the vignette about schizophrenia, and up to 1.37 in total.

Qualitative data collected by asking some questions during the second administration of the AMIQ revealed that participants appreciated the experience of meeting the EBEs, following which they were able to identify some key concepts for social work practice.

Students' answers confirmed that they had improved their personal attitudes towards service users:

Table 1. Pre-test and post-test scores.

Vignette	Pre-test mean (SD)	Post-test mean (SD)	Change score
John (cocaine)	−1.51 (2.84)	−.68 (3.15)	+.83
Tom (depression)	+.52 (2.74)	+.84 (2.69)	+.32
Stefano (alcohol)	+.05 (3.63)	+.96 (3.42)	+.91
Robert (law problems)	−5.43 (2.53)	−4.39 (2.82)	+1.04
Michael (schizofrenia)	−1.39 (3.29)	−.17 (3.35)	+1.22
Claude (disability)	+5.22 (2.75)	+5.17 (2.61)	−.05
Paul (birth parent of a child in foster care)	+.4 (3.93)	+1.07 (4.09)	+.67
Luke (gambling addiction)	−1.42 (2.75)	−.81 (3.53)	+.61
Total	−.45	+.25	+.70

Table 2. Pre-test and post-test scores for students who initially had a high level of prejudice.

Vignette	Pre-test mean (SD)	Post-test mean (SD)	Change score
John (cocaine)	−3.14 (2.39)	−2.32 (2.52)	+.82
Tom (depression)	−.82 (2.77)	+.36 (2.51)	+1.18
Stefano (alcohol)	−2.46 (3.40)	−.61 (3.63)	+1.85
Robert (law problems)	−6.96 (1.68)	−5.39 (2.48)	+1.57
Michael (schizofrenia)	−3.89 (2.85)	−1.18 (3.18)	+2.71
Claude (disability)	+3.96 (3.34)	+4.46 (2.60)	−.50
Paul (birth parent of a child in foster care)	−1.68 (3.67)	−.68 (3.36)	+1.00
Luke (gambling addiction)	−3.43 (2.50)	−2.11 (3.24)	+1.32
Total	−2.30	−.93	+1.37

> I have learnt more about drug addictions, revising my wrong ideas
>
> I found out that these people have a problem, but are not a problem.

The answers to the qualitative questions suggested that students' stigmatizing views of service users as bad or lacking people were questioned after meeting them:

> Prior to the meeting I was worried, but now I have to say that service users are strong and brave people.
>
> When I will become a social worker it will be important for me to treat each service user as a unique person, giving him/her the chance to change and avoiding to focus on past events.
>
> Service users are people who take on the challenge of starting a new life. They are people from whom we can and we have to learn.

This change in the image of service users requires to be further elaborated in a critical perspective, following the idea that each user, just as each person, could have both strengths and vulnerabilities. However, for a young student at the first step of the education way this change of perspective could represent a promising starting point. For future practitioners engaged in human relationships, these statements are meaningful, because being able to suspend one's own conjectures and judgements, and to set aside one's own feelings and free associations in order to recognize the otherness will be essential for them (Sevenhuijsen, 1998).

Furthermore, students underlined that they needed to improve their personal reflexive abilities:

> I learned that prior to expecting other people to change I have to question myself.
>
> To become a good social worker I need to work deeply on myself, coping with my worries, understanding my limits and my resources.

Analysing these answers appeared from the same students the danger to run into a stigmatizing attitude and at the same time the wish to avoid it. This idea represents an important issue for the young would-be social workers. The experience opens the way to get to the core of the matter during the educational pathway.

Finally, to the question 'Was the meeting a positive, negative or neutral experience for you?', none of the students answered 'negative', two students answered 'neutral' and most of them expressed enthusiasm and satisfaction.

Discussion

Overall, the findings of the present study are encouraging. Data suggest that meeting face-to-face with people who are expert in coping with their own life difficulties had positive effects on social work students. Change scores show a reduction of stigma for almost all the vignettes presented in the AMIQ.

The only exception showing no improvement was the situation of a man with disability (Claude). It is possible that the students who talked with people with disability or their relatives during the meeting had already a good understanding of the everyday difficulties of living with a disability, so their attitudes did not change significantly.

Interestingly, stigmatizing attitudes seem to have decreased not only with reference to the problems of which the EBEs had a personal experience (and about which, then, they talked with the students during the meeting) but also with reference to the situation of

Robert (offender), that had no correspondence to any of the self-help and mutual-aid groups involved.

Despite the pre-/post-improvement, Robert was by far the most stigmatized character in the opinions expressed by our sample of students. Therefore, particular attention will have to be paid in addressing prejudice towards offending people and, if possible, it may be useful to involve in future meetings also EBEs who have experienced this kind of difficulty.

For the students of our sample, the full-day meeting with the EBEs was one of the first opportunities to interact with service users. Qualitative findings of the present study suggest that this encounter has some characteristics of a relational and dialogical practice culture. It is a brief intervention that may have a significant impact on students. The students of our sample pointed out how this kind of experience could help them recognize users' value, respect their identities and facilitate empowerment and participatory approaches.

Limits

The most obvious limitation of the present study is the lack of a comparison group. Therefore, it cannot be claimed that the decrease in students' stigma was entirely or mainly due to the meeting with the EBEs, though it may be reasonably assumed.

Moreover, it was not assessed if and how long the changes in students' attitudes last. In their framework for evaluation of educational programmes, Robinson and Webber (2013) have highlighted eight levels of evaluation, based on: learners' perceptions (1a), service users' or carers' perceptions (1b), staff perceptions (1c), modification in learners' attitudes and perceptions (2a), acquisition of knowledge and skills by learners (2b), changes in learners behaviour (3a), changes in organizational practices (3b), benefits to users and carers 84). The research presented placed at the level 2a (modification in students attitudes and perceptions). With reference to level 3a, at the present it's not possible to prove if the effects of this experience persist in the students. In the same way, from this study there are no elements to prove that this experience could influence their behaviour in future social work practices. Future studies would be needed to scrutinize if an experience like this could produce long-term effects.

It would be both interesting and important, for future research, to gather EBEs' opinions and perceptions about their engagement. The vast and enthusiastic participation by service users and carers that has been observed over the years suggests that this activity benefits EBEs too.

AIMQ was used earlier in social and clinical studies (Galletly & Burton, 2011; Luty, Kumar, & Stagias, 2010; Luty, Maducolil, & Mendes, 2011; Luty et al., 2006; Onesirosan, Ohiole, & Osemudiamen, 2012) from which the problem of role expectation has never mentioned. However, it's not possible to exclude that this could be occurred. Furthermore, it's important to note that the positive effects generated thanks to the experience with EBEs are general, not only related to the single problem encountered. The design of the study had not allowed to identify the factors associated with positive changes in students' attitudes. In this sense, the change may have occurred due to the nature of shared experience, rather than the core views held regarding the subject matter. The change could be strongly connected to the nature and the structure of the experience that aimed to create a social climate in which experiences and expertise were reciprocally exchanged. For all these limits, this has been an exploratory study without statistical claims.

Conclusions

Participants to the meeting expressed satisfaction and appreciation about this initiative. Besides, data suggest that the full-day meeting was effective in reducing stigmatizing attitudes and mistrust towards people who have personal and social problems.

Stigmatizing attitudes towards people with mental illness, drug addiction or offenders is commonly reported among professionals. It is widely recognized that in order to become effective and morally upright social workers, it is essential to develop some abilities related to human, relational and personal skills (Banks, 2008; Barnes, 2006; Braye & Preston-Shoot, 1995; Schön, 1983; Thompson, 2002; Trevithick, 2005; Wilkes, 1985). Promoting face-to-face contact with experts by experience may be an effective strategy to reduce dangerous feelings of anger, mistrust and discrimination.

To think of people who are living life problems as 'experts by experience' it is necessary to recognize their power, their abilities and their feelings, irrespective of the resolution of problems. Furthermore, for social work professionals, the obligatory way to 'create' power is to take a step back and relinquish some of their own power (Folgheraiter & Raineri, 2012). Social work education has the responsibility of encouraging students' awareness about the need to establish fully collaborative relationships with service users, co-creating help interventions. The reciprocity of help—letting the user be an equal and help the social worker—is not an empty slogan or a luxury. It is a radical turning point (Folgheraiter, 2012) because, if this reciprocity is absent, the help withers and dies (Beresford & Croft, 2008).

This study confirms that social work education can be enhanced through the participation of service users as 'experts by experience'. Given that in a true helping relationship both human agents aid each other (Pettersen & Hem, 2011) and that both experts and interested parties should work together in a synergic search for a common good (Folgheraiter & Raineri, 2012), learning from service users is for would-be social workers a valuable educational opportunity at the first steps on their path.

Disclosure statement

No potential conflict of interest was reported by the authors.

References

Agnew, A., & Duffy, J. (2010). Innovative approaches to involving service users in palliative care social work education. *Social Work Education, 29*, 744–759. doi:http://dx.doi.org/10.1080/15433714.2014.939382

Allegri, E. (2015, June). *Service users and carer involvement in social work education: Lessons from an innovative Italian experience*. Paper presented at EASSW biennial conference 'Social work education: Towards 2025', Milan.

Anghel, R., & Ramon, S. (2009). Service users and carers' involvement in social work education: Lessons from an English case study. *European Journal of Social Work, 12*, 185–199. doi:http://dx.doi.org/10.1080/13691450802567416

Askheim, O. P. (2012). Meeting face to face creates new insights: Recruiting persons with user experiences as students in an educational programme in social work. *Social Work Education, 31*, 557–569. doi:http://dx.doi.org/10.1080/02615479.2011.590972

Baldwin, M., & Sadd, J. (2006). Allies with attitude! Service users, academics and social service agency staff learning how to share power in running social work education courses. *Social Work Education, 25*, 348–359. doi:http://dx.doi.org/10.1080/02615470600593543

Banks, S. (2008). Critical commentary: Social work ethics. *British Journal of Social Work, 38*, 1238–1249. doi:http://dx.doi.org/10.1093/bjsw/bcn099

Barnes, M. (2006). *Caring and social justice*. Basingstoke: Palgrave.

Benbow, S. M., Taylor, L., Mustafa, N., & Morgan, K. (2011). Design, delivery and evaluation of teaching by service users and carers. *Educational Gerontology, 37*, 621–633. doi:http://dx.doi.org/10.1080/03601277.2011.559849

Beresford, P. (2000). Service users' knowledge and social work theory: Conflict or collaboration? *British Journal of Social Work, 30*, 489–503. doi:http://dx.doi.org/10.1093/bjsw/30.4.489

Beresford, P., & Boxall, K. (2012). Service users. Social work education and knowledge for social work practice. *Social Work Education, 31*, 155–167. doi:http://dx.doi.org/10.1080/02615479.2012.644944

Beresford, P., & Croft, S. (2008). Democratising social work—A key element of innovation: From "client" as object, to service user as producer. *The Innovation Journal: The Public Sector Innovation Journal, 13*, 5–22. Retrieved from http://www.innovation.cc/scholarly-style/beresford_2_democrat_sw.pdf

Branfield, F. (2009). *Developing user involvement in social work education*. London: Social Care Institute for Excellence.

Braye, S., & Preston-Shoot, M. (1995). *Empowering practice in social care*. Buckingham: Open University Press.

Brown, K., & Young, N. (2008). Building capacity for service user and carer involvement in social work education. *Social Work Education, 27*, 84–96. doi:http://dx.doi.org/10.1080/02615470701381491

Burke, P., & Parker, J. (2007). *Social work and disadvantage: Addressing the roots of stigma through association*. London: Jessica Kingsley.

Cabiati, E. (2016). Teaching and learning: An exchange of knowledge in the university among students, service users and professors. *European Journal of Social Work, 19*, 247–262. doi:http://dx.doi.org/10.1080/13691457.2015.1024615

Cooper, H., & Spencer-Dawe, E. (2006). Involving service users in interprofessional education: Narrowing the gap between theory and practice. *Journal of Interprofessional Care, 20*, 603–617. doi:http://dx.doi.org/10.1080/13561820601029767

Corrigan, P. W., & Penn, D. L. (2015). Lessons from social psychology on discrediting psychiatric stigma. *Stigma and Health, 1*, 2–17. doi:http://dx.doi.org/10.1007/s10464-008-9189-5

Coulter, S., Campbell, J., Duffy, J., & Reilly, I. (2013). Enabling social work students to deal with the consequences of political conflict: Engaging with victim/survivor service users and a 'pedagogy of discomfort'. *Social Work Education, 32*, 439–452. doi:http://dx.doi.org/10.1080/02615479.2012.668180

Covarrubias, I., & Han, M. (2011). Mental health stigma about serious mental illness among MSW students: Social contact and attitude. *Social Work, 56*, 317–325. doi:http://dx.doi.org/10.1093/sw/56.4.317

Cree, V. E. (2013). Stigma in health and social work. In L. Beddoe & J. Maidment (Eds.), *Social work practice for promoting health and wellbeing: Critical issues* (pp. 76–85). London: Routledge.

Cunningham, J. A., Sobell, L.C., & Chow, V. M. C. (1993). What's in a label? The effects of substance types and labels on treatment considerations and stigma. *Journal of Studies on Alcohol, 54*, 693–699. Retrieved from http://dx.doi.org/10.15288/jsa.1993.54.693

Doel, M. (2009). *Social work palcements: A traveller's guide*. London: Routledge.

Dominelli, L. (2002). *Anti oppressive social work theory and practice*. London: Palgrave Macmillan.

Dominelli, L. (2008). *Anti-racist social work*. London: Palgrave Macmillan.

Donati, P. (2010). *Relational sociology: A new paradigm for the social sciences*. London: Routledge.

Duffy, J., Das, C., & Davidson, G. (2013). Service user and carer involvement in role-plays to assess readiness for practice. *Social Work Education, 32*, 39–54. doi:http://dx.doi.org/10.1080/02615479.2011.639066

Edwards, C. (2003). The involvement of service users in the assessment of diploma in social work students on practice placements. *Social Work Education, 22*, 241–249. doi:http://dx.doi.org/10.1080/02615470309138

Folgheraiter, F. (2004). *Relational social work: Toward networking and societal practices*. London: Jessica Kingsley.

Folgheraiter, F. (2007). Relational social work: Principles and practices. *Social Policy and Society, 6*, 265–274. doi:http://dx.doi.org/10.1017/S1474746406003526

Folgheraiter, F. (2012). *The mistery of social work*. Trento: Erickson.

Folgheraiter, F., & Raineri, M. L. (2012). A critical analysis of the social work definition according to the relational paradigm. *International Social Work, 4*, 473–487. doi:http://dx.doi.org/10.1177/0020872812440588

Folgheraiter, F. (2015). Relational social work. In J. D. Wright (Ed.), *International encyclopedia of the social & behavioral sciences* (2nd ed.) (Vol. 20, pp. 221–226). Oxford: Elsevier.

Fook, J. (2012). *Social work: A critical approach to practice*. Thousand Oaks, CA: Sage.

Galletly, C., & Burton, C. (2011). Improving medical student attitudes towards people with schizophrenia. *Australian and New Zealand Journal of Psychiatry, 45*, 473–476. doi:http://dx.doi.org/10.3109/00048674.2011.541419

Gee, M., Ager, W., & Haddow, A. (2009). The caring experience: Learning about community care through spending 24 hours with people who use services and family carers. *Social Work Education, 28*, 691–706. doi:http://dx.doi.org/10.1080/02615470802404200

Gregor, C., & Smith, H. (2009). I'm not a performing monkey: Reflections of the emotional experience of developing a collaborative training initiative between service users and lecturer. *Journal of Social Work Practice, 23*, 21–34. doi:http://dx.doi.org/10.1080/02650530902723290

Gupta, A., & Blewett, J. (2008). Involving services users in social work training on the reality of family poverty: A case study of a collaborative project. *Social Work Education, 27*, 459–473. doi:http://dx.doi.org/10.1080/02615470701380261

Health and Care Professions Council. (2014). *Regulating health, psychological and social work professionals*. London. Retrieved from http://www.hcpc-uk.org/

Heijnders, M., & Van Der Meij, S. (2006). The fight against stigma: An overview of stigma-reduction strategies and interventions. *Psychology, Health & Medicine, 11*, 353–363. doi:http://dx.doi.org/10.1080/13548500600595327

Irvine, J., Molyneux, J., & Gillman, M. (2015). Providing a link with the real world: Learning from the student experience of service user and carer involvement in social work education. *Social Work Education, 34*, 138–150. doi:http://dx.doi.org/10.1080/02615479.2014.957178

Judkins, B. M., & Lahurd, R. A. (1999). Building community from diversity: Addressing the changing demographics of academia and society. *American Behavioral Scientist, 42*, 786–799. doi:http://dx.doi.org/10.1177/00027649921954525

Lebel, T. P. (2008). Perceptions of and responses to stigma. *Sociology Compass, 2*, 409–432. doi:http://dx.doi.org/10.1111/j.1751-9020.2007.00081.x

Levin, E. (2004). *Involving service users and carers in social work education*. London: Social Care Institute for Excellence (SCIE).

Luty, J., Fakuda, F. W., Umoh, O., & Gallagher, J. (2006). Validation of a short instrument to measure stigmatised attitudes towards mental illness. *Psychiatric Bulletin, 30*, 257–260. doi:http://dx.doi.org/10.1108/17570980200900011

Luty, J., Kumar, P., & Stagias, K. (2010). Stigmatised attitudes in independent pharmacies associated with discrimination towards individuals with opioid dependence. *The Psychiatris, 34*, 511–514. doi:http://dx.doi.org/10.1192/pb.bp.109.028951

Luty, J., Maducolil, Easow J., & Mendes, V. (2011). Stigmatised attitudes towards the 'stressed' or 'ill'models of mental illness. *The Psychiatris, 35*, 370–373. doi:http://dx.doi.org/10.1192/pb.bp.110.032136

McCusker, P., MacIntyre, G., Stewart, A., & Jackson, J. (2012). Evaluating the effectiveness of service user and carer involvement in post qualifying mental health social work education in Scotland: Challenges and opportunities. *The Journal of Mental Health Training, Education and Practice, 7*, 143–153. doi:http://dx.doi.org/10.1108/17556221211269956

McLaughlin, H. (2009). What's in a name: 'Client', 'patient', 'customer', 'consumer', 'expert by experience', 'service user'—What's next? *British Journal of Social Work, 39*, 1101–1117. doi:http://dx.doi.org/10.1093/bjsw/bcm155

Molyneux, J., & Irvine, J. (2004). Service user and carer involvement in social work training: A long and winding road? *Social Work Education, 23*, 293–308. doi:http://dx.doi.org/10.1080/0261547042000224047

Morgan, A., & Jones, D. (2009). Perceptions of service user and carer involvement in healthcare education and impact on students' knowledge and practice: A literature review. *Medical Teacher, 31*, 82–95. doi:http://dx.doi.org/10.1080/01421590802526946

Nordt, C., Rössler, W., & Lauber, C. (2006). Attitudes of mental health professionals toward people with schizophrenia and major depression. *Schizophrenia Bulletin, 32*, 709–714. doi:http://dx.doi.org/10.1093/schbul/sbj065

Onesirosan, James B., Ohiole, Omoaregba J., & Osemudiamen, Okogbenin E. (2012). Stigmatising attitudes towards persons with mental illness: A survey of medical students and interns from Southern Nigeria. *Mental Illness, 4*, 32–34. doi:http://dx.doi.org/10.4081/mi.2012.e8

Pettersen, T., & Hem, M. (2011). Mature care and nursing in psychiatry: Notions regarding reciprocity in asymmetric professional relationships. *Health Care Analysis, 19*, 75–66. doi:http://dx.doi.org/10.1007/s10728-011-0167-y

Preston-Shoot, M. (2007). Whose lives and whose learning? Whose narratives and whose writing? Taking the next research and literature steps with experts by experience. *Evidence & Policy: A Journal of Research, Debate and Practice, 3*, 343–359. doi:http://dx.doi.org/10.1332/174426407781738056

Quinney, L., & Fowler, P. (2013). Facilitating shared online group learning between carers, service users and social work students. *Social Work Education, 32*, 1021–1031. doi:http://dx.doi.org/10.1080/02615479.2012.734801

Raineri, M.L. (2011). Il valore delle conoscenze esperienziali. In P. Donati, F. Folgheraiter, & M. L. Raineri (Eds.), *La tutela dei minori. Nuovi scenari relazionali* (pp. 87–101). Trento: Erickson.

Reynolds, J., & Read, J. (1999). Opening minds: User involvement in the production of learning materials on mental health and distress. *Social Work Education, 18*, 4417–4431. doi:http://dx.doi.org/10.1080/02615479911220411

Robinson, K., & Webber, M. (2013). Models and effectiveness of service user and carer involvement in social work education: A literature review. *The British Journal of Social Work, 43*, 925–944. doi:http://dx.doi.org/10.1093/bjsw/bcs025

Saleebey, D. (1996). The strengths perspective in social work practice: Extensions and cautions. *Social Work, 41*, 296–305. doi:http://dx.doi.org/10.1093/sw/41.3.296

Scheyett, A., & Kim, M. (2004). Can we talk? *Journal of Teaching in Social Work, 24*, 39–54. doi:http://dx.doi.org/10.1300/J067v24n01_03

Schön, D. (1983). *The reflective practitioner. How professionals think in action*. New York, NY: Basic Books.

Sevenhuijsen, S. (1998). *Citizenship and the ethics of care: Feminist considerations of justice, morality and politics*. London: Routledge.

Sewpaul, V., & Jones, D. (2005). Global standards for the education and training of the social work profession. *International Journal of Social Welfare, 14*, 218–230. doi:http://dx.doi.org/10.1111/j.1468-2397.2005.00362.x

Shor, R., & Sykes, I. J. (2002). Introducing structured dialogue with people with mental illness into the training of social work students. *Psychiatric Rehabilitation Journal, 26*, 63–69. doi:http://dx.doi.org/10.1080/09638231000118276

Skilton, C. J. (2011). Involving experts by experience in assessing students' readiness to practise: The value of experiential learning in student reflection and preparation for practice. *Social Work Education, 30*, 299–311. doi:http://dx.doi.org/10.1080/02615479.2010.482982

Skokandić, S., & Urbanc, K. (2009). Participation of service users in social work education: Teachers' perspective. *Ljetopis Socijalnog Rada, 16*, 327–354. Retrieved from http://hrcak.srce.hr/file/71645

Skoura-Kirk, E., Backhouse, B., Bennison, G., Cecil, B., Keeler, J., Talbot, D., & Watch, L. (2013). Mark my words! Service user and carer involvement in social work academic assessment. *Social Work Education, 32*, 560–575. doi:http://dx.doi.org/10.1080/02615479.2012.690388

Smith, M. (2013). Involving child protection service users in social work education. *The Journal of Practice Teaching and Learning, 11*, 77–91. doi:http://dx.doi.org/10.1921/175951511X661255

Steinberg, D. M. (2010). Mutual aid: A contribution to best-practice. *Social Work With Groups, 33*, 53–68. doi:http://dx.doi.org/10.1080/01609510903316389

Taylor, I., Braye, S., & Cheng, A. (2009). *Carers as partners (CaPs) in social work education*. London: Workforce Development Report.

Thompson, N. (2002). *Loss and grief: A guide for human services practitioners*. Basingstoke: Palgrave Macmillan.

Thompson, N. (2006). *Anti-discriminatory practice*. Basingstoke: Palgrave Macmillan.

Thompson, S., & Thompson, N. (2008). *The critically reflective practitioner*. Basingstoke: Palgrave Macmillan.

Trevithick, P. (2005). *Social work skills*. Berkshire: Open University Press.

Tyler, G. (2006). Addressing barriers to participation: Service user involvement in social work training. *Social Work Education, 25*, 385–392. doi:http://dx.doi.org/10.1080/02615470600593394

Waterson, J., & Morris, K. (2005). Training in 'social' work: Exploring issues of involving users in teaching on social work degree programmes. *Social Work Education, 24*, 653–675. doi:http://dx.doi.org/10.1080/02615470500185093

Weiss, M. G., Ramakrishna, J., & Somma, D. (2006). Health-related stigma: Rethinking concepts and interventions 1. *Psychology, Health & Medicine, 11*, 277–287. doi:http://dx.doi.org/10.1080/13548500600595053

Wilkes, R. (1985). Social work: What kind of profession? In D. Watson (Ed.), *A code of ethics for social work: The second step* (pp. 40–58). London: Routledge/Kegan Paul.

Wilson, A., & Beresford, P. (2000). Anti-oppressive practice: Emancipation or appropriation? *British Journal of Social Work, 30*, 553–573. doi:http://dx.doi.org/10.1093/bjsw/30.5.553

Zavirsek, D., & Videmsek, O. (2009). Service users involvement in research and teaching: Is there a place for it in Eastern European social work? *Ljetopis Socijalnog Rada, 16*, 207–222. Retrieved from http://hrcak.srce.hr/file/71599

Zellmann, K. T., Madden, E. E., & Aguiniga, D. M. (2014). Bachelor of social work students and mental health stigma: Understanding student attitudes. *Journal of Social Work Education, 50*, 660–677. doi:http://dx.doi.org/10.1080/10437797.2014.947900

The Meaningful Involvement of Service Users in Social Work Education: Examples from Belgium and The Netherlands

Kristel Driessens, Hugh McLaughlin and Lia van Doorn

ABSTRACT

This article links the development of service user involvement championed in the United Kingdom to two examples in Dutch-speaking qualifying social work programmes: one from Belgium and one from the Netherlands. In both projects, a longer lasting cooperation with more marginalised service users was established. The Belgium project highlights social work lecturers and service users living in poverty, working in tandem to deliver a module to social work and socio-educational care work students. The example from the Netherlands involves young people from a homeless shelter as peer-researchers, working together with social work students.

Both projects, one focusing on social work education and on social work research, highlight striking similarities in the positives and challenges of working with service users including how this challenges both groups preconceptions of the other, deepens learning but also creates greater potential for confrontations which need to be managed creatively. The article also identifies the pre-requisites for this to be effective including appropriate resourcing, training, facilitative skills and acknowledges that collaborations can be extremely fragile. However, such projects need further investment, experimentation and implementation on an international scale to share learning and promote creative approaches for the development and learning of social work students.

1. Introduction

Social work has a proud tradition of involving service users in practice but it has taken longer to develop in social work education. In 2003, in England, it was identified as a key requirement for the approval of all programmes providing the new social work degree (Department for Health [DoH], 2002). In addition, such a requirement is now underpinned by a new standard of education and training (SET) introduced by the Health and Care Professions Council (HCPC) the regulatory body for social work. This standard states that 'service users and carers must be involved in the programme' (Health & Care Professions Council (HCPC), 2014). Service user and carer involvement in social work education is also being championed in other countries (Wikler, 1979; Zavirsˇek & Videmsˇek, 2009). In this article, we link primarily the English experiences to lessons learned through projects in two university colleges, one in Antwerp (Belgium) and one in Utrecht (the Netherlands). This does not negate that there has been other important contributions to service user involvement in the other UK nations including N Ireland (Agnew & Duffy, 2010; Duffy, Chaitali, & Davidson, 2013); Scotland (Ager, Dow, Ferguson, et al., 2005; Scottish Social Services Learning Networks West & South West, 2009) and Wales (Biskin, Barcroft, Livingston, & Snape, 2013; Morris, Prankard, & Lefroy, 2013). We discuss the projects highlighting collaboration with service users in the provision of a module in the professional bachelor's degree programme of social work and of socio-educational care work and another experiment, in which service users and students carried out a project as co-researchers.

2. The Development of a Mandated Practice in England

Since 2003 in England, there has been a requirement for service users to be involved in all the differing aspects of social work education including admissions process, curriculum design, curriculum delivery, assessment and programme management. To aid the development of service user involvement, the General Social Care Council (GSCC) (the regulator at the time) provided all registered social work programmes with a grant to support and facilitate the involvement of service users in social work education. Service users have also been involved in the assessment of social work programmes as members of the approval teams for the HCPC who visit and assess social work courses as part of their approval and reapproval processes.

2.1. Considerations on the Concept of 'Service Users'

First we should clarify what we mean by a service user. Social work has referred to those who have been in receipt of its services in a number of different ways including viewing them as patients, clients, customers and as service users (McLaughlin, 2009a). The term service user can be criticised for focussing solely on one aspect of a person, that is that they are someone who is in receipt of social services. This neglects that they may also be a parent, a football coach or even a university professor! Each of these roles may be deemed to be a more desirable role than merely a service user. As McLaughlin (2009a, p. 1115) notes, the 'language we use is imbued with meaning and power'.

We should also avoid the danger of bifurcation, in that it is possible to be both a service user and a service provider. Certainly, a service provider may not be a service user at present, but this is not to suggest that they have not been in the past or will be in future. To further complicate matters, Smith (2014) (a pseudonym), who was sexually abused as a child, writes about bringing this experience into the social work classroom as a social work student. We should therefore not automatically assume that all student social workers have no service user experience.

2.2. Lessons from a Literature Review

In a recent review of the literature, Robinson and Webber (2013) found that there was a widespread support amongst service users, student social workers and lecturers for the involvement of service users in social work education. In response to this University, social work departments have adopted a variety of methods to incorporate service user involvement in their programmes.

> Methods include developing long-term relationships with service user networks (e.g. Baldwin & Sadd, 2006); involving a large number of local service user and carer groups (e.g. Ager, Dow, & Gee, 2005); and creating a pool of service user and carer consultants (e.g. Anghel & Ramon, 2009), often co-ordinated by service user involvement development workers. (e.g. Robinson & Webber, 2013, p. 936; Stevens & Tanner, 2006)

It is important to engage with a range of organisations and diverse service user groups to not only avoid the charge of only using the 'usual suspects' but also ensure that student social workers are exposed to a range of perspectives. This diversity of views is important; service users like social work students are not a homogenous group.

To actively promote the involvement of service users in social work programmes, the active support of staff members is essential (McLaughlin, 2009a). Service users cannot be expected to make effective contributions to the education of social workers if they are not supported or encouraged to develop the necessary skills. We should not assume that the participation of service users will always be positive. Edwards (2003) has noted that that the involvement of service users in practice learning has often led to feedback that has been too ambiguous and inconsistent. This reinforces the need for training, clear criteria of assessment, clarity of roles and the need for service user training to make their involvement in assessment meaningful (Advocacy in Action with Staff & Students from University of Nottingham, 2006). Farrow (2014) refers to the need for clear objectives and explanation of the reasons why educators are involving service users in their programmes, as well as the need to prepare both students and service users for this mutual contact and the importance of a debriefing session for service users.

Ambivalence to service user views is also possible and is best highlighted in the assessment process. Whilst many students find service user feedback helpful Crisp, Lister, and Dutton (2006, p. 729) there are also reported concerns that service users:

> may be overly positive about the student and consequently service user feedback may reflect a student's popularity rather than their competence.

The opposite is also possible whereby the student may be marked too harshly. Duffy et al. (2013) in their study of involving service users in role plays to assess social work qualifying student's fitness to practice also reminds us that we should not assume that social work academics will be keen to share their power with service users.

The involvement of service users in social work programmes is generally seen as a 'good thing' providing a balanced education to potential practitioners and to modelling good practice for the future (Baldwin & Sadd, 2006). Sustainability and resources have also been key themes in the literature (e.g. Baldwin & Sadd, 2006; Gutteridge & Dobbins, 2010). However, there are also organisational issues that can present barriers to involvement including access to universities, paperwork, the inflexibility of university payment systems, the support and training of service users and working with academic staff to ensure the meaningful involvement of service users (Branfield, Beresford, & Levin, 2007; Brown & Young, 2008). McLaughlin (2009b) also notes that service users' previous negative experience of involvement/consultation can also be a barrier.

Whilst, social work students and lecturers are supportive of service user involvement in social work education, this is primarily focused on processes rather than outcomes. The meaningful involvement of service users in education has potential impacts for both students and educators and the possibility of new pedagogic approaches which Beresford and Boxall (2012) claim can lead to new forms of professional knowledge challenging traditional power structures. Robinson and Webber (2013, p. 939) in their review of the literature, however, concluded that there is 'a dearth of outcome-focused research on service user involvement in social work education'. This article seeks to begin to address this shortfall. We describe two projects in Dutch-speaking qualifying social work programmes. The challenge was to set up meaningful collaboration with marginalised service users, one in education and one in research projects with social work students. A comparative analysis on the evaluation reports showed us striking similarities in the benefits from the perspectives of the students and service users involved, in the specific facilitating role of the lecturers and the organisational conditions to support the cooperation with these extra vulnerable clients. Thus, whilst the two projects were conducted independently, both used similar methods and add to our understanding and repertoire of meaningful service user involvement in social work education.

3. Service Users as Tandem Partners in an Educational Module

A project on educational innovation was conducted with service users living in poverty undertaken by the social work and socio-educational care work programmes at the Karel de Grote University College in Antwerp (Driessens & De Clerck, 2014). In the past, service users had been invited in as guest speakers to give their 'testimony' for one-off lectures. In this experiment, a lecturer assisted by a service user provided the entire module in tandem. This was done with the conviction that the development of a deeper, more advanced dialogue would provide additional understanding of and insight into the client perspective, whilst also contributing to the development of a respectful attitude towards service users. Two programme components were selected. In social work, the project was conducted in the second-year training course in social work practice with individuals, which was taught in groups of approximately 15 students. In socio-educational care work, it was conducted in the second-year substantive course in 'family-centred practice in youth care', which is taught in groups of approximately 32 students. The project was supported by Bind-Kracht (Bonding/Bridging Strengths), a collaborative partnership of service users, who were living in poverty and academic researchers. Various Bind-Kracht trainers and service users with years of experience in providing educational programmes for professional service providers participated in the project. In all, eight lecturers, five service users and 315 students were involved in the project during the 2013–2014 academic year.

Given the differences between the two projects, they were evaluated separately using a mixed methods approach (Cresswell, 2013). Neither project required ethical approval by their university nor Government although both projects faced ethical issues including informed consent, assured anonymity of respondents and safe interviewing of research respondents which are discussed in this article.

The students at Karel de Grote were surveyed using a web-based anonymous questionnaire; informed consent to involvement was assumed by the completion of the questionnaire. There were no adverse implications for students in non-completion of the survey. These quantitative data were supplemented through focus groups with students and an evaluation meeting involving all staff members. Lecturers and service users were also interviewed.

3.1. Academic Achievement Influenced by the Participation of Service Users

The response rate for the web-based questionnaire was high. The questionnaire was based on the ET37-questionnaire for students' evaluation of teaching used by the University of Antwerpen (Spooren, Mortelmans, & van Loon, 2012), some extra questions were introduced about working with service users in education. It was completed by 72% ($n = 43$) of the social work students and by 92% ($n = 235$) of the students of the socio-educational care work.

The students perceived the participation of the service users as a benefit. Although it seemed somewhat strange at first, a climate of openness and willingness to listen eventually emerged. The service users offered a glimpse into the worlds in which they were living, which enhanced the students' respect for their survival strategies, perceptions and experiences. The students learned a new way of looking at people living in poverty: as powerful people and as fighters.

> 'It opens your eyes, you get a view on the field, you can hear it from a different perspective, a different voice.'

Students of social work observed that the project had enhanced the realism of the course: the theories started to come to life, the cases gained a personal face and the students were able to practise working with real-life practical situations. Students gave additional consideration to their manner of interviewing (92% $n = 35/38$[1]), and they became more aware of pitfalls and strengths in communication (90% $n = 34/38$). They also learned to conduct a respectful dialogue with people who had experienced exclusion (84% $n = 32/38$) to suspend judgement and identified the importance of a respectful and authentic attitude. The exercises with service users also taught them to focus their questions more (see also Skilton, 2011), even when sensitive information was required.

The socio-educational care students reported that they had heard striking and captivating stories that had made them rethink about the potential meaning of social services to those involved.

> Their stories helped me to see that there are many pitfalls in counselling clients, often due to inadequate communication or because the service providers failed to listen to the clients' stories.

The majority of the students (80% $n = 184/230$) reported that they had become more aware of pitfalls and the power imbalance of working with families in the delivery of services. They also learned to ask for and respect the opinions of parents. They gained insight into the ways in which youth services are perceived, in addition to acquiring more understanding for the reactions of parents (see also Gupta & Blewett, 2008; Krumer-Nevo, 2008).

The feedback provided by service users was appreciated: they noticed different things, pointed out errors, stimulated discussion and showed how things could be done differently. Students observed their attitudes and the manner in which they expressed their ideas.

> This different way of looking at what you take for granted as a student was captivating. These confrontations are going to stay with you.

The transdisciplinary working methods and the connection of various types of knowledge—theoretical frameworks, practical professional knowledge and the experience-based knowledge of clients—were explicitly mentioned as benefits (see also Driessens, Saurama, & Fargion, 2011). Obvious assumptions were broken and different frames of reference became tangible, thereby strengthening the empathetic capacities of the students.

3.2. A Combination of Roles that Promotes Learning

> We asked all of the parties about the roles assumed by the various actors: what is the role of the service users and what do you expect of the lecturer?

3.2.1. Role of the Service Users

The students noted that service users bring practice into the classroom. They revealed the worlds in which they live and thus the consequences of exclusion. They spoke from personal experience about their views of 'good social work'. They contributed real-life case studies, which were captivating due to the emotion, amazement and indignation that they invoked. They were able to bring theoretical frameworks to life, and they applied their own emphases to the interpretation of these frameworks. They shared their desire for involvement in the delivery of services, expressing frustration when they were not given these opportunities.

Students were reluctant to impose conditions on the service users. They felt that service users should be social and open to other opinions and penetrating questions. It was important for them to take the initiative, to talk about relevant issues and to relate positive, hopeful stories. Students expected the service users to be able to recognise their efforts and provide affirmation of their work. From their perspective, the service users identified opportunities that the students had missed and provided them with recommendations. In role-play exercises, they assumed the role of the client in a realistic manner and offered students safe opportunities to practise. Service users reported that they needed to be able to get along with students, to react to offensive statements and to be cautiously confrontational in some cases. Both groups of students appreciated the fact that the service users did not assess work or assign marks. This ensured an open and safe dialogue. In one of the programme components, however, they did participate in the assessment and provided feedback on a role-play exercise. The results indicated that they had found it difficult to look at the students critically (Skilton, 2011).

3.2.2. Role of the Lecturer

Students noted that lecturers who work with service users had an entirely different presence in the classroom. They emphasised the importance of the facilitating role of the lecturer. In the beginning, it was important to introduce the service users properly, specifying their role and expectations clearly and identifying ground rules for cooperation. Lecturers offered theory, frameworks and vision, in addition to securing the objectives of the programme component. They also encouraged dialogue, framing the stories of the service users and bringing structure to these stories. They provided sufficient space, posed focused questions and continually involved the service users and the students. They supported the service users and enhanced their strengths. One of the service users formulated it as follows:

> 'This lecturer always found new inroads; she could really respond to me. She could always find the right words to restart the conversation. I truly admired her, and I thought, "Wow! Nice job!"'

Lecturers also needed additional skills in coaching and diplomacy, in interviewing, mediation, caring, flexibility and integrity to work in tandem with service users whilst some of these may have been developed in their time as practitioners they may not have been practiced recently or been developed for an educational setting. Their roles were essential for keeping the delicate interaction on the right track.

3.3. Organisational Conditions for Successful Collaboration

The ability to transform collaboration with service users into a high-quality pedagogical method is subject to several conditions. Participants in the focus groups and interviews were asked about the organisational conditions for the success of such processes.

Comparison of the organisational structure of the programme components revealed a major difference in group size. The size of the training groups in the social work programme (maximum 15 students per group) proved ideal as it allowed for an in-depth dialogue. There was sufficient space for practice and feedback. This posed an obstacle in groups of approximately 32 students. Not all of the students exhibited commitment, and it was more difficult to guarantee safety or support an open dialogue. In some groups, this was addressed by placing the chairs in a circle, thereby allowing for more eye contact.

For lecturers and service users, additional time was required for preparation and debriefing. For tandem teaching, it is important for both actors to be well attuned to each other, to be sufficiently familiar with each other and to be able to trust each other (Baldwin & Sadd, 2006). In addition, the support from Bind-Kracht proved essential. Bind-Kracht provided a pool of service users. In Bind-Kracht, the service users had the opportunity to participate and practice in training programmes in small groups, in which they could support each other. Bind-Kracht also ensured that all of the service users received volunteer contracts, permission to perform volunteer work and insurance during their activities, in addition to making sure that their volunteer payments were paid as quickly. Studies in other countries have identified this support as an important success factor (Gupta & Blewett, 2008).

3.4. Evaluation by the Parties Involved and Lessons from the Project

The students were extremely positive with regard to the input provided by the service users. Their openness, honest input and experiences enhanced the realism of the course, brought the theoretical insights to life and contributed captivating examples. Students were introduced to 'people living in another world', and they had the opportunity to feel the effects that exclusion can have and to see how social services can lead to either negative reinforcement or positive change. A few students offered critical remarks: they would like to have heard more positive, hopeful stories about services. The service users could have been more proactive and the feedback on their actions and manners of communication could have been stronger.

The service users felt that they had been treated with respect, in addition to receiving recognition and appreciation. They considered it worthwhile to help beginning service providers find their way, and they empathised with the students. They nevertheless expressed a desire to do better the next time, by knowing more about the programme, the course objectives and the substantive topics, as well as about the requirements for good feedback (Beresford et al., 2006). The lecturers expressed a great deal of ambivalence and uncertainty.

Some were concerned about the service users. They were satisfied about student attendance, the authentic dialogues and the stimulating teachable moments. All of the parties involved were convinced of the benefits of this type of collaboration, and the programme remains committed to continuing with the project.

4. On the Trail of Homeless Young People: Social Work Students as Co-researchers in Utrecht.

In 2013, fourth-year students in the social and community work programme at the University of Applied Sciences Utrecht (HU) collaborated on a research project with young people from the Pension Singelzicht[2] homeless shelter. In this project, four female students and four male homeless young people—who were of the same age—went in four pairs to interview twelve former male residents of Pension Singelzicht. Each interview was structured by a topic list and lasted about an hour. The interviews took place at a location of preference by the interviewees. Each interview was audio recorded and transcribed by the students. (Franchimont & Haarsma, 2013).

4.1. Academic Achievements Influenced by the Cooperation with Service Users

The primary beneficiaries of the research project were the four students. It allowed them to practise their research skills within the turbulent professional practice domain of homelessness services and to acquire knowledge about homeless young people and themselves.

> 'Before the project, I had held several prejudices about homeless young people – that they often used alcohol and drugs, and that they were violent and aggressive. They obviously have a lot of problems, but they are also simply peers who share our concerns and dreams for the future'. Student Suze (p. 25)

The research project was also beneficial for the residents of Singelzicht. For the homeless young people, it was an important experience collaborating with the students from the HU, whose lives were quite different from their own. It provided them with the opportunity to expand their social networks and broaden their horizons. Another aspect that they considered valuable was the interview training, in which they worked with students to practise engaging others, interviewing techniques and other skills.

> 'Participating in such a study is certainly educational. You can earn a little pocket money. It's helpful in two ways: it allows you to learn something, and you get to help someone else'. He added, 'What I learned from the student was perseverance: things don't always go the way you plan. But now I know that I just have to keep going. The student helped me to see this, and it's made me more serious in some respects'. (Co-researcher Daryll, p. 18)

Another co-researcher, Brian (p. 19), stated what he had learned as follows: '*Just good co-operation. That at some point in the interviews, I just started talking more and taking charge. That's what I learned*'.

Another benefit of the research project for the homeless young people—most of whose experiences with education had been negative and most of whom had ended their school careers prematurely—was that it offered them the opportunity to gain new experiences at the HU and to adjust the images that they had of themselves, higher education and training. At the end of the study, the young people received certificates from the HU. This was a special moment for the homeless young people: some had never completed any type of diploma or certificate. Several were even inspired to enrol in a university degree programme.

A third benefit is that the study provided insight into the course of the rehabilitation processes of former residents of Singelzicht. This knowledge was valuable to the co-researchers. Former residents who had brought semblance of order to their lives became role models for them.

> 'It was remarkable to see how much the homeless young people and the former residents found that they had in common. The contact with the former residents provided the homeless young people with food for thought regarding their futures. As a student, I was also a role model for them'. (Student Suze (p. 25)

Moreover, the reflections of the former homeless shelter residents on their rehabilitation processes provided valuable information for the professionals and the management of Singelzicht. There was, however, considerable variation amongst the former residents in terms of satisfaction. Some former residents expressed great appreciation for the assistance that they had received from Singelzicht. They reported that, without the help and support of Singelzicht, they would still be homeless. In contrast, others were critical of the assistance and services provided: stating they had survived because of their own strengths. On the one hand, their statements indicated that they had indeed received little support from Singelzicht. On the other hand, they might also indicate that the professionals had succeeded in reinforcing their autonomy and independence, thereby helping them to take control over their own lives. The co-researchers also had difficulty understanding the meaning of these critical voices of former residents. They interpreted the statements of dissatisfied former residents as evidence of the failure of the services provided by Singelzicht, and they regarded this as a threat to their own situations. After the interviews, these co-researchers wondered whether they should be at Singelzicht. The lecturer-researchers discussed this topic at length with both students and co-researchers, but without satisfying results. This reverse side of the research project and the question of how it should be addressed deserve further consideration.

A fourth benefit of the participation of the co-researchers was the enhanced quality of the study (see also Driessens et al., 2011; McLaughlin, 2010). As an illustration, the co-researchers were closely involved in the process of drafting the list of items for the topics to be addressed in the interviews. They made many valuable suggestions. For example, in addition to asking their age, some of the homeless young people proposed asking the former residents the question, 'How old do you feel?' The co-researchers emphasised the importance of asking this question, as experience had taught them that homeless young people often feel younger or older than their actual ages. This question on the perception of age provided additional depth to the study. The co-researchers were also less reluctant than the students were to follow up when interviewees gave contradictory answers. The students also considered it instructive to reflect on the interviews with the co-researchers. During the interviews, the co-researchers sometimes noticed things that had escaped the students' attention, for example that an interviewee who had been sleeping rough for ten years, now spent the nights in his apartment sleeping on his couch instead of in his bed.

An additional benefit became apparent after the study was completed. The affinity between several pairs of students and homeless young people had been so strong that they remained in touch with each other expanding and enriching the social networks of both the students and the homeless young people.

4.2. Lessons from the Project

The researchers and lecturers of the HU identified a number of lessons from the research project. It had offered them the opportunity to experiment with the form and content of the interview training for students and co-researchers. After the interim evaluation, they concluded that the optimal form would be to offer a training course consisting of two sessions covering, introductions, the goal and design of the study, the specification of mutual expectations and developing interviewing expertise through role-play exercises. A list of ground rules for the interviewers was compiled during the training that both parties committed to—partly because they had developed the rules themselves. Nevertheless, some of the interview pairs encountered problems. One of the homeless young people had become involved in a conflict at Singelzicht and was suspended for one month. In consultation with all parties involved, this person's participation was also suspended for one month. The pair resumed the interviews a month later. This resulted in a slight delay for the student in the completion of her studies.

During the training, all students and co-researchers worked collaboratively and at the end of the second training day, they were asked to choose the partners with whom they would prefer to work. The preferences coincided and the interviews were conducted by these pairings. One practical lesson was that the co-researchers, who where all chain-smokers needed to take periodic smoking breaks during the training. The research project and the reflection on the research methods of the lecturers and the researchers resulted in a manual, thus rendering the method transferable (Franchimont & Haarsma, 2013).

4.3. The Role of Lecturer-researchers

The lecturer-researchers were charged with facilitating the project. This posed the recurring question of when they should direct the students and co-researchers and when they should relinquish control and trust the pairs.

To ensure that the project would proceed smoothly, the lecturer-researchers established ground rules with the students and the homeless young people with regard to do's and don'ts during the research project. For example, they adopted the rule that the interviews would be conducted only during the day (during daylight hours) and that they would be held in the homes of the former residents or at a mutually agreed location. It was also agreed that the interview would be discontinued if the former resident was not responsive (e.g. due to being under the influence of drugs). Another rule required both the student and the co-researcher to be present during the interview. De-briefing sessions were held at the end of each interview, and both researchers called the project leader with a report. It was also agreed that the student, in consultation with the co-researcher, would make the appointments. The day before the interviews, students would remind their co-researchers of the appointments, and they would meet them at Singelzicht the following day. The lecturer-researchers also reached agreements with the pairs regarding privacy and confidentiality (Farrow & Fillingham, 2012).

4.4. Organisational Conditions for Successful Collaboration

The research identified several organisational conditions that must be met in order to allow research with students and co-researchers to succeed. Such research requires flexibility on the part of the educational institution (e.g. the institute had to improvise an area where the co-researchers where allowed to smoke) and lecturers. Second, it is advisable to reserve additional funds in the budget to cover unforeseen expenses, expect the unexpected (McLaughlin, 2009b). Another recommendation is to schedule additional time for research projects involving the participation of co-researchers. Such projects require additional preparation time on the part of lecturer-researchers. For the fourth-year students, this was part of the final examination assignment. The co-researchers also had much at stake. Failure or disappointment would once again damage their self-respect and, as argued by McLaughlin (2009b), it could prevent them from participating in such projects in the future. For this research, an ethical approval was not required under the Dutch law and code of conduct for research.

5. Conclusion

Academics in various countries are conducting experiments with the involvement of service users in social work degree programmes. In the United Kingdom, such involvement has been mandatory for 10 years and this article connects British experiences to recent experiments in the Netherlands and Flanders where the findings were similar.

The results from the two projects in Dutch-speaking social work programmes, collaborating with very vulnerable service users (people in poverty and homeless youngsters) indicate that all the parties involved tended to regard the experience as beneficial. Both gained additional insight into differing life experiences; sensing the limitations of one's own frame of reference; reflecting on one's own first impressions; communicating and acting; developing a respectful, positive basic attitude; and daring to engage in dialogue and learn from the experience of the other.

Nevertheless, the various projects have indicated that such collaboration is extremely fragile. It requires lecturers to adopt a more facilitatory role, whilst service users are expected to have a certain level of stability in their lives, in addition to openness, communication skills, diplomacy and resilience. Organisational support is also of fundamental importance, in terms of training, coaching and supporting both the service users and the lecturers. The additional time that lecturers and service users must invest in relationship building, preparation, delivery and debriefing requires additional resources, as does the practical organisation of such collaboration. Even if such resources are available, however, the balance is tenuous: confrontations, necessary survival strategies and collisions between contrasting life experiences are highly likely in any authentic collaboration. Such confrontations can be captivating and instructional to all parties, if managed properly. The collaboration transcends the professional, brings ethical dilemmas to the surface and touches the essence of the profession that we are training students to enter. It is the authors' contention that despite the time and reframing that it demands; the benefits of these educational innovations deserve further investment, experimentation and implementation on an international scale. In particular, we need to build more robust evidence on the impact of such service user involvement in educating the social workers of tomorrow (Irvine, Molyneux, & Gillman, 2014).

Notes

1. We only counted the answers 'completely agree' and 'agree'. The answers 'somewhat agree' we didn't include.
2. Stichting Singelzicht provides 24-h care to homeless people between the ages of 17 and 23 years in Utrecht.

References

Advocacy in Action with Staff & Students from University of Nottingham. (2006). Making it our own ball game: Learning and assessment in social work education. *Social Work Education: The International Journal, 25*, 332–346.

Ager, W., Dow, J., Ferguson, I., Gee, M., MacPhail, M., & McSloy, N. (2005). *Service user involvement in social work education: Good practice guidelines*. IRISS.

Ager, W., Dow, J., & Gee, M. (2005). Grassroots networks: A model for promoting the influence of service users and carers in social work education. *Social Work Education: The International Journal, 24*, 467–476.

Agnew, A., & Duffy, J. (2010). Innovative approaches to involving service users in palliative care social work education. *Social Work Education, 29*, 744–759.

Anghel, R., & Ramon, S. (2009). Service users and carers' involvement in social work education: Lessons from an English case study. *European Journal of Social Work, 12*, 185–199.

Baldwin, M., & Sadd, J. (2006). Allies with attitude! Service users, academics and social service agency staff learning how to share power in running social work education courses. *Social Work Education: The International Journal, 25*, 348–359.

Beresford, P., Branfield, F., Taylor, J., Brennan, M., Sartori, A., Lalani, M., & Wise, G. (2006). Working together for better social work education. *Social Work Education, 25*, 326–331.

Beresford, P., & Boxall, K. (2012). Service users, social work education and knowledge for social work practice. *Social Work Education: The International Journal, 31*, 155–167.

Biskin, S., Barcroft, V., Livingston, W., & Snape, S. (2013). Exploring service user and carer involvement on a social work degree programme. *Social Work Education: The International Journal, 32*, 301–316.

Branfield, F., Beresford, P., & Levin, E. (2007). *Common aims: A strategy to support service user involvement in social work education*. London: Social Care Institute for Excellence.

Brown, K., & Young, N. (2008). Building capacity for service user and carer involvement in social work education. *Social Work Education: The International Journal, 27*, 84–96.

Cresswell, J. W. (2013). *Research design: Qualitative, quantitative, and Mixed methods*. London: Sage.

Crisp, B. R., Lister, P. G., & Dutton, K. (2006). Not just social work academics: The involvement of others in the assessment of social work students. *Social Work Education: The International Journal, 25*, 723–734.

Department for Health. (2002). *Requirements for social work training*. London: Department of Health.

Driessens, K., Saurama, E., & Fargion, S. (2011). Research with social workers to improve their social interventions. *European Journal of Social Work, 14*, 59–76.

Driessens, K., & De Clerck, W. (2014). Ervaringsdeskundigen als tandempartners in hogeschoolopleidingen (experts by experience as tandem partners in professional bachelor programmes in University colleges). *Welwijs, 25*, 30–33.

Duffy, J., Das, C., & Davidson, G. (2013). Service user and carer involvement in role-plays to assess readiness for practice. *Social Work Education: The International Journal, 32*, 39–54.

Edwards, C. (2003). The involvement of service users in the assessment of diploma in social work students on practice placements. *Social Work Education, 22*, 341–349.

Farrow, K. (2014). Involving service users in social work management education: What makes it meaningful according to the 'experts'? *Social Work Education: The International Journal, 33*, 805–818.

Farrow, K., & Fillingham, J. (2012). Promises and pitfalls: Involving service users and carers in social work manager education. *Social Work Education: The International Journal, 31*, 835–847.

Franchimont, M., & Haarsma, L. (2013). *Leren van medeonderzoekers. Medeonderzoekers leren. Dubbelparticipatief onderzoek door zwerfjongeren and HBO-studenten* [Learning from fellow researchers/Fellow researchers learning: A dual participation study of homeless young people and university-college students]. Project management: Lia Van Doorn. Utrecht: Kenniscentrum Sociale Innovatie, Hogeschool Utrecht.

Gupta, A., & Blewett, J. (2008). Involving service users in social work training on the reality of family poverty: A case study of a collaborative project. *Social Work Education, 27*, 459–473.

Gutteridge, R., & Dobbins, K. (2010). Service user and carer involvement in learning and teaching: A faculty of health staff perspective. *Nurse Education Today, 30*, 509–514.

Health and Care Professions Council. (2014). *Service user and carer standard and guidance (SET3.17)*. Retrieved September 23, 2014, from http://www.hcpc-uk.org/assets/documents/10001A9DStandardsofeducationandtrainingguidanceforeducationproviders.pdf

Irvine, J., Molyneux, J., & Gillman, J. (2014). 'Providing a link with the real world': Learning from the student experience of service user and carer involvement in social work education. *Social Work Education: The International Journal, 34*, 138–150.

Krumer-Nevo, M. (2008). From noise to voice: How social work can benefit from the knowledge of people living in poverty. *International Social Work, 51*, 556–565.

McLaughlin, H. (2009a). What's in a name: Client, patient, customer, consumer, service user, service user: What's next? *British Journal of Social Work, 19*, 1101–1117.

McLaughlin, H. (2009b). *Service user research in health and social care*. London: Sage.

McLaughlin, H. (2010). Keeping service user involvement in research honest. *British Journal of Social Work, 40*, 1591–1608.

Morris, G., Prankard, S., & Lefroy, L. (2013). Animating experience: Bringing student learning to life through animation and service user and career experience. *Journal of Practice Teaching and Learning, 12*, 17–28.

Robinson, K., & Webber, M. (2013). Models and effectiveness of service user and carer involvement in social work education: A literature review. *British Journal of Social Work, 43*, 925–944.

Scottish Social Services Learning Networks West and South West. (2009). *Effective engagementin social work education: A good practice guide to involving people who use services and cares*. IRISS. Retrieved December 31, 2015, from http://www.iriss.org.uk/sites/all/files/SCLD-Effective-Engagement.pdf

Skilton, J. K. (2011). Involving service users in assessing student's readiness to practise: The value of experiential learning in student reflection and preparation for practice. *Social Work Education: The International Journal, 30*, 299–311.

Smith, J. (2014). The resilient survivor – A student social worker's journey on placement. *Social Work Education: The International Journal, 33*, 861–873.

Spooren, P., Mortelmans D., & van Loon F. (2012). Exploratory structural equation modeling ESEM: An application to the SET37-questionnaire for students evaluation of teaching. *Procedia: Social and Behavioral Sciences, 69*, 1282–1288.

Stevens, S., & Tanner, D. (2006). Involving service users in the teaching and learning of social work students: Reflections on experience. *Social Work Education The International Journal, 25*, 360–371.

Wikler, L. (1979). Consumer involvement in the training of social work students. *Social Casework, 60*, 145–149.

Zavirsˇek, D., & Videmsˇek, P. (2009). Service users involvement in research and teaching: Is there a place for it in Eastern European social work? *Ljetopis Socijalnog Rada, 16*, 207–222.

Mend the gap – strategies for user involvement in social work education

Ole Petter Askheim, Peter Beresford and Cecilia Heule

ABSTRACT
A major strand in social work's history has been its paternalistic character, partly due to a philanthropic tradition, but also to the tendency to import an individualist expert model into social work practice. As a result, gaps have arisen between expert and experiential knowledge. In this article, so called 'gap mending strategies' developed by the international network PowerUs are discussed. PowerUs consists of teachers and researchers from schools of social work and representatives from service user organizations in nine European countries. The gaps as the network identifies them are presented and we share some processes within our practices that mend or maintain gaps between service users and professionals. Two main strategies will be explored in more detail—a strategy that has been developed in the UK of mainstreaming service user participation in all stages of social work education, and a strategy that has been developed in Scandinavia of developing joint courses for social work students and students from service user organizations. A main conclusion is that alliances between educational institutions and service user organizations will be important to get a fuller understanding of what gaps we are facing and how they best could be mended.

Introduction

Service user involvement is an objective of increasing importance in social policy generally, as well as in the education of social workers specifically. The concept is fundamental in the international definition of social work adopted by the International Association of Schools of Social Work, IASSW and the International Federation of Social Workers (IFSW)[1]:

> The social work profession's core mandates include promoting social change, social development, social cohesion, and the empowerment and liberation of people./.../ The uniqueness of social work research and theories is that they are applied and emancipatory. Much of social work research and theory is co-constructed with service users in an interactive, dialogic process and therefore informed by specific practice environments.

In a European Framework for Quality Assurance of the Social Professions developed by the IFSW, the involvement of service users in the running and development of social services is identified as a key element in the social work role (Anghel & Ramon, 2009; Beresford, 2016). However, despite the good intentions, the achievement of the goal of increased user involvement and empowerment as a result of social work appears to remain distant. A major strand in social work's history has been its paternalistic character, partly due to a philanthropic tradition, but also to the tendency to import an individualist medicalized expert model into social work practice. As a result service users are mainly conceived of as persons with deficiencies and problems. The attitudes are transferred to the students of social work. Students mainly learn about user involvement and empowerment through theory and mainly meet service users as clients during their placement periods or when service users give isolated lectures. The cooperation with the 'practice field' is mainly limited to contact with the professionals (Beresford et al., 2006; Börjeson, Denvall, Heule, & Kristiansen, 2008).

In this article, so called 'gap-mending strategies' developed by the international network PowerUs to reduce the gaps between the declared aims and the experienced realities are discussed. PowerUs consists of teachers and researchers from schools of social work and representatives from service user organizations in nine European countries (www.powerus.se). Firstly, the gaps as the network identifies them will be presented and we will then share some processes within our practices that mend or maintain gaps between service users and professionals. Two main strategies will be explored in more detail—a strategy that has been developed in the UK of mainstreaming service user (and carer) participation in all stages of social work education, and a strategy that has been developed in Scandinavia of developing joint courses for social work students and students from service user organizations. We will finally discuss to what degree the gap-mending strategies represent approaches to renew social work in a radical transformative way.

Relationships and roles in social work education and practice

Policy documents have prioritised service user participation in recent years (Beresford, 2011; Eriksson, 2015). Beresford and Croft (2003) identify two different traditions of service user participation, with different goals and philosophical roots. The first, they call consumerist/managerialist, and comes from management strategies. It sees service users as customers that can help develop more effective services. Its approach emerged under neo-liberalism and was put in place in service systems. Here the concern has been to include the views and ideas of people as public service users, in the same way that they have been in market research in the provision of mainstream commercial goods and services. The aim is to provide market intelligence rather than to bring about any transfer of control or increased say in decision-making. The other model is called a democratic/citizenship one. Its goal is delivery from different kinds of exclusions and oppression and the redistribution of power. The democratic/citizenship model emphasizes the importance of active service user participation in all aspects of support and services (Cameron, 2014; Priestly, 1999).

Many social scientists agree that specific methods are of less importance than the relationships that are developed in social work practice (Hasenfeldt, 1992; Parton, 2000; Trevithick, 2003). However what roles the service users should take in relation to social workers differs greatly between different social work models. The professionalization of social work practice has led to an increasingly common view of the social worker as an expert in other people's problems. Social work has sought to develop its own body of knowledge, with social workers seen as having specific expert professional knowledge to validate their activities. The tendency is reinforced since the social workers generally are employed in organizations characterized by certain ways of defining and understanding the problem. The institutions have a certain repertoire of measures and benefits at their disposition, which influences how practitioners identify the problems and the persons seeking help. The Danish researchers Järvinen and Mik-Meyer (2003), p. 15) describe the development in social work as the 'standardisation of human problems'. Consequently, categories and roles are constructed, and individuals reduced to cases. The tendency has gained further strength as manageralism and New Public Management (NPM) ideas have gained ground (Beresford, 2009; Lavalette (ed.), 2011; Rogowski, 2010). The users are reduced to passive consumers. At the same time, strong elements of control in the NPM model to secure the efficiency and cost-effectiveness of the services express lack of confidence to both the users and the producers of the services.

Research has also shown that social workers often share negative views of social problems that are widespread among the wider population. Stigmatizing attitudes are not only present in society at large, but also among helping professionals and students in areas as psychiatry, psychology and social work (Mittal et al., 2014; Nordt, Rössler, & Lauber, 2006; Svensson et al., 2014; Trevithick, 2012). A consequence of all this can be that the experiences and contributions of people with direct experience as social work service users are devalued or ignored. Reports from service users also show that they often feel humiliated and oppressed as a result of their contact with people who are employed to help them (Johansson, 2006; Oliver, Sapey, & Thomas, 2012; Rønning, 2005).

In contrast to this paradigm stands a model based on reciprocal relationships and co-production of knowledge, which reflects the referred goals of social work expressed by the IFSW and the IASSW. The participatory model suggests that social workers should see vulnerable and disadvantaged groups as their allies in mutual efforts to change and better society. To include service users in developing society and its services is a political matter, as well as a matter of human rights. Additionally, empirical studies from different service user groups show that service users' satisfaction with the services, and also their recovery processes and positive solutions of their problems, are strongly associated with a positive reciprocal relation between the users and the services, with the basis in the users' own values and preferences (e.g. Davidson, Andres-Hyman, Fry, & Kirk, 2008; McCormack & McCane, 2010).

Mending the gaps

The gap-mending concept can be characterized as a reflective tool that helps teachers and researchers to consider what, in their practices increases, maintains or mends gaps between policies, services and professionals—as well as service users. Gaps always exist in a context. Gaps can develop and be maintained because of prejudices based on social work's categorization of people, because of language barriers, because of institutional hierarchies and the roles we have created for people within them. They can also exist because of lack of knowledge. Contextual knowledge is therefore essential in gap-mending reflections, as well as a good understanding of existing gaps.

An essential component of the gap-mending concept is co-production. Co-production is defined as a particular form of partnership between people who use social care services and the people and agencies who provide them (Hunter & Ritchie, 2007, p. 9). Bowers and Wilkins (2012, p. 100) declare that 'as a concept co-production is renowned for its 'excessive flexibility in terms of the ways in which it has been defined and interpreted'.

Needham and Carr (2009) distinguish between three levels of coproduction: at the lowest level, co-production is simply used as a *description* of how all services rely on some productive input from the users. This approach simply restates existing approaches to public services as co-productive, and fails to acknowledge the potential for more effective use of productive capacities among service users or for creating social capital. At an intermediate position, Needham and Carr describe co-production as a tool of *recognition* for the people who use services and their carers, acknowledging their input, valuing and harnessing the power of existing informal support networks and creating better channels for people to shape services. This level of co-production offers a way to acknowledge and support the contributions of service stakeholders, although without necessarily changing fundamental delivery systems. There is therefore a danger that it can be a device to legitimize existing approaches, helping people who use services better to understand the strains that providers face, rather than changing organizational cultures and improving service provision. At its most effective, Needham and Carr describe co-production as an approach, which involve a *transformation* of the services. The transformative level of co-production requires a relocation of power and control, through the development of new user-led mechanisms of planning, delivery management and governance. It involves new structures of delivery to entrench co-production, rather than simply ad hoc opportunities for collaboration and brings service users and practitioners together in new ways.

It is important that these different levels of co-production are remembered and acknowledged when we talk about co-producing methods in social work, and that existing power mechanisms have to be challenged. When we speak of gap-mending strategies, it is essential to emphasize that it is co-production at a transformative level we have in mind. Beresford (2011, p. 109) reminds us of this when he describes social work as co-production: 'What it means is that understanding and construction of social work practice comes to be seen as a joint activity between service user and worker, in which the former can play an active part in structuring and shaping in accordance with their rights and needs'.

An important ingredient in transformative co-production is the concept of empowerment. The concept of empowerment originates from the literature on marginalized people and the process through which marginalized people can mobilize and raise awareness, in order to draw on their own abilities and resources to solve their own problems. Empowerment has been important as an organizing concept for the disabled people's and service users' movements. Vital sources of inspiration have been the Black civil rights movement in the USA in the 1950s (Solomon, 1976) and not least, Paulo Freire's book 'Pedagogy of the Oppressed' (1970). Two related aspects of empowerment are personal and political empowerment. This acknowledges the importance of both personal and political change and their inter-relation. Thus, service users highlight *personal empowerment*—meaning the need for change within us—if we are to be actively and meaningfully involved in making change. Otherwise we may only serve as a stage army. Such personal empowerment is likely to include gaining confidence, knowledge and skills. But *political empowerment* is also of importance—and this is understood as the need for making change at wider structural and political levels. This model of empowerment places an emphasis on the need to address both of these elements if people are to be truly rather than tokenistically involved in making change. Disabled people and service users have seen developing their self-organization through their own 'user led organisations' (ULOs) as the major method of doing this. Such organizations can support people's personal empowerment as a first step to them becoming actively collectively involved to achieve change. This can be gained through the greater strength that comes from developing collective ideas and agendas and working together to achieve them in their own organizational space (Campbell & Oliver, 1996; Jacks, 1995; Oliver & Barnes, 2012; Shera & Wells, 1999). A gap-mending practice should be empowering for service users as well as professionals and they should help empowering each other.

The PowerUs network

The concept of gap-mending was developed by the PowerUs network,[2] which started in 2011 through an EU-funded project consisting of social work teachers and service users from three countries—Sweden, Norway and the UK. The purpose of the network was to share good experiences of service user participation in social work education and research. Participants of the original network had developed different strategies aiming to reduce the distance between social workers and service users and to enhance the experiences of the service users. In Scandinavia (Lund (Sweden) and Lillehammer (Norway), this had been done by creating university courses that included both students from the social work programme, as well as students recruited from different service user organizations. In the UK, the development had taken a different turn. Service users had, in collaboration with researchers and teachers of social work, succeeded responding to a new requirement of mainstreaming service user participation in all aspects and stages of planning and execution of social work professional education.

In five years, the PowerUs network has grown to include new participants from countries like Denmark, Germany, Switzerland, The Netherlands, France and Belgium. The requirement to join the network is an active practice of collaboration between service users and academics in developing methods that the network has come to call 'gap-mending' methods. Theoretical approval of service user participation is thus not enough. There is a growing European interest in methods developed within the network, which was demonstrated at the international conference organized by the European Association of Schools of Social Work (EASSW) in Milan 2015, in which PowerUs was a partner. The conference was introduced with a film produced by PowerUs.[3] The EASSW has expressed a desire to disseminate the values and methods of PowerUs to its 300 member schools. In some European countries, service user involvement in social work education has become a requirement, however, there are still many European countries where the inclusion of users of social services is still considered as a 'taboo' issue and it has been ignored.

The Swedish experiences

There is no legislation in Sweden that regulates service user influence in municipal social services or in the education of social work. However, the National Board of Health and Welfare has published several publications to provide the municipality's advice and guidance to develop service user participation in their activities. This has not resulted in a considerable change in the practice. When it comes to social work educations in Sweden, the importance of service users' perspectives was pointed out 2009 in an evaluation made by the Swedish National Agency for Higher Education (Högskoleverket, 2009). Although the schools of social work in Sweden have courses about service users, it is very rare to involve them as partners in planning or development of the curriculum.

In 2005, teachers at Lund University launched a new pedagogical concept, including a group of service users in a 75 ects (European Credit Transfer and Accumulation System) credit course that had normally been an elective course for social work students in their last semester. Since then, 18 such Mobilization courses have been undertaken, with approximately 400 social work students and a little over 200 service users involved. The service users study along side with the social work students and achieve university credits. The teachers have been inspired by many social theorists and pedagogues throughout the years, among them Freire (1970), Levinas (1998), the work of Joan Tronto (2009) as well as the writings of the recovery-movement (Deegan, 1988; Topor, 2001; Wilken, 2010).

One important goal of the experimental course was to shift a focus that there often is, on the needs, or the problems of the individual, to the need for reciprocal relationships and a strengthened community in society. This can be seen as a paradigm shift, as the organization of social work in Sweden is mainly structured around the categorization of individuals according to their problems. The change can also be understood as an attempt to shift social work activity from regulation to inclusion.

An important lesson learned in the early years was to deconstruct categories that are dominant in social work practice and that tend to cause tension between the two student groups. Not until methods that required a more personal input from the students were developed did the teachers experience a breakthrough in their aim of creating community and solidarity between the student groups. One method of developing this reciprocity is by initial personal presentations, where every student gets 15 min in front of the others to talk about who they are, and what matters to them in social work practice. For social work students, an important boundary is crossed as they share both doubts and weaknesses with each other and with the other student group. This works as an icebreaker and makes it possible for the students from service user organizations to face the social work students outside their prejudices, built on earlier experiences.

Social work students experience empowerment, as they can draw from earlier life experiences, including hardships, and become more personal in their future practice, with a better ability to resist bureaucratic demands of conformity. It is unlikely that they would choose to be so generous in showing themselves from a vulnerable side, were it not for the presence of the students from service user organizations. In the reflections from the social work students, they share that they normally experience university courses as being more competitive and encouraging them to show sides of themselves that could leave them vulnerable or disadvantage them in that competition. Service user students also say that they are relieved to be able to talk freely and on equal terms about the need for a changed social work practice. Many of them have earlier thought of university studies as something unapproachable. Some continue to study, in some cases, to become social workers.

The vision of the course has been to reconstruct a better and more inclusive practice. The students spend most of the time developing project ideas that are often both innovative and close to the needs expressed earlier in the course through the presentations of the participants. A difficulty is, though, that although these projects have great importance and value, they are often not compatible with the rigidity of the social service organization in Sweden. However, some of the projects have been realized, and some new service user organizations have been launched with the help of the platform and network that is created by the mobilization course. We have also seen further empowerment within the local service user movement, as many of their members have been challenged and further equipped through university studies. Students network with each other on social media and in public lectures that are held in the School of Social Work in Lund, also with students that have taken the course in other semesters than themselves.

For the teachers the platform of the mobilization course have been an ideal structure for testing research hypothesis in practice, and with the help of students–developing new knowledge about community principles and mechanisms (Angelin, 2015; Heule & Kristiansen, 2011, 2013, in press, Kristiansen & Heule, 2016).

Reflections from Norway

In the Norwegian Act of Social Services, it is stated that the services as far as possible should be designed in cooperation with the service users.[4] The curriculum for social work education declares that the services users' needs should be at the centre of the work and that the social workers should show respect for the service users' knowledge and choices.[5] Still, there are weak traditions for involving service users in the social work and social education courses in Norway. Traditionally people with user experiences are used in single lectures; otherwise the students mainly meet them as clients in their practice placements.

Inspired by the mobilization course in Lund the course 'Empowerment: meeting face to face creates new insights' (5 ECTS-points) since 2009 has been organized at Lillehammer University College as a joint course for undergraduate/bachelor students in social work and social education together with students with experiences as users of welfare services (Askheim, 2012). About 120 internal and 70 external students have since taken part in the course.

The title of the course, 'Empowerment: Meeting face to face gives insights', declares the goal: to create new insights for both groups. The intention is to give the participants new knowledge about the possible implications of marginalization and powerlessness and how they could be challenged when service user knowledge and professional 'expertise' are regarded as equally valid approaches to these problems. More specifically the goals are to give the students insight into:

- How power and powerlessness are created in the relationship between service users and professionals
- What empowerment can involve at different levels (individual/systemic level)
- How service user competence and professional competence can complement each other
- How empowerment can be realized in practice

Most of the external students have experiences connected to mental-health problems and are recruited through their service user organization or a user-led regional centre Another main group has service user experiences relating to drug misuse. Additionally some students have service user experiences relating to physical impairments, sensory impairments, as well as problems that are more mixed.

During the course, the students work intensely together four days every week during a three-week period. One day each week is reserved for individual studies. The course starts with a seminar located outside the college. On this seminar the students work together through experience based and creative methods derived from art and expressive therapy (Levine & Levine, 1999). These are methods well suited for promoting community, building trust and creating a safe learning environment. The second part consists of lectures that aim to illuminate the concept of empowerment. Discussion groups composed of students with different backgrounds then follow and the students then meet in plenary sessions. Finally, the students conduct a group project, which the groups present in plenary. The presentation takes place in a variety of ways, as role-plays, video productions, and as oral and written presentations. This presentation is a final exam.

The immediate evaluations of the courses are very positive. Both internal and external students say that they have come to new understandings about each other and about the use of theoretical concepts in practice (Askheim, 2012; Askheim, Altmann, & Hasvold, 2014). At the same time the relationship challenges established attitudes and roles. The course makes both parties reflect upon their roles and attitudes. The 'us-and-them' distinction between the parties dwindles.

A crucial criterion of whether such a course is successful or not, is nonetheless if the course has a lasting effect, if it adds values to programs, and enhances and changes professional practice, as well as improving service users' outcomes. A comprehensive literature review of projects with service user involvement in social work education concludes that there is no sufficient empirical evidence that service user involvement improves outcomes for students, nor that it has an effect on social work practice or on outcomes for future service users (Robinson & Webber, 2013). The conclusion further that in order to get meaningful service user involvement it is urgent to define specifically what the overarching aims should be. They refer to Beresford (2005) who defines meaningful involvement as evidence of change or improvements.

To investigate further whether our course seems to have a more lasting effect, we did a follow-up study with a selection of former students in 2014 (Altmann & Hasvold, 2015). What the students express four to five years after the complementation of the course correspond strongly with their immediate feedbacks. What the former students emphasized as valuable by the end of the course was repeated and elaborated. Former internal students felt that participating in the course had changed their attitudes and perceptions of the social worker's as well as of the service user's role, and as a consequence their practice. The external students described increased awareness about suppression mechanisms, self-worth and status as equal participants, and how this had affected how they today act in the role as service user.

Two of five former external students said that participation in the course has been a crucial factor for them to start further education. Having good experiences as students on the Face-to-Face course, and having their competences recognized, seems to be of great significance. This suggests that each of them has gained a greater degree of control of their own future.

The differences between Robinson and Webber's (2013) and our findings, can be related to the fact that their data were mainly based on service user's participation in admission interviews for studies, service users' assessment of students' assignments, and service user lectures. These are measures well suited to clarify and recognize a service user perspective, but differ from our course where internal and external students are *learning together.* Our study is based on the gap-mending pedagogy that reflects a partnership between the student and the service user This cooperative learning seems to have brought change or improvements in the way as Beresford (2005) refers to as meaningful service user involvement.

The British model

The UK is probably the country where the importance of user involvement in social work has been most clearly recognized officially and where it has the longest history. The new degree in social work, which was introduced in England and Wales in 2003, has made these countries the only ones in Europe where educational institutions are obliged to involve service users actively in the implementation, practice and evaluation of social work programmes at all levels (Department of Health, 2002). The Department of Health in addition provided special grants from central funding in order to support higher education institutes (HEIs) to develop and resource strategies to involve service users and carers (Levin, 2004). Government guidance does not prescribe the exact form of inclusion and participation to be pursued.

However, the British model can be summed up historically as primarily focusing on involving service users and carers (it has always involved both) in the process of social work education, in order to add their perspectives and input to the learning and knowledge provided for the students taking part (Branfield, 2009; Branfield, Beresford, & Levin, 2007). Projects documenting user involvement show that people with service user experiences are involved as lecturers and consultants in the development of programmes and curriculum, in the process of recruiting and assessing students and in the evaluation and quality assurance of the programmes (Anghel & Ramon, 2009; Baldwin & Sadd, 2006; Gupta & Blewett, 2008; Humphreys, 2005; Levin, 2004). Some courses have developed relationships with local 'user controlled organisations' (ULOs) to take forward this task; others have set up their own groups to work with the students. Students value the input of service users in their training because they provide a unique and valuable perspective, and people who rely on various services find their involvement in professional education to be worthwhile and beneficial (Beresford, 2014; Evaluation of Social Work Degree Qualification in England Team, 2008).

The involvement of service users in the design and delivery of the social work programmes does not necessarily imply that they take an active part as students. However, in some English projects, people with user experiences have been specially recruited as students and have obtained academic credits (Barnes, Carpenter, & Dickingson, 2006; Taylor & Le Riche, 2006) Increasingly when students are recruited to social work courses, there also seems to be recognition that their own lived experience—as both service users and carers—is something to be valued rather than viewed as a deficit.

More recently two developments have taken place which have had an impact on user involvement in UK social work education. First, building on the activities and experience gained by PowerUs, courses based on the Scandinavian model have also begun to emerge in Britain. Both London South Bank University and New College, Durham, have developed such courses. What has been especially interesting about the Durham course is that it has broken new ground, involving as students' mothers whose involvement with the social work service has related to child care and child protection issues (Casey, 2016). Secondly, there has been an increasing political and policy interest in England in so-called 'elite' social work graduate courses, including Frontline, Step Up To Social Work and Think Ahead. All have been concerned with 'improving the quality' of candidates for social work, but have tended to interpret this in terms of perceived improvements in their academic ability interpreted in terms of their qualifications and the status of their undergraduate universities. This has raised concerns that this devalues lived experience and limits diversity and reflects a desire to tailor social work training to a neoliberal agenda and to restrict undergraduate routes to qualification (SWAN, 2014).

Concluding remarks

There is increasing urgency to develop systematic and effective user involvement in social work and social work education. Without it, social work's values and goals are likely to be subverted because of the paternalistic traditions of social work and the dominating political climate in the contexts where social work is to be practised.

As the title indicates, the gap-mending concept has been developed as a reflective tool for mending the gaps between the declared goals of social work as, for example, stated in IASSW and IFSW-definition and between policies, services, professionals–and service users. The aim is to renew social work in a transformative way, consistent with its declared goals. The experiences from the gap-mending approaches referred to in this article and the growing interest in different countries is promising. How the gap-mending strategies more concretely should be developed is likely to vary and will have to take into account national and local considerations. Alliances and networks between educational institutions and service user organizations as well as across national borders will be important to disseminate the values and methods and learn from each other, inspire each other and discuss with each other to get a fuller understanding of what gaps we are facing and how they could best be mended. The growth of the PowerUs network and the growing cooperation between PowerUs and the EASSW is a promising start for such a development. The EASSW conference in Paris in June 2017 will be an important event to reinforce the gap-mending principle further and to spread it to new partners within Europe.

Notes

1. http://www.eassw.org/global-social-work/2/gdsw-a-global-definition-of-social-work-.html.
2. www.powerus.se.
3. https://www.youtube.com/watch?v=QExM_aA2Mus seen 2016-01-15.
4. https://lovdata.no/dokument/NL/lov/2009-12-18-131#KAPITTEL_1.
5. https://www.regjeringen.no/globalassets/upload/kilde/kd/pla/2006/0002/ddd/pdfv/269389-rammeplan_for_sosionomutdanning_05.pdf.

References

Altmann, L., & Hasvold, T. (2015). Brukerinvolvering i sosialfaglig utdanning. Hva kan «gap-mending» pedagogikk bidra til? [User involvement in social work education. What can be the contribution of gapmending pedagics?] *Fontene Forsking, 2*, 77–89.

Angelin, A. (2015). Service user integration into social work education: Lessons learned from nordic participatory action projects. *Journal of Evidence Informed Social Work, 12*, 124–138.

Anghel, R., & Ramon, S. (2009). Service users and carers' involvement in social work education: Lessons from an English case study. *European Journal of Social Work, 12*, 185–199.

Askheim, O. P. (2012). 'Meeting face to face creates new insights': Recruiting persons with user experiences as students in an educational programme in social work. *Social Work Education, 5*, 557–569.

Askheim, O. P., Altmann, L., & Hasvold, T. (2014). «Ansikt til ansikt gir innsikt» - brukere som medstudenter i sosialfaglig utdanning [Meeting face to face creates new insights] . In G. Bjørke,

H. Jarning, & O. Eikeland (Eds.), *Ny praksis—ny kunnskap: om utviklingsarbeid som sjanger* [New practice - new knowledge: Developmental work as a new genre] (pp. 190–201). Oslo: AMB-media.

Baldwin, M., & Sadd, J. (2006). Allies with attitude! Service users, academics and social service agency staff learning how to share power in running social work education cources. *Social Work Education, 25*, 348–359.

Barnes, D., Carpenter, J., & Dickingson, C. (2006). The outcomes of partnerships with mental health users in the interprofessional education: A case study. *Health and Social Care in the Community, 14*, 426–435.

Beresford, P. (2005). Theory and practice of user involvement in research: Making the connection with public policy and practice. In L. Lowes & I. Hulatt (Eds.), *Involving service users in health and social care research* (pp. 6–17). London: Routledge.

Beresford, P. (2009). Differentiated consumers? A differential view from a service user perspective. In R. Simmons, M. Powell, & I. Greener (Eds.), *The consumer in public services* (pp. 197–218). Bristol: The Policy Press.

Beresford, P. (2011). Radical social work and service users: A crucial connection. In M. Lavalette (Ed.), *Radical social work today. Social work at the crossroads* (pp. 95–114). Bristol: The Policy Press.

Beresford, P. (2014, June 3). Social work education leads the way on involving service users. *The Guardian*, Social Care Network. Retrieved from http://www.theguardian.com/social-care-network/2014/jun/03/social-work-education-leads-way-involving-service-users

Beresford, P. (2016). *All our welfare: Towards participatory social policy*. Bristol: The Policy Press.

Beresford, P., & Croft, S. (2003). Involving service users in management: Citizenship, access and support. In J. Reynolds, J. Henderson, J. Seden, J. Charlesworth, & A. Bullman (Eds.), *The managing care reader* (pp. 21–28). London: Routledge/The Open University.

Beresford, P., Branfield, F., Taylor, J., Brennan, M., Sartori, J., Lalani, M., & Wise, G. (2006). Working together for better social work education. *Social Work Education, 25*, 326–331.

Börjeson, B., Denvall, V., Heule, C., & Kristiansen, A. (2008). *Vi och dom, Om att ifrågasätta en gränssättning* [We and them. About questioning boundaries]. Stockholm: Ersta Sköndal University College.

Bowers, H., & Wilkins, A. (2012). Co-production in evaluation and outcome. In P. Beresford & S. Carr (Eds.), *Social care, service users and user involvement* (pp. 96–119). London: Jessica Kingsley Publishers, Research Highlights in Social Work.

Branfield, F. (2009). *Developing user involvement in social work education* (Workforce Development Report 29). London: Social Care Institute for Excellence.

Branfield, F., Beresford, P., & Levin, E. (2007). *Common aims: A strategy to support service user involvement in social work education* (Position paper 7). London: SCIE.

Cameron, C. (Ed.). (2014). *Disability studies: A student's guide*. London: Sage.

Campbell, J., & Oliver, M. (1996). *Disability politics: Understanding our past, changing our future*. London: Routledge.

Casey, H. (2016). *Mending the gap in professional education*. London: Research And Scholarship Journal, Association of Colleges.

Davidson, L., Andres-Hyman, R., Fry, J., & Kirk, T. (2008). From double trouble to dual recovery: Integrating models of recovery in addiction and mental health. *Journal of Dual Diagnosis, 4*, 273–290.

Deegan, P. (1988). Recovery: The lived experience of rehabilitation. *Psychosocial Rehabilitation Journal, 11*, 11–19.

Departement of Health. (2002). *Requirements for social work education and training*. London: Author.

Eriksson, E. (2015). *Sanktionerat motstånd. Brukarinflytande som fenomen och praktik* [Sanctioned resistance. User influence as phenomenon and practice]. Lund: Lund University.

Evaluation of Social Work Degree Qualification in England Team. (2008). *Evaluation of the new social work degree qualification in England. Volume 1: Findings*. London: Kings College Social Care Workforce Research Unit.

Freire, P. (1970). *Pedagogy of the oppressed*. New York, NY: Herder & Herder.

Gupta, A., & Blewett, J. (2008). Involving service users in social work training on the reality of family poverty: A case study of a collaborative project. *Social Work Education, 27*, 459–473.

Hasenfeldt, Y. (1992). *Human services as complex organizations*. London: Sage.
Heule, C., & Kristiansen, A. (2011). Språk och begrepp som stigmatiserande eller mobiliserande faktorer [Language and concepts as stigmatizing and mobilizing factors]. In V. Denvall, C. Heule, & A. Kristiansen (Eds.), *Social Mobilisering En utmaning i socialt arbete* [Social mobilization. A challenge for social work] (pp. 33–41). Gleerups: Lund.
Heule, C., & Kristiansen, A. (2013). Vem är en brukare? [Who is the user?] Kan en brukare representera andra brukare än sig själva? *Socialpolitik* nr 1/2013. Retrieved from http://www.socialpolitik.com/2013/12/01/vem-ar-brukare/
Heule, C., & Kristiansen, A. (in press). Gap mending as an additional concept in analytical reflections about service user involvement. In C. Spatscheck, S. Ashencaen Crabtree, & J. Parker (Eds.), *Methods and methodologies of social work – Relecting professional interventions*. Bremen: Whiting & Birch.
Högskoleverket. (2009). *Utvärdering av socionomutbildningen vid svenska universitet och högskolor* [Evaluation of the social work studies at Swedish Universities]. Stockholm: Högskoleverket.
Humphreys, C. (2005). Service user involvement in social work education: A case example. *Social Work Education, 24*, 797–803.
Hunter, S., & Ritchie, P. (2007). *Co-production and personalisation in social care*. London: Jessica Kingsley.
Jacks, R. (Ed.). (1995). *Empowerment in community care*. London: Chapman and Hall.
Järvinen och Mik-Meyer. (2003). *At skabe en klient* [Creating a client]. Copenhagen: Hans Reitzels Förlag.
Johansson, T. (2006). Mötets många ansikten—när professionella möter klienter [The meeting's many faces. When professionals meet clients]. In A. Meeuwisse, S. Sunesson, & H. Swärd (Eds.), *Socialt arbete* [Social work] (pp. 149–165). Stockholm: Natur och kultur.
Kristiansen, A., & Heule, C. (2016). Sweden: Power, experiences and mutual development. Using the concept of gap-mending in social work education. In E. Chiapparini (Ed.), *The service user as a partner in social work projects and education. Concepts and evaluations of courses with a gap-mending approach in Europe* (pp. 37–56). Berlin: Barbara Budrich Publishers.
Lavalette, M. (Ed.). (2011). *Radical social work today. Social work at the crossroads*. Bristol: The Policy Press.
Levin, E. (2004). *Service users and carers in social work education*. London: Social care Institute for Excellence.
Levinas, E. (1998). *Entre nous. Thinking of the other*. London: The Athlone Press Ltd.
Levine, S. K., & Levine, E. G. (1999). *Foundations of expressive arts therapy*. London: Jessica Kingsley.
McCormack, B., & McCane, T. (2010). *Person-centered nursing. Theory and practice*. Oxford: Wiley-Blackwell.
Mittal, D., Corrigan, P., Shermann, M. D., Chekuri, L., Han, X., Reaves, C., … Sullivan, G. (2014). Healthcare providers' attitudes towards persons with schizophrenia. *Psychiatric Rehabilitation Journal, 37*, 297–303.
Needham, C., & Carr, S. (2009). *Co-production: An emerging evidence base for adult social care transformation* (Research Briefing 31). London: Social Cers Institute for Excellence.
Nordt, C., Rössler, W., & Lauber, C. (2006). Attitudes of mental health professionals towards people with schizophrenia and major depression. *Scizophrenia bulletin, 32*, 709–714.
Oliver, M., & Barnes, C. (2012). *The new politics of disablement*. Basingstoke: Palgrave Macmillan.
Oliver, M., Sapey, B., & Thomas, P. (2012). *Social work with disabled people* (4th ed.). Basingstoke: Palgrave Macmillan.
Parton, N. (2000). Some thoughts on the relationship between theory and practice in and for social work. *British Journal of Social Work, 30*, 449–463.
Priestly, M. (1999). *Disability politics and community care*. London: JKP.
Robinson, K., & Webber, M. (2013). Models and effectiveness of service user and carer involvement in social work education: A literature review. *British Journal of Social Work, 43*, 925–944.
Rogowski, S. (2010). *Social work. The rise and fall of a profession*. Bristol: The policy Press.
Rønning, R. (2005). Den institusjonelle ydmykingen [Institutional humiliation]. *Nordisk Sosialt Arbeid, 2*, 111–121.

Shera, W., & Wells, L. M. (Eds.). (1999). *Empowerment practice in social work: Developing richer conceptual foundations*. Toronto: Canadian Scholars' Press.
Solomon, B. H. (1976). *Black empowerment. Social work in oppressed communities*. New York, NY: Columbia University Press.
Svensson, B., Brunt, D., Bejerhold, U., Eklund, M., Gyllensten, A. L., Leufstadius, C., … Hansson, L. (2014). Health care students' attitudes towards people with schizophrenia – A survey of eight university training programs. *Open Journal of Psychiatry, 4*, 309–316.
SWAN (Ed.). (2014). *In defence of social work: Why Michael Gove is wrong*. London: Author.
Taylor, I., & Le Riche, P. (2006). What do we know about partnership with service users and carers in social work education and how robust is the evidence base? *Health and Social Care in the Community, 14*, 418–425.
Topor, A. (2001). *Managing the contradictions: Recovery from severe mental disorders*. Stockholm: Stockholm University Press.
Trevithick, P. (2003). Effective relation-based practice: A theoretical exploration. *Journal of Social Work Practice, 17*, 163–176.
Trevithick, P. (2012). *Social work skills*. Berkshire: Open University Press.
Tronto, J. (2009). *Moral boundaries. A political argument for an ethic of care*. New York, NY: Routledge.
Wilken, J. P. (2010). *Recovering care. A contribution to a theory and practice of good care*. Amsterdam: SWP Publishers.

Social work undergraduates and service users as co-learners and researchers

Merav Moshe Grodofsky and Carolyn Gutman

ABSTRACT

The article presents an analysis of the process and content of an undergraduate social work research seminar conducted with service users in Israel. The seminar focused on human rights and the experiences of service users as they attempted to access their rights. Analysis of the seminar process revealed three classroom phases, similar to normative group stages of development. Discourse content analysis revealed two major themes. The first focused on role relationships between the students, the service users and the institutions responsible for provision of rights and entitlements. The analysis exposed power imbalances as experienced by the service users in their relationships with social work professionals and the institutions responsible for rights provisions. Moreover, students' experiences of powerlessness in their roles within those institutions were articulated. The second theme addressed the significance of the joint service user and student platform and the importance of meeting within the academic context. Students and service users expressed their sense that the seminar partnership was a meaningful experience. The analysis sheds light on the process of engaging students and service users in partnership work and on those areas that may contribute to advancing our understanding of the role of service users in social work education.

This article presents an analysis of the process and content of an undergraduate social work research seminar conducted together with service users in Israel. Eight students and three service users participated in the seminar. Students chose the seminar from among eight research seminars in the undergraduate programme. Service users were recruited through a local rights-based community practice centre and through organizations for the physically disabled and mental health service users. Service users were interviewed prior to the commencement of the seminar. Of the total number of service users interviewed, three chose to participate.

The seminar focused on human rights and the experiences of service users as they attempted to access their rights. The seminar addressed two issues of interest to the social work profession; service users and research and service users and professional education.

Service users and research

Social work professionals are directed to use research to inform their practice. They are also directed to contribute to its production (Krysik & Finn, 2013). Furthermore, they are expected to analyse and evaluate the quality and outcomes of their practice together with people who use social work services (BASW, 2014).

Despite the call to involve service users in research (Beresford, 2002), until fairly recently, the greater part of health and social care research was conducted within a positivist tradition. Service user involvement in research was primarily passive and user voices were largely absent from the research discourse.

With the development and presence of both top-down and bottom-up models of user involvement in civil society (Beresford & Croft, 2008), an increasingly complex array of research methods such as service user research, emancipatory research, participatory action research (PAR) and user-led research have emerged (Beresford, 2002; Ramon, 2003) leading to recognition of the user's role in the development of research agendas.

Growing evidence suggests that collaboration with service users in health and social care research may result in richer and more relevant methodologies and findings (Maglajlic, 2010). Their active involvement in the research is seen as a powerful tool to 'improve the relevance, quality, and impact, and thus the social value, of the research' (Delman & Lincoln, 2009, p. 140).

Favourable findings have emerged with different groups of service user researchers in different countries; for example, older people (Gutman et al., 2014; Munn-Giddings, McVicar, Boyce, & O'Brien, 2009), mental health service users (Gillard, Turner, & Neffgen, 2015; Hutchinson & Lovell, 2012), young carers (McLaughlin, 2006) and people with learning disabilities (Nind & Vinha, 2014). These are positive developments, yet dilemmas remain, particularly 'power imbalances and interpersonal dynamics between the "researcher" and the "researched"' (Ray, 2007, p. 80) and the additional expense and time required to conduct the study (Delman & Lincoln, 2009).

PAR is recognized as a relevant methodology to ensure service user collaboration (Maglajlic, 2010). It builds on principles of inclusion and reciprocity and values the lived experience of the individuals and communities who participate in the research. It is consistent with service user participation in professional education (Barnes, Taylor, & Ward, 2013; Beresford, 2002; Maglajlic, 2010). It 'refers to research in which the subjects participate, are involved, and have their knowledge given validity and voice' (Krumer-Nevo & Barak, 2006, p. 776).

PAR is based upon a number of critical principles; it begins with a problem that is identified by the study participants; study participants act as co-researchers; it is goal-oriented in the sense that the research is conducted in order to advance change vis-à-vis the identified problem (Hacker, 2013; Maglajlic, 2010).

This type of research can engage service users at different stages of the process including initiation of the research, defining the research question, accumulating and analysing data and advancing social change action resulting from the research (Krumer-Nevo & Barak, 2006; Schahar & Shemer, 2012). The process promotes principles of dialogical praxis; those engaged have opportunities to influence and to be influenced. This is consistent with a service user participation approach focused on transfer of power from those who traditionally hold it to those traditionally excluded from it (Biskin, Barcroft, Livingston, & Snape, 2013).

Moreover, PAR is a method that involves a 'systematic group process of assessment, learning, and a spiral movement towards transformation' (Schahar & Shemer, 2012, p. 559) as it relates both to the individual and the broader context of social change (Krumer-Nevo & Barak, 2006).

Service users and social work education

In the UK, service user and carer involvement has been a formal requirement for social work programmes since 2003, conducted through various means including participation in the admissions process, in teaching modules and in student evaluations (Waterson & Morris, 2005). The most commonly reported aspect of user and carer involvement is in teaching (Robinson & Webber, 2013).

There are increasing reports from other countries on the involvement of users as participants in social work classes (Biskin et al., 2013; Kjellberg & French, 2011; Scheyett & Diehl, 2004; Shor & Sykes, 2002). In Sweden, older adults collaborated with younger students in a social policy course (Kjellberg & French, 2011). In Israel and the US, mental health service users participated intermittently in structured classroom dialogues (Scheyett & Diehl, 2004; Shor & Sykes, 2002).

Service user involvement in social work education in Israel is in its very early stages, largely limited to guest speakers in single classroom sessions but also involving service users as co-teachers in professional and in occupational therapy programmes (Gutman, Kraiem, Criden, & Yalon-Chamovitz, 2012). Service user involvement in social work education is not a recognized requirement by The Israel Council for Higher Education and therefore is not funded.

There is a growing body of literature that suggests that user involvement in social work education may impact positively on student learning and practice (Higgins, Maguire, Watts, Rani, & Alexander, 2011; Morgan & Jones, 2009). Evidence compiled by Higgins et al. (2011) from the fields of social work, psychology and nursing, states that user participation impacts on 'students' communication, partnership and advocacy skills, challenging professional orthodoxies and power, and enabling practitioners to be more conscious and reflective of the implications of treatments and approaches used' (p. 520).

Morgan and Jones (2009), studied user involvement strategies in healthcare education reporting that 'students found the experience of user involvement rewarding and felt that it had a positive impact… and it enhanced their understanding and promoted learning about the user's perspective'. They note that 'students agreed with user-centred values… and reported a desire to change services' (p. 11).

Current literature supports both user involvement in research as well as user involvement in education for the helping professions. However, there is limited work that addresses user involvement as co-researchers in research modules in undergraduate social work education. Existing studies focus on user involvement in research that evaluates their involvement in practice courses (Gutman et al., 2012) or in the overall social work programme (Biskin et al., 2013).

In parallel, there is a body of research that reports on social work undergraduates' lack of enthusiasm for research throughout their training (Bell & Clancy, 2013; Blakemore & Howard, 2015; Langer, Lietz, & Furman, 2007; Secret, Ford, & Lewis Rompf, 2003). However, in courses where students undertake research projects that integrate research and practice, they report on more positive attitudes as well as an appreciation of the research (Blakemore & Howard, 2015; Hostetter, Williamson Sullenberger, & Wood, 2013; Morgenshtern, Freymond, Agyapong, & Greeson, 2011).

The desire to encourage positive and confident attitudes towards research knowledge and skills among the students, together with the recognition of the value of service user involvement in research and in social work education, led to the development of a joint service user and undergraduate social work student PAR pedagogy in the field of human rights. Following McNicoll (1999), the authors believed that this type of PAR course '... would provide social work students with needed training in non-oppressive and social change-oriented research strategies, which are consistent with the pursuit of emancipation and equity' (p.51).

Method

Research objective and context

The research was conducted in Israel with students and service users in an undergraduate social work research seminar during the 2014–2015 academic year. Students and users partnered in learning about social rights and access to rights, particularly as they related to the Israel National Insurance Institute (NII). The objectives of the research were twofold:

(1) To explore the process between students and users as they developed and implemented a joint research project.
(2) To identify key themes that arose in the seminar discourse.

Participants and procedure

Eight senior social work students in their final year of study and three service users participated in the course. As noted, users were recruited through local organizations for the physically disabled and mental health service users and through the rights-based community practice centre. Service users ranged in age from 45 to 65 and had a variety of physical and/or mental health disabilities. Both female and male users participated in the course. They were not paid for their participation.

The research protocol was approved by the ethics committee of the academic institution. Prior to course commencement, users met individually with the first author to discuss course aims, methods and motivations. Of the total number of service users interviewed, three expressed consent to participate. In parallel, social work students whose ages ranged between 23 and 27 chose the seminar from among eight offered in the undergraduate programme.

Participants signed informed consent forms, and agreed to the transcription of the seminar sessions. Participants were informed that transcriptions would be incorporated into scholarly articles and presented at professional conferences. They were notified that identities would not be revealed to ensure anonymity.

Fourteen sessions were transcribed by the research assistant and analysed to understand the process and learning content of the research seminar.

Content analysis

Content analysis of the transcribed narratives was conducted by the researchers and the research assistant in three stages. Initially, the research assistant and the researchers read the entire text to identify predominant processes and voices. In the second stage the researchers and research assistant individually identified meaningful content units. In the third stage the researchers met and identified the main themes reflected in the text (Patton, 2002; Unrau & Coleman, 1997). Based upon the analysis the authors determined how to present the study findings.

Content analysis pinpointed two foci. The first focused on the learning process enabling the researchers to identify the flow of the seminar. Three distinct learning phases were identified.

The second aspect of the analysis revealed themes of the seminar discourse enabling the authors to pinpoint key issues in student–service user research partnership.

Findings

The learning process

The classroom process entailed three different stages: the initial stage, the working stage and the final stage of the course.

Initial stage

The first goal in the initial stage was to create a learning environment based on partnership and symmetry between students and users within a safe space for group process and communication. This setting was unique because typically service providers and service users meet in the context of hierarchical relationships. In the seminar the objective was to work together to create a joint research initiative.

Part of furthering the dialogical process within the classroom entailed exploration of the right of users to determine how they would be named. In traditional social service settings users are referred to as 'clients', 'consumers' and 'patients'. Class discussion led to the service users' decisions to choose the names 'service users', 'copers' and 'social change agents'.

The second goal of this stage was to discuss the research framework. Participants were introduced to major concepts and components of human rights and PAR. Service users and students learned that the goal of the research was to promote social change. They were excited about the possibility that their research would lead to change. By the end of this stage, the group created a working environment essential to the research process.

The working stage

The goals of the working stage were also twofold. The first was to develop the research question and methodology which focused on service user experience as they attempted to access rights and entitlements. The second goal was to use the classroom context and relationships between users and students to process the experiences of the participants in relation to rights and entitlements.

Processing personal experiences promoted movement from a sense of chaos and uncertainty to the crystallization of the research question. As the participants shared their experiences the instructor assisted in framing them into potential research questions.

In essence, two group processes evolved simultaneously: participants engaged in discussion about service user and professional experiences as they relate to rights and entitlements and participants began to see the potential for the development of research questions that reflected their experiences. Research questions were defined and circulated among participants for review. In the subsequent session, the research question was finalized.

During this stage students and service users identified relevant literature. For example one user shared material including websites that addressed user rights. Students borrowed materials and asked to exchange phone numbers for further contact. The group decided to create a common email list to share materials. Excitement about group development undermined ethical considerations that in retrospect should and could have been discussed regarding exchange of personal contact details.

The methodology to examine the research question was defined during the working stage. Sessions were devoted to creating the interview protocol and testing it through simulations. Together participants decided that students would be responsible for the research interviews. Thirty-two service users, other than those in the course, were interviewed about their experiences as they attempted to access rights through the NII.

Final stage

The seminar's final stage had three foci. The first was to analyse results of the 32 interviews that comprised the sample. The second was to determine how the findings could be transformed into a plan for action that would benefit service users as they attempted to access rights through the NII. Finally, the third focus was to evaluate the course and student–user partnership.

Data analysis carried out jointly by students and users revealed user experiences as they attempted to access rights through the NII. Results of the analysis of the 32 interviews will be reported in a future paper. Based upon the analysis, course participants prepared and implemented a meeting with the local NII director and staff. Students and users introduced the seminar content and goals, the research methodology and findings. They conducted simulations with the NII director and staff to illustrate the experiences of services users as identified through their research. A proposal for the development of joint future research and intervention with the NII were discussed.

Finally, this last and final stage of the course was used to evaluate the course concept and pedagogy, research outcomes and the student–user partnership.

The classroom discourse content

Analysis of the discourse content revealed two themes. The first theme focused on role relationships between students, service users and the institutions responsible for the provision of rights and entitlements ('Us and Them'). The second theme addressed the significance of joint user and student partnership and the importance of meeting within the academic context.

The relationship between 'us' and between 'us' and government institutions

The classroom setting and processes provided opportunities to experience roles of both service provider and service user. Early on in the course, users and students were invited to address their experiences with the social service system. The course instructor noted that while users spoke about themselves, students adopted the role of active listeners and initiating questions.

The instructor asked the participants why users told their stories, while students refrained from telling theirs. She reiterated the goal of the course which was to have students and users work together on human rights focused research and not to assume traditional roles as implemented in social service agencies. This led one user to criticize social workers. A. said,

> I feel like you have information about my rights and how I can access them and that you hide this from me in your notebooks. That information is critical in order to enable me to access my rights. However you are not willing to share it with me.

The instructor asked the user and the students to reflect on what they sensed during this interaction. Focused on the 'here and now' they spoke about discomfort, a power imbalance and lack of transparency.

Later on in the academic year class participants were invited to reverse traditional roles. Students adopted service user roles and users became service providers. In the discussion that followed, service users, in their role as service providers, reflected on their frustration in hearing painful stories. They addressed the gap between what they *felt* should be done to assist service users to access their rights and the limitations of the service provider mandate.

> I was in the role of the service provider. It was odd for me to be in this role. I was more comfortable in the role of the service user. In the beginning I was asked many questions . . . I felt very strong . . . when I have power I feel badly for more vulnerable people. I presented myself as a rehabilitation social worker. This is a difficult role because not everyone receives his rights and entitlements . . . there are criteria. (S., service user)

> I thought that I was strong . . . king of all the universe that I could control . . . but in fact you cannot . . . (A., service user)

> It doesn't matter how nice or wonderful the social worker or the service provider is . . . in the end if the person doesn't receive what he needs he won't be satisfied . . . his experience will not be satisfactory. (L., service user)

Discussing their position as service users within the role-play, students reflected on their concern as to how they would behave once they completed their studies and became social service agency employees. The role-play enabled them to share concerns that they too would become part of the power hierarchy of the social service structure oftentimes preventing rather than assisting service users to access rights.

> It was difficult for me to see the other side and to put myself into her shoes and to understand what she experiences. (E., student)

> It reminds me of the first time that social work students sit on the chair . . . you have a lot of power. It didn't feel to me that S. was being vicious . . . rather you were displaying the difficulty that you have within your institution that doesn't allow you to give . . . (H., student)

> You said something amazing about the therapist chair . . . there is something overly powerful in what we do . . . There are people that have to sit across from you and not by choice . . . (Y., student)

> I understand the importance of the research and all . . . it just seems to me that we are once again putting out fires and not really making change . . . (Z.; student)

> I think that as social workers we experience obstacles … there are policies that restrict me and if I am not successful in helping my client-in the end he'll criticize me … we're always subject to this kind of criticism. (I., student)

> We can't always help to access rights … but we can try to make the process more pleasant. (A., student)

Analyses of classroom discourse shed light not only on the nature of power relationships between future professionals and users, but also on their relationships with government institutions responsible for social rights and entitlements.

> If we believe that the change will come from within us … we're wasting our time …

> I think that things have to change from the bottom up but we have to figure out the system. The service users have to hear that we are very small, insignificant people and no one takes us into account …. We are second rate people in this country. I'll be the first to take to the streets with the service users. (H., student)

> At the top of the pyramid sits someone with a lot of money and status and he determines our future. (A. student)

> There is a definite division between what is possible to change and the approach and desire of those who sit in the chair to help … (I., student)

> It's true … there is something in the public service that is falling apart … there's no trust and they cannot stand social workers. (T., student)

One student remarked that perhaps the inclusion of service users in the research had in fact impacted negatively on the study.

> What you share with us influences us and what is said here is difficult for me and it is important that you know that … It is hard for me to think that soon I will step out into the work market knowing that there are social workers in the NII who might act bureaucratically. In fact maybe the fact that you are here actually hurt the research because we didn't come in with a clean slate. (A., student)

A. attempted to convey her sense that service user participation in the course biased the researchers and the research itself. User participations had oftentimes led to 'siding' with them against the NII and social services. For some students this created a sense of discomfort. After all, they would join these systems upon graduation.

A.'s comment pinpointed acritical issues in user–student partnership; that is the move away from hierarchic to more symmetric relationships. As relationships become more symmetrical students are challenged to critically reflect on traditional power relationships that they abide by.

The significance of the relationship between service users and students and the importance of meeting within the academic context

A second theme that resonated from classroom discussion analysis was the significance of the platform to meet together within the academic setting. For all participants the joint work was meaningful.

> I am happy to be here together with you. This course helps me to feel that I have power. (S., service user)

> There is a very different atmosphere here than in other places. We're glad to be here. My excitement grows from the moment that I reach the college gate... (L., service user)

> This has been the best year of my life... I will never be able to thank you enough for believing in me and assisting me to continue to work for my rights. (L., service user)

> Throughout the year you (the students) may have thought that you weren't really helping- but I see how we have changed and more importantly how the approach of the NII can change. I know because I have known them for over twenty years. This time they were listening. (A., service user)

> The research seminar, together with the service users enabled me to experience how the power relationships between the social worker, the course instructor and the service user were broken down. That means that we were able to converse based upon principles of equality. Service users were not afraid to share their experience as they attempt to access their rights and they were able to speak critically about their experiences. At first I felt like I had to defend and justify myself but throughout the year I learned to put my pride aside and to listen, to really listen... The course enabled me to turn theory and the idea of rights into a rights-based practice approach. (H., student)

Analysis

The pedagogy that emerged from student–service user partnership and the themes that dominated the course discourse suggest a step forward in service user involvement in social work education and research, and a step forward in research pedagogy. The pedagogy enabled participants to transform their knowledge and experiences into research that encouraged intervention; in this case in the NII. A number of key foci contributed to these developments.

First, power hierarchies were addressed throughout the course. Power hierarchies are a major component of traditional social work practice (Gutman et al., 2012; French & Swain, 2001) and were apparent early on in the classroom. They were deconstructed (Molyneux & Irvine, 2004) through dialogical praxis and alternative forms of interaction developed between the authors, students and service users. This enabled participants to identify and try out new ways of interacting in manners that were more symmetrical and less hierarchical. This experience was different from bureaucratic hierarchies that users encounter, and social workers conform to and that serve as barriers to benefits (Lipsky, 2010; Peleg, 2013).

Second, classroom partnership involved critical reflection upon participants' lived experiences. This was evidenced during interview simulations and through reverse role plays that emphasized lived experiences of both groups within rights and entitlement transactions. Empathy was reinforced between participants through recognition of common experiences of frustration and bureaucratic disentitlement in the quest to access services in daily interactions.

The ambiguous nature of 'partnership work' is discussed in the literature (e.g. Barr, Freeth, Hammick, Koppel, & Reeves, 2000). Sometimes partnership is seen as nothing more than rhetoric or an end in itself. We therefore need to identify those components that demonstrate genuine collaboration. Despite advancements noted, certain issues as they pertained to partnership were not sufficiently addressed or alternatively, did not alter power imbalances among participants. While service users were active in the seminar, they did not fully take part in all aspects of the research, and as such were not fully equal partners. For example, they did not interview service users or write research papers.

Classroom time was spent debating these issues. The decision to restrain from participating in the interviews was made by service users. Their decision was based upon two considerations; first, concern that their involvement might influence the ability of the interviewees to speak honestly about their experience with the NII. Second, concern that if the NII staff were to identify them with the research that this might negatively impact on future decisions regarding their entitlements. Certainly, these issues could have been constructively challenged in the spirit of co-learning.

One might argue that concerns about partnership and power balances were addressed in joint discussions among seminar participants. In fact, participatory action methodology allows for flexibility as it relates to issues of participation. However, by not tackling these concerns the seminar may in parallel have neglected an opportunity to attend to the power imbalance between the NII and service users.

In retrospect, not enough attention was paid to questions regarding user participation in writing the research reports. Early on services users stated that they did not want to write reports. The desire to respect their wishes, together with time constraints and methodological considerations led to acceptance of user statements on this matter as opposed to advancing a process to cope with the complexities that writing entails.

Students received course credit for participation. Service users did not receive compensation for participation, and in fact questions of payment were never raised. Service users participated in the course as an opportunity to advance their rights and to promote the education of future social work professionals who would be more aware of the rights and needs of service users.

One could argue that the satisfaction that users expressed at the end of the academic year in regard to the impact of their work on the NII staff and the development of the students as future professionals was a form of reward for their labour. In the authors' opinion this is not sufficient.

One final issue that emerged revolved around different knowledge bases that drove the course work. Questions arose regarding the value of service users' experiential knowledge and how this knowledge could be better integrated into social work's knowledge base. Trevithick's (2008) discussion on the topic draws attention to the notion that a key area of professional knowledge may be drawn from users who, through their need to make sense of their lives, attempt to explain what is happening and why. In other words, these efforts at explanation may, in the academic arena, be viewed as attempts to theorize about their situation. This knowledge is more than experiential knowledge as it attempts to bring experience into some kind of coherent understanding. This coherence provides an invaluable contribution to the variety of knowledge-based sources available to the social work professional. In the current setting, this need to 'make sense of reality' was useful in enabling students to gain particular understanding of processes of disentitlement.

Furthermore, as Trevithick (2008) notes, users may often have direct, personal and current knowledge in areas such as legislation, social and agency policies, as well as benefits and limitations. This knowledge is oftentimes relevant to others who experience personal and social disentitlements and rights-related abuses. This knowledge can be an invaluable resource. For the students in the course, it expanded their knowledge base as it related to the service users and human rights.

Conclusion

The article presents a unique research training pedagogy. Its uniqueness is expressed through the combination of two approaches, each of whose necessity has been recognized in earlier literature, yet which have not been fully tested and analysed as a joint educational approach; they are, involvement of service users in undergraduate social work research and student–user participation in the implementation of a PAR methodology in the undergraduate curriculum.

The experience of the students and service users who participated in the research seminar suggests that this pedagogy is useful in training undergraduate social work students in research. Nonetheless, a number of suggestions for future initiatives of this kind are in line.

First, it is important that service users receive some form of payment for their participation. One option is certainly monetary payment. We suggest specific service user training in PAR methods and writing in order to enhance their skills and confidence in these areas. While this is a time-consuming undertaking, it is an important contribution to service users and can contribute to the advancement of future collaboration.

The seminar's multi-focus on research, service user–student partnership and human rights made it jam-packed. Future efforts need to consider the balance between the different foci of the course content to ensure that each receives appropriate attention. The course necessitates attention to both learning content and process. Here too, it is important to balance between the two. Finally, we suggest additional research to follow this emerging research pedagogy.

Disclosure statement

No potential conflict of interest was reported by the authors.

Acknowledgments

We would like to thank our students and service users for their insights and wisdom. We also thank the manuscript assessors for their extremely helpful feedback.

References

Barnes, M., Taylor, D., & Ward, L. (2013). Being well enough in old age. *Critical Social Policy, 33*, 473–493.

Barr, H., Freeth, D., Hammick, M., Koppel, I., & Reeves, S. (2000). *Evaluations of interprofessional education: A United Kingdom review for health and social care.* London: CAIPE/British Educational Research Association.

BASW. (2014). *The code of ethics for social workers: Statement of principles.* Retrieved from http://cdn.basw.co.uk/upload/basw_95243-9.pdf

Bell, L., & Clancy, C. (2013). Postgraduate students learning about research: Exploring the attitudes of social work and mental health students in an English university setting. *Social Work & Social Sciences Review, 16*, 37–50.

Beresford, P. (2002). User involvement in research and evaluation: Liberation or regulation? *Social Policy and Society, 1*, 95–106.

Beresford, P., & Croft, S. (2008). Democratising social work – A key element of innovation: From "client" as object, to service user as producer. *The Innovation Journal: The Public Sector Innovation Journal, 13*, 1–22.

Biskin, S., Barcroft, V., Livingston, W., & Snape, S. (2013). Reflections on student, service user and carer involvement in social work research. *Social Work Education, 32*, 301–316.

Blakemore, T., & Howard, A. (2015). Engaging undergraduate social work students in research through experience-based learning. *Social Work Education, 34*, 861–880.

Delman, J., & Lincoln, A. (2009). Service users as paid research workers: Principles for active involvement and good practice guidance. In J. Wallcraft, B. Schrank, & M. Amering (Eds.), *Handbook of service user involvement in mental health research* (pp. 139–151). Oxford: Wiley.

French, S., & Swain, J. (2001). The relationship between disabled people and health and welfare professionals. In G. Albrecht, K. Seelman, & M. Bury (Eds.), *The handbook of disability studies* (pp. 735–738). Thousand Oaks, CA: Sage.

Gillard, S., Turner, K., & Neffgen, M. (2015). How does who we are shape the knowledge we produce?: Doing collaborative research about personality disorders. In P. Staddon (Ed.), *Mental health service users in research: Critical sociological perspectives* (pp. 53–68). Bristol: Policy Press.

Gutman, C., Hantman, S., Criden, W., Ben-Oz, M., Anghel, R., & Ramon, S. (2014). Involving service users in social work education: Developing a bi-national participatory action research framework. *Educational Gerontology, 40*, 186–197.

Gutman, C., Kraiem, Y., Criden, W., & Yalon-Chamovitz, S. (2012). Deconstructing hierarchies: A pedagogical model with service user co-teachers. *Social Work Education, 31*, 202–214.

Hacker, K. (2013). *Community-based participatory action research*. Los Angeles, CA: Sage.

Higgins, A., Maguire, G., Watts, M., Rani, S., & Alexander, J. (2011). Service user involvement in mental health practitioner education in Ireland. *Journal of Psychiatric and Mental Health Nursing, 18*, 519–525.

Hostetter, C., Williamson Sullenberger, S., & Wood, L. (2013). The key to learning: Engaging undergraduate students in authentic social work research. *The Journal of Baccalaureate Social Work, 18* (Special issue), 47–62.

Hutchinson, A., & Lovell, A. (2012). Participatory action research: Moving beyond the mental health 'service user' identity. *Journal of Psychiatric and Mental Health Nursing, 20*, 641–649.

Kjellberg, G., & French, R. (2011). A new pedagogical approach for integrating social work students and service users. *Social Work Education, 30*, 948–963.

Krumer-Nevo, M., & Barak, A. (2006). Service users' perspectives on the benefits system in Israel: A participatory action research. *Social Policy & Administration, 40*, 774–790.

Krysik, J., & Finn, J. (2013). *Research for effective social work practice*. New York, NY: Routledge.

Langer, C. L., Lietz, C. A., & Furman, R. (2007). A model for teaching qualitative research methods to undergraduate social work students. *The Journal of Baccalaureate Social Work, 12*, 70–82.

Lipsky, M. (2010). *Street level bureaucracy: Dilemmas of the individual in public services*. New York, NY: Russell Sage.

Maglajlic, R. A. (2010). "Big organisations" supporting "small involvement": Lessons from Bosnia and Herzegovina on enabling community-based participation of children through PAR. *American Journal of Community Psychology, 46*, 204–214.

McLaughlin, H. (2006). Involving young service users as co-researchers: Possibilities, benefits and costs. *British Journal of Social Work, 36*, 1395–1410.

McNicoll, P. (1999). Issues in teaching participatory action research. *Journal of Social Work Education, 35*, 51–62.

Molyneux, J., & Irvine, J. (2004). Service user and carer involvement in social work training: A long and winding road? *Social Work Education, 23*, 293–308.

Morgan, A., & Jones, D. (2009). Perceptions of service user and carer involvement in healthcare education and impact on students' knowledge and practice: A literature review. *Medical Teacher, 31*, 82–95.

Morgenshtern, M., Freymond, N., Agyapong, S., & Greeson, C. (2011). Graduate social work students' attitudes toward research: Problems and prospects. *Journal of Teaching in Social Work, 31*, 552–568.

Munn-Giddings, C., McVicar, A., Boyce, M., & O'Brien, N. (2009). Older people as researchers – Why not? An overview of a partnership project to train older people to be researchers. *Working with Older People, 13*, 16–19.

Nind, M., & Vinha, H. (2014). Doing research inclusively: Bridges to multiple possibilities in inclusive research. *British Journal of Learning Disabilities, 42*, 102–109.

Patton, M. Q. (2002). *Qualitative research and evaluation methods*. Thousand Oaks, CA: Sage.

Peleg, E. (2013). *The poverty challenge of administrative law*. Tel Aviv: Resling (in Hebrew).

Ramon, S. (Ed.). (2003). *Users researching health and social care: An empowering agenda?* Birmingham, AL: Venture Press.

Ray, M. 2007. Redressing the balance? The participation of older people in research. In M. Bernard and Scharf, T. (Eds.), *Critical perspectives on ageing societies* (pp. 73–87). Bristol: The Polity Press.

Robinson, K., & Webber, M. (2013). Models and effectiveness of service user and carer involvement in social work education: A literature review. *British Journal of Social Work, 43*, 925–944.

Schahar, E., & Shemer, O. (2012). We'll learn with the community: A narrative approach and learning in partnership through dialogue in community work, *Society and Welfare, 4*, 553–577 (in hebrew).

Scheyett, A., & Diehl, M. J. (2004). Walking our talk in social work education: Partnering with consumers of mental health services. *Social Work Education, 23*, 435–450.

Secret, M., Ford, J., & Lewis Rompf, E. (2003). Undergraduate research courses. *Journal of Social Work Education, 39*, 411–422.

Shor, R., & Sykes, I. (2002). Introducing structured dialogue with people with mental illness into the training of social work students. *Psychiatric Rehabilitation Journal, 26*, 63–69.

Trevithick, P. (2008). Revisiting the knowledge base of social work: A framework for practice. *British Journal of Social Work, 38*, 1212–1237.

Unrau, Y., & Coleman, H. (1997). Qualitative data analysis. In M. Grinnell (Ed.), *Social work research and evaluation: Quantitative and qualitative approaches* (pp. 512–514). Itasca, IL: Peacock.

Waterson, J., & Morris, K. (2005). Training in "social" work: Exploring issues of involving users in teaching on social work degree programmes. *Social Work Education, 24*, 653–675.

A critical examination of the knowledge contribution service user and carer involvement brings to social work education

Kieron Hatton

ABSTRACT

Service user/carer involvement in social work education is supported by the Health Care Professions Council and currently, by the Department of Health. It is generally seen as beneficial but the reasons why this may be the case are often under-theorised and seen as un-problematic. This article seeks to provide a theoretical justification for an approach which values involvement as central to educational practice. It begins by looking at models of participation and how they can help us understand processes of involvement. It suggests that to move beyond tokenistic approaches we need to develop an approach which is based on equality and partnership. Drawing on European approaches to social pedagogy, particularly those utilising 'the Common Third', and debates around creativity and social power the article articulates an approach based on the co-production of curricula and assessment artefacts. This, the paper suggests, tests the students ability to empathise and communicate with people using services and utilises the latters' personal expertise to bring the curricula alive. The article outlines a theory of creativity, inclusion and power which the author believes validates the approach developed and which provides a model for evaluating the real level of recognition given to the service user/carer voice within the educational process, particularly in social work education. It is suggested that such an approach is consistent with the social work professions' commitment to the promotion of social justice and social change.

Introduction

From somewhat limited beginnings service user/carer involvement has become central to the accreditation and validation of social work programmes (Hatton, 2015). The introduction of degree and Masters level qualifications in 2003 and the support of service user/carer involvement by grant monies from the Department of Health (admittedly at a relatively low level of £7500 per annum) has been maintained so far following the demise of the General Social Care Council and its replacement by the new Health Care Professions Council (HCPC) regime in 2013. However, the extent and depth of service user/carer involvement varies widely across the country and in many, but not all, cases focuses on the involvement of service users/carers in the more traditional elements of the programme – admissions interviews, guest teaching, as an expert speaker. This paper suggest that if we are to make service user/carer involvement meaningful we need to develop a more holistic and complex way of understanding how service users/carers can contribute to social work education. This will involve seeing this involvement not as a way of legitimising our commitment to inclusion but seeing service users/carers as co-producers and partners in the educational experience. To achieve this the paper argues we need a more developed analysis of power, agency, imagination and creativity. The paper uses the phrase service users/carers for clarity although it fully recognises that (a) service users/carers are not a homogenous grouping and (b) that the very words are themselves contentious (McLaughlin, 2009). The author also recognises that service users/carers have multiple identities beyond their status as service users/carers. For example, looked after children, parents, carers themselves, advocates, stakeholders (particularly in Third Sector organisations) service deliverers, etc. and that many of these roles intersect (Goodley, 2011) and cause contradictions/conflicts. This is the content of a companion piece and will be dealt with in a separate article.

The development of service user involvement

Over the last 10–15 years, service users/carers have at last been recognised as having a significant role in the delivery, management and development of welfare services. This is reflected in the attention given to service user involvement in both the legislative and policy contexts. These debates cut across all service boundaries and raise questions about service user representation (Payne, 2014; Stepney & Popple, 2008; Warren, 2007), the efficacy of current initiatives (Social Care Institute for Excellence [SCIE], 2004) and the usefulness of the service user perspective across a range of service user areas: young people (Children's Rights Alliance & National Youth Council of Ireland's, 2002; Hayden, Goddard, Gorin, & Van Der Spek, 1999); people in poverty (Bennett & Roberts, 2004; Beresford & Hoban, 2005); evaluating community outcomes (Jakes and Cassidy, n.d.); homeless people (FEANTSA, 2009); and with traditional service user groups such as people with mental distress, people with disabilities and older people.

The drivers behind these initiatives have often been service users themselves. The role of disability activists in creating the political climate to support anti-discriminatory legislation around disability is well known (Shakespeare, 2013), as was their role in ensuring that the Disability Discrimination Act 1995 was amended to give disabled people the right to enforcement action if their entitlements were not met. Equally, the voice of the service user can be seen in the *Valuing People* White Paper (Department of Health, 2001; 2009) and subsequent policy developments which grew out of that, including *Valuing People Now* (HM Government, 2009). The White Paper enshrined the concepts of rights, independence, choice, inclusion, and argued that:

> people with learning disabilities have little control over their lives … .The Government's objective is to enable people with learning disabilities to have as much choice and control as possible over their lives and the services and support they receive. (Department of Health, 2001, p. 4)

Recently the development of services incorporating personalisation and co-production have provided an important motor for this enhanced move towards empowering people in the adult social care sector. The seven core principles for self-care promoted by Skills for Care and Skills for Health in 2009 suggested that services should ensure that people are able to make informed choices, communicate their needs effectively, develop skills in self-care, be supported to access other networks and 'support and enable risk management and risk taking to maximize independence and choice' (Department of Health, 2010, p. 44). This is supported further by Local Authority Circular/Department of Health which says that personalisation is about 'every person across the spectrum of need, having choice and control over the shape of his or her support, in the most appropriate setting' (2008, p. 2).

Such an approach was further developed in the proposals around co-production which placed the emphasis on users and user-led organisations. Ramsden (2010) cites the Personal Communications Toolkit, which describes co-production as occurring when:

> [y]ou as an individual influence the support and services you receive, or when groups of people get together to influence the way that services are *designed, commissioned and delivered*. (Ramsden, 2010; emphasis added)

The SCIE (2013) has produced a guide to co-production which, suggests that it is possible to identify some key features that are present. Co-production they suggest:

- define(s) people who use services as assets with skills and breaks(s) down the barriers between people who use services and professionals;
- build(s) on people's existing capabilities and include(s)reciprocity (where people get something back for having done something for others) and mutuality (people working together to achieve their shared interests); and
- (enables people to) work with peer and personal support networks alongside professional networks while facilitating services by helping organisations to become part agents for change rather than just being service providers (SCIE, 2013, p. 7).

One of the organisations consulted on the development of the guide *Think Local Act Personal* is quoted as saying:

> Co-production is not just a word, it's not just a concept, it is a meeting of minds coming together to find a shared solution. In practice, it involves people who use services coming together to find a shared solution. In practice it involves people who use services being consulted, included and working together from the start to the end of any project that affects them. (Ramsden, 2010, p. 7)

Three features of personalisation – design, commission and delivery – are critical to our ability to distinguish whether involvement has any meaning. Equally the key elements of co-production involve promoting people's strengths, reciprocity and mutuality, and the idea of people as change agents. All of these ideas resonate with the key debates with which we will need to engage if we are to take forward discussions around service user/carer involvement. Ideas of co-production, in particular, link closely to the concerns within this paper about how we develop 'meaningful' ways of securing the involvement of service user/carers in the delivery of social work education.

Service user/carer involvement in social work education

There has been a developing literature around the involvement of service users/carers in higher education. Lathlean et al. (2006) have looked at the challenges health care education faces involving service users and suggest that previous poor experience of participation by service user participants led to feelings of tokenism which, 'devalues user initiatives and reinforces "institutional userism" which leads to exclusion and disempowerment' (2006, p. 736). They suggest that there needs to be a commitment to service and organisational change to counteract these tendencies. Townend, Tew, Grant, and Repper (2008) argue that the training of psychological therapists could be enhanced through, 'greater engagement from people who have experience of using psychological therapy services' (2008, p. 75). They suggest that this could occur at a number of levels including interviewing for programmes, assessment, direct delivery commissioning and planning and by promoting alternative models of distress, risk and recovery. However they warn that such interventions are not always experienced positively and warn that, 'confrontation, lack of support and not being valued can lead to emotional distress' (p. 71). It is with these issues in mind that we advocate in this paper supportive, co-produced and creative approaches to involvement.

Over 10 years ago SCIE (2004b) suggested that service users should be involved at a strategic and management level with universities social work programmes. This may include involvement at programme management and partnership levels (although this is an area of collaboration and partnership which remains underdeveloped at present). It is more likely to focus on, selecting students; teaching and learning provision; placement learning opportunities – the opportunity to work with and within service user-controlled organisations assessment of students; quality assurance. SCIE noted the connection between values underpinning service user organisations and social work. They argued:

> The service user movement emphasises the importance of models of participation that are based on human rights, equalities, inclusion and the social model of disability. Their approaches seek to empower people and counter oppressive and discriminatory practice. There is overlap between the values of service user-controlled organisations and those of social work and social care. (SCIE, 2004b, p. 11)

Beresford argued that to achieve such a level of involvement entails a focus on values – treating service users with honesty, openness, respect, equality and of course commitment, and strategy, which will involve 'a fundamental culture change. We will all need to do things differently and changes in practice – supporting service user training, developing user-controlled organisations, addressing diversity, research, evaluation and payment' (SCIE, 2004b, pp. 13, 14).

Involvement across the curricula

Wilson and Beresford (2000) have warned against a simplistic attempt to suggest that a commitment to anti-oppressive values of itself ensures that service users' views are heard and respected. Instead they argued that:

> [s]uch a theory [of anti-oppressive practice] is by definition reliant upon user knowledge and ideas. Social work's adoption of a façade of "anti-oppressive practice" which in reality appropriates and incorporates the knowledge and experiences of service users, whilst retaining the power to determine just what it is that counts as 'anti-oppressive' is for us the most oppressive aspect of its anti-oppressive stance. (2000, p. 565)

They concluded that anti-oppressive practice needed to be re-evaluated to ensure that it properly reflects service users' views and aspirations. One way of ensuring this in the academic environment is, they suggest, to recognise that service user involvement should be across the curriculum and not just in those areas where the service users are deemed to be experts because of their experience of a particular service. Davis and Wainwright (2005) provide a useful reminder that even within the protected environs of academia a focus on social work's potential to change the life chances of the poorest sections of society should not be forgotten. This is an important reminder of how service user involvement needs to be mainstreamed rather than regarded as an add-on, even if a value add one, of social work education.

Within social work there has been a clear articulation of the importance of securing service user/carer involvement, (Anghel & Ramon, 2009). This is reflected in teaching (Waterson & Morris, 2005), assessment and peer review (Humphreys, 2005; Skoura-Kirk et al., 2013), 'face to face' interactions between service users/carers and students and the use of video and other tools (Waterson & Morris, 2005). As Irvine, Molyneux, and Gillman (2015) argue the students they looked at had a, 'strong perception that their practice was improved by the input they had been given from service users and carers' (p. 148).

Different models of involvement

Webber and Robinson (2012) have rightly stressed that service user/carer involvement in social work education should be 'meaningful'. They suggest that models of involvement can be characterised in four ways: as a process of consultation; as a partnership in which the service user/carer contribution is 'equal to other contributors' (p. 1268); as being political and contributing to wider political change or through a model of 'user control'. They suggest that more empowerment focused programmes will gravitate towards the latter models while those that see service user/carer involvement as bringing added value to the educational experience will be characterised by an emphasis on consultation and partnership. Robinson and Webber (2012) were not able to evaluate which of these models was the most effective although they suggest that the use of Arnstein's model of citizen participation can over-simplify complex considerations of how 'meaningful involvement is'/can be (Arnstein, 1969). One example of an attempt to use Arnsteins model as an evaluative tool is that provided by Allain et al. (2006). Their conclusion was that they entered the process of involvement at the lowest phase (one of manipulation), that they succeeded in moving up Arnstein's ladder to rung five (placation) but that they had not reached a level which could really be regarded as partnership, delegation or control. This raises important questions about the efficacy of service user/carer involvement which, in this paper, and in much of the literature, is posited as a good. A review of the evidence supporting this position is beyond the scope of this paper which focuses on attempting to develop a new theoretical framework for exploring this involvement. However such a review is the focus of a separate piece of work which will evaluate not only the effectiveness, but also the sustainability, within education and professional practice, of such work.

Clearly the ability to exercise control within a modern, often neo-liberal, university environment would be a difficult task. It does raise important issues however as to how the power differentials between people using social work services and universities can be articulated. These issues will form an important element of the discussion of how we can conceptualise the involvement of service user/carers in our work which will be developed below. Before that however an outline of the ways in which service user/care involvement has been developed at the University of Portsmouth will be provided to contextualise this debate.

The University of Portsmouth – Social Work Inclusion Group: an example

Social Work Inclusion Group (SWIG) has been established in slightly different forms since June 2004 with support of money provided by the General Social Care Council to secure the

Table 1. Service user/carer involvement at the University of Portsmouth.

• Interviewing and admissions procedures.	• Teaching—the group was one of the pilot groups chosen by Skills for Care to deliver a training programme to train service users to teach on the Portsmouth social work degree programme.
• Redesigning the curricula.	• Assessing students 'Readiness for Practice' at the end of the first year (UG) or first semester (PG).
• Producing a video, 'What I want from a social worker' and a series of DVDs for Palgrave's Social Work Toolkit.	• Assessing student presentations.
• Developing a range of drama and cultural activities for use in social work training, particularly around (a) a *CREATE* day in which people who use social work services work with groups of social work and creative arts students to produce a creative artefact such as a photographic exhibition, a piece of drama or film, a poem, etc. (b) the *Black and White/ Perspectives* project which involves service users/cares co-producing a series of photographic representations of the service user/carer experience(for more detail see Hatton, 2013, Ch. 4, see also Pauvels, 2010) (c) *Debate Days* for first-year students.	• Assessing presentations by applicants seeking academic positions.
• Small-scale research around homelessness, working with ex street homeless people and homelessness organisations as co-researchers.	• Auditing work placements—the group is currently designing an audit tool to assess whether placement agencies meet students' learning needs.
• Attend and contribute to team meetings.	• Attend, and contribute to, course validation and other events.

Source: see www.swig.uk.net.

involvement of service users in the delivery of social work education. Since its formation the group has been involved in the following activities (Table 1).

SWIG's experience illustrates the point made by Foucault about the pace at which we seek to secure meaningful change. He spoke of the need to proceed a little at a time. Yet many agencies, in the desire to be seen to be ticking all the right boxes, treat service user involvement as if it is an immediate imperative and the service user should sublimate their own needs to achieve it. In 2005, the Service User Inclusion Group, (SUIG, the precursor of SWIG), along with a number of other service user organisations, were commissioned by the Training Organisation for the Personal Social Services (TOPSS; now Skills for Care) to undertake training of service users to enable them to teach on the new social work degree. SUIG was encouraged to pilot a training programme in two cities in the South. When the agreed start date for the training arrived, TOPSS had not produced the relevant training material and the group needed to develop their own. TOPSS appeared to think that training could be easily rescheduled. They appeared to have had no understanding that service users were themselves extremely busy people, with their own schedules, and they also appeared to be unaware that SUIG members had their own expectations and aspirations, which they had invested in the programme (SUIG, 2005). The hard copies of the training material arrived only after the project had finished. This illustrates the point made by Wilson and Beresford (2000) when they spoke of how there was a real danger that service users' views and aspirations could be appropriated by larger, more powerful, professional or sectoral organisations (see also Allain et al., 2006).

Conceptualising the involvement of people using services in social work education

The theoretical underpinning for such an approach has frequently been under-conceptualised. Generally involvement has been seen as good and part of a broader inclusion agenda which seeks to engage with the empowerment of people using social work services (users and carers). It has focused on the importance of power relationships (Dominelli, 2010; Tew, 2006), the need for service user 'voice' (Beresford, 2013) and has been critical of managerialist and procedural approaches to engagement with people using social work services (Jordan, 2011) particularly in the age of austerity (Jordan & Drakeford, 2012).

However even these areas, although often highlighted, could be further developed. Power discourses have drawn on a range of writers from sociology, political philosophy and from within the social work and community work literature. Lukes (1975) suggested that power needs to be understood in three ways: as the capacity to act ((A) having the power to make (B) do something against their wishes); as the management of dissent by the prevention of issues being placed on the public agenda; and by the lack of recognition on the part of powerless groups that their interests are being threatened (Hindess, 1996; Lukes, 1975, 2004).

Foucault (1991) reminds us that power operates in a complex way and that we need to interrogate our understanding of power at macro and micro levels. He argues that:

> [T]he problems which I try to address … which involve daily life, cannot be easily resolved. It takes many years, decades of work carried out at grass roots level with the people directly involved, and *the right to speech and political imagination must be returned to them (my emphasis)* … the complexity of the problem will be able to appear in its connection with people's lives … the object is to proceed a little at a time, to introduce modifications that are capable of, if not finding a solution, then at least changing the givens of a problem. (pp 158, 159)

While Foucault was addressing issues of political power in the broad sense, his comments can just as easily be seen as a prime legitimation for our concern with involving people who use social work services. Work with service users and carers is specifically about releasing people's *political imagination* so that they can envision an alternative experience, a different way of experiencing and delivering welfare and social work services. It is also about focusing on the particular daily experience of those people most directly involved in delivering social work services. It is concerned with changing the way issues are framed so that service users are not seen as 'problems' or 'clients' but rather as active partners in changing the services they directly experience. As Castells argues, we need to:

> *live with the tension, and the contradiction, between what we find and what we would like to happen.* I consider social action and political projects to be essential in the betterment of a society that clearly needs change and hope. (2000, p. 389, emphasis added)

This suggest that engaging and creating partnerships with people who use social work services has a change dimension, it is essentially political, which means that when examining service user/carer involvement we need to ask, (Webber & Robinson, 2012) whether the involvement we are discussing is real or tokenistic. This is a key focus of this paper where it is argued that to achieve this we need to have a multi-dimensional concept of power which incorporates a range of variables as illustrated in Figure 1.

This concept of power includes inclusion/participation, the link between theory and practice, the actualisation of personal and political power through creativity and artistic action and an underpinning commitment to the recognition of agency as the determining factor in people realising their potential.

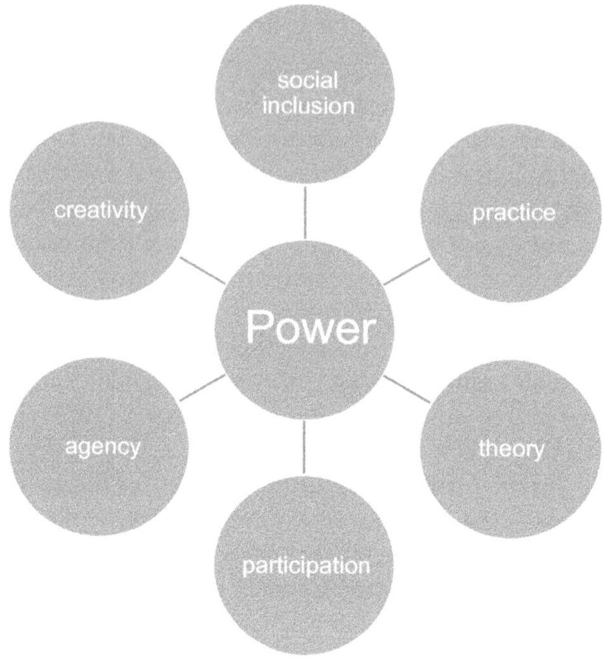

Figure 1. A dynamic view of power.

Service users/carers attribute great importance to their having a significant role in training and educating social workers. Their concern is not just to highlight issues but to contribute to the development and improvement of services. Such an involvement is essential if services are to be able to meet the demands placed on them in the new welfare mix.

Values

This raises a question about how we can create sets of values which challenge existing power relationships, particularly in view of the fact that these relationships are not always as obvious or visible as might be expected. Gramsci (1971) maintained that ruling classes dominate through a mixture of force and consent, where the consent is gained through assuming the political, moral and intellectual leadership in society. He argued that civil society (political parties, churches, cultural, charitable and voluntary groups) are central in maintaining hegemony. Civil society is the place where democratic struggles can be linked together. The ruling class maintains control by making their rule and the legitimacy of state rule appear like 'common sense'. It is then the role of external agents, such as intellectuals, union organisers and community leaders, to challenge this common sense. He believes that an oppressed group needs its own organic intellectuals (those that emerge from within their own ranks) to challenge these dominant ideas. He argues that:

> "everyone" is a philosopher ... it is not a question of introducing from scratch a scientific form of thought into everyone's individual life, but of renovating and making "critical" an already existing activity. (Gramsci, 1971, pp. 330, 331, cited in Allman, 2001, p. 114)

There is a danger that without an analysis of the way in which ideas are mediated we re-produce an analysis which suggests that service users are passive in the face of the institutional power of large social work or professional agencies. Yet from this reading of Gramsci when can see service users/carers struggling to have their voices heard are themselves 'organic intellectuals'.

How can we acknowledge the capacity of service users to take action to gain power rather than have power handed to them (which must in any case be an unlikely scenario)? We can do this by seeing service users as people with the capacity to bring about change not only in their own, individual circumstances, but in the broader institutions and structures against which they struggle. As such empowerment becomes central to the service user/care experience. In this sense we can see empowerment as essentially a strategy to bring about personal and political change (Hatton, 2015).

Promoting meaningful change

To make involvement and participation real, we need to look not just at how power can be exercised but also at how it can be resisted. How can we develop strategies to promote meaningful change? Giddens' analysis of agency and structure can provide some pointers as to how this may occur. He refers to power as 'the transformative capacity of human action' (Cassell, 1993, p. 109). This, Giddens (1979) suggests, following Marx, is the key element in the notion of praxis. The creation of a radical practice, based on notions of overcoming oppression, tackling discrimination/oppression and the creation of new cooperative social relationships, is at the heart of any theory of social action. Similar ideas can also be seen in Freire's idea of 'conscientisation', the notion that when the person becomes aware of the way their oppression is determined they develop the capacity to take action to change their situation (Burr, 1995; Freire, 1972; Gramsci, 1971).

Foucault (1980) points to the way in which power is:

> localised, dispersed, heteromorphous and accompanied by numerous phenomena, of inertia, displacement and resistance, so that, one should not assume a massive and primal condition of domination, a binary structure with "dominators" on the one side and "dominated" on the other. (p. 142)

Power should be viewed as a dynamic concept in which individuals 'are always in the position of simultaneously undergoing and exercising ... power [they] are the vehicles of power, not its application' (p. 98). Foucault suggests that 'the mechanisms of power [need to be analysed] on the basis of daily struggles at grass roots level, among those whose fight was located in the fine meshes of the web of power' (p. 116). This is the agency that we, as social workers, academics and users/carers, are looking for, the sense that service users can resist and reframe their experience in a way that can change the way services are delivered. However, it is necessary to avoid an outcome in which the organisation benefits more than the service user. As Jordan noted, outcomes can be seen in significantly different ways:

> the agencies' goal is to get target groups to bear as much of the costs of social care as possible, without sacrifice of professional power or significant material resources; the groups' to gain relevant resources and influence policy. (1996, p. 185)

There is a need to identify why people act or fail to act to redress any disadvantage they experience. Underpinning the need for a focus on participation/inclusion is a commitment to recognise the agency of service users. Giddens' concept of agency, is characterised by 'human action' or what Fook has characterised as a 'sense of responsibility, of agency, an appreciation of how each player can act upon it to influence a situation' (2002, p. 200). Central to this, Fook suggests, is the development of a consciousness, which can imagine another different way of doing things, a point similar to that attributed to Foucault earlier in this paper (Foucault, 1981). Hatton (2015) has suggested that this would enable, 'the creation of a radical practice based on notions of overcoming oppression, tackling discrimination/ oppression and the creation of new cooperative social relationships, (which are) at the heart of any theory of social action' (p. 113).

Service user involvement and social pedagogy

The importance of such an approach is evidenced by Akcelrud Durao (2006) who argues that it is essential that for social action to be effective arguments for change need to emerge from excluded communities or in our case from service users/carers themselves (p. 93). One way in which this can be seen is through the prism of the European concept of social pedagogy (Hatton, 2013) which is defined by Hamalainen (2003) as 'the basic idea … (of social pedagogy) is to promote people's social functioning, inclusion, participation, social identity and social competence as members of society' (p. 76). This commitment to social action is recognised as a central tenet of social pedagogy by a number of writers including Hamalainen (2003). This is also reflected in Vygotsky's idea of the 'creative imagination' which occurs 'whenever a person imagines, combines, alters and creates something new' (2004, p. 11). This will involve setting agendas for change, not just responding to the agenda of those with power (Jordan & Drakeford, 2012) and developing new participatory organisations and practices which signify real and lasting change. This would clearly illustrate Foucault's point about individuals simultaneously undergoing and exercising power and would help us understand the way power operates (Foucault, 1980).

Lorenz (1994) argues that social pedagogy 'signifies a concept which pays attention to the formation of society as a whole' (p. 92) and suggests that one alternative is to take on 'the critical conscience of pedagogy, the thorn in the flesh of the official agenda, an emancipatory programme for self- directed learning processes inside and outside the education system geared towards the transformation of society' (p. 93).

Central to a pedagogues activity is the use of *head, heart and hands*. The former enables the pedagogue to develop an understanding of the reasons for their intervention, the heart indicated the regard for and empathy with the person or group with whom the pedagogue is intervening and the hands indicate the range of practical and creativity which the pedagogue uses in any intervention (Boddy & Statham, 2009).

Hamalainen, argues that social pedagogy:

> aims to alleviate social exclusion. It deals with the processes of human growth that tie people to the systems, institutions and communities that are important to their well being and life management. (Hamalainen, 2003, p. 76)

'The *Common Third*'

Similar to social work, social pedagogy has a varied theoretical and practical tradition. An example is the Danish tradition of social pedagogy which draws on a range of sources from Freire to Kierkegaard (Hatton, 2001). Central to this approach is the 'Common Third' which Aabro describes as a descriptive project or ambition within the pedagogical tradition of 'relations in social work in which there is a "deliberate focus on the object as something outside the subject. The object being a "common thing" which both parts in the relation" can connect with' (see Hatton, 2006, 2015). Aabro describes the work of Husen who sees the key element of social pedagogy as being:

> To be sharing something, to have something in common, implies in principle to be equal, to be two (or more) individuals on equal terms, with equal rights and dignity (subject–subject relation). In a community you don't use or exploit the other (subject-object relation). (Husen, 1996, p. 231, translated by Aabro, 2004 in Hatton, 2015, pp. 135, 136)

At the core of this relationship are notions of equality and respect and the eradication of unequal power relations. Cacinovic Vogrincic (2005) argues that the social pedagogue or social worker needs to develop a new language and concepts but makes, 'the co-creation of solutions together with the client possible' (p. 336). He suggests that such an approach is based on an agreement to work, common understandings, a focus on participation, a focus on strengths rather than weaknesses and finally what he calls co-presence, which he says is about, 'confrontations, understanding, agreements … (as) … sources of new experience and possible changes' (p. 338). He suggests that the key to these elements is the transfer of professional knowledge into professional action.

As Aabro suggests it is 'through a common or joint activity (that) the users and the social workers enter a subject-subject relation. (in which) … the professional is meant to "forget himself" and the things around him – and devote entirely to the process and activity … the pedagogical challenge is to be able to realise activities which don't reflect the interests and needs of only one part, but instead seek to establish a *common* and *productive* activity.' (Aabro's emphasis in Hatton, 2006). One respondent to the review of social pedagogy in Essex undertaken by Eischteller and Holthoff (2012) commented positively on their experience of using the 'Common Third', saying:

> I now give great emphasis to using the "Common 3rd approach" to building relationships with the young people. Seeking out opportunities via a seemingly endless scope of activities will allow for valuable bonding between two individuals or groups ... I decided to utilise my time and get out of my comfort zone ... I made the most of building positive relationships with all the young people. I remarketed myself as accessible and traded admin for activities.

From understanding to action

Diesterweg, a German educationalist, a contemporary of Kant, Froebel and Pestalozzi argued that it was important to emphasise the democratic nature of education, with a particular focus on the social context within which education took place. He argued that, 'all (educational) theory separated from practice' is ineffectual and inappropriate (Gunther, 1993, p. 296) and regarded equality as the key to educational provision. He saw education as a means of improving people's situation and promoting self-development.

A more recent influence on Danish pedagogy has been the work of Freire (Eriksson & Markstrom, 2003; Hatton, 2001, 2015). Freire (1972) argues that a key way in which people without power are marginalised is through a process in which their behaviour becomes pathologised and their human nature is constructed in a distorted way through what he describes as processes of indoctrination, manipulation and 'dominated consciousness'. He argues that as a result people lack the consciousness or understanding to decode their situations. He argues therefore that we should encourage people to see the commonality of their situation, that this focus on the common interest can only be achieved through a process which he describes as *conscientanzo*. This is a process through which people not only become aware but act on that awareness.

Noting the influence of Freire, Eriksson and Markstrom (2003) suggest that the key contribution of Freire to social pedagogy is his emphasis on social mobilisation and emancipation. In this context they see social pedagogy as a means of initiating a process through which people mobilise their own resources. Marynowicz-Hetka (2007) suggests that social pedagogy can orientate practitioners towards the field of social action. She suggests that, an important part of the social pedagogic approach, are what she characterises as:

> reflection on the possibilities of learning ... to act in/through and for communities ... analysis of other solutions outside the traditional areas of social pedagogy, and their application to optimise and transform social practice. (2009, p. 4)

The role of creativity

An important element of this approach is a focus on creativity and art. Vygotsky's focus on creativity and imagination suggests a way forward. Our creative actions are, he argues, based on our use of imagination which is:

> The basis of all creative activity, ... an important component of all aspects of cultural life, enabling artistic, scientific, and technical creation alike ... whenever a person imagines, combines, alters and creates something new, (they are engaging their creative imagination). (p. 11)

Vygotsky sees this creative process as being dependent on both current environmental context and previous historical development. Creative developments then can be linked to processes of structural and class oppression. To free the creative imagination is to challenge the organisation of the society in which we live and to improve the life chances of the people we work with. Finally he reminds us of the 'agonies of creation'. As he says, 'creation is difficult, the drive to create does not always coincide with the capacity to create, and this is the origin of the agonizing feeling of suffering caused by the fact that the word does not capture the thought' (p. 39). Despite this he concludes by advocating the particular importance of cultivating creativity (p. 87).

Hacking, Secker, Spandler, Kent, and Shenton (2009) describe the way in which an arts project in the UK sought to engage with people with mental health needs. They found small but significant increases in social inclusion and indications that people were building stronger immediate networks and significant improvement in the overall empowerment of participants. They suggest that there were five processes which could be seen to be linked to the increased empowerment of the participants. These included:

- Getting motivated – they describe this as the participants developing inspiration and pride in their art work which in turn gave them a sense of purpose.
- Expressing self –through creating art the participants began to discover and accept themselves, this was particularly true of those participants with complex mental health issues, difficult past experiences and those who self-harmed.
- Connecting with abilities, rebuilding identities and changing peoples' perceptions of themselves.
- Expanding horizons – they suggest that people began to see themselves as having an identity as an artist rather than of a mental health service user. They quote one

> participant who says; 'It's not just something that someone with mental health problems has produced, its something that an artist has produced and it just so happens that they have got mental health problems as well'. (FEANTSA, 2009, p. 12/13)

Youth Music, a UK charity focusing on transforming the lives of marginalised and disadvantaged young people in the UK see music as a means of enabling young people and allowing them to take control of their lives. Their work, 'explores the outcomes that can be achieved through music-making projects for looked after children, and the barriers and facilitators to the effective delivery of these projects' (Dillon, 2009, p. 4). They maintain that, 'music-making can contribute to the development of a wide range of social and personal development outcomes for looked after children'.

Gray and Webb (2008) warn however of the danger of sentimentalising the use of creativity, intuition and a focus on the aesthetic side of social work in that it can also be:

> indicative of a reactionary sentiment that partly relates to a sense of mourning, or a loss progressively engendered by the deskilling of the task, the degradation of work, the reduction of professional autonomy, the break-up of professional identities and the consumerist marketisation of clients as "service users". (p. 184)

Gray and Webb (2008) argue instead for the idea of 'art as struggle' or of 'an art in the service of a politics of liberation' (p. 184) as being based on a sense of mutuality, partnership and equality. Lymbery (2003) suggest a solution may be found by recognising, but seeking to resolve, the contradiction between competence and creativity in social work. Lymbery (2003) suggests that in practices which involve assessment and/or evaluation skills the competence underpinning this work is insufficient and needs to be enhanced by 'the creativity that characterises best social work practice' (p. 114). Indeed Fazzi (2016) has pointed to the way the focus on the professionalisation of social work and the increased focus on specialisation are likely to, 'reduce the creativity and innovation' in our work.

To summarise a creative approach can have relevance across the helping professions. Play, music, drama, awareness of the body can be employed in work with siblings, mental health users, people with physical and intellectual disabilities and in the care of older people. An understanding of the theory behind creative activity can promote, reflection and learning in a variety of contexts.

The CRISP model

A model which suggests a way of linking these divergent thoughts together is the one which lies behind the service user/care involvement work in Portsmouth. The Creativity, Inclusion, social pedagogy (CRISP) model is an attempt to build a model of social theory and practice which makes explicit the need for creativity and inclusion to be part of the pedagogic/social work task (Hatton, 2013). The approach advocated suggests that the missing link between the creativity, which it is suggested is essential to good, empowering practice and social pedagogy is the notion of inclusion. Creativity suggests a way of realising the potential of people working in and making use of welfare services. Social pedagogy is predicated on equal partnerships between people working in and using welfare services. Both are central to the idea of inclusion. Inclusion provides the philosophical, practical and professional rationale for joining together creativity and social pedagogy and achieving a 'politics of liberation' as suggested by Gray and Webb (2008).

It is now widely accepted that a focus on inclusion is central to good social professional practice (Beresford & Hoban, 2005; Hatton, 2015). Those involved with radical social and community work will appreciate the difficulty of achieving real inclusion rather than the often tokenistic attempts at inclusion which agencies seek to perpetuate (Arnstein, 1969; Ferguson & Woodward, 2009: Hatton, 2015; Stepney & Popple, 2008). However, one of the reasons for adopting such an approach is that it can produce a sense of localism which can connect us to the people with whom we work. Such an approach should be at the centre of any involvement strategy.

Heikkila and Junkunen (2003) suggest that a number of key principles should underpin this commitment to inclusion. These include:

- Involvement as a right and responsibility – there should be a democratic right for service users to be involved …
- All service users should have access to services of sufficient quantity and quality …
- All services should have a culture of service user involvement.
- Users should be seen as recipients and actors – they should play a full role in decisions and debates around social care.
- Full accounts should be taken of users networks as a way of maximising user involvement.

Inclusion and choice

However, it is important to recognise that the encouragement of involvement or inclusion is not the same as the way choice is presented in current prevailing social policy discourses. Jordan points to the potentially contradictory ways in which the question of choice is framed. He argues that an emphasis on *choice* and the user as consumer typifies the way the welfare state is developing, suggesting that 'the public infrastructure is redesigned so as to promote choice, giving citizens information (for instance in the form of league tables) about the performance of hospitals, school and care homes, so that they can switch to the best amenities' (Jordan, 2006, p. 142). Yet the reality is that within this scenario those without the material resources to make these choices real, lose out in a marketised form of welfare.

Inclusion and participation should therefore not be confused with a choice agenda which as currently expressed in the discourses of the current government can be seen as a neo-liberal attempt to mask the inequalities in existing provision and ensnare people into believing that they exercise control over the welfare services and welfare agencies with which they are involved.

A holistic view of our social interventions is reflected in some of the educational programmes offered at the University of Portsmouth. Social pedagogy and creativity are integrated into the social work curriculum at the University. Pete Shepherd (2012 quoted in Hatton, 2013), a senior lecturer on the social work programme, says:

> In the teaching of a creativity and empowerment unit the author and the students have worked alongside artists, poets and filmmakers who are engaged in changing perceptions and mainstreaming perspectives that have previously occupied the position of being "outside" most institutions. (We seek to) critically evaluate how such a curriculum has been developed with the involvement of service users and been delivered to student groups over the last two years. We use creative artefacts to assess student's knowledge and their ability to embrace the principles

of participation in their consultative work with service users and carers. (Shepherd, 2012 quoted in Hatton, 2013, p. 38)

Conclusion

It is now generally accepted by the institutions of the state (Government departments and the HCPC), Higher Education Institutions, academics, students and users of social work services that the involvement of service users/carers in social work education is a good thing. This paper reflects this view but questions whether we need a more rigorous theoretical underpinning to this work. Clearly there is evidence of a recognition of power relationships, of the need for inclusion and for an understanding of the importance of the service user/carer 'voice'. This paper seeks to build on these insights to suggest a conception of involvement which develops these concerns and provides a deeper conception of power, the importance of involvement, inclusion and participation and the need for us to embrace creativity as a way of enhancing such involvement.

The paper draws on European debates around creativity, models of social pedagogy and the experience of delivering a creative agenda at the University of Portsmouth. It is suggested that we need to fuse together a multi-dimensional analysis of power, (with a particular focus on the idea that we co-produce learning activities and experiences), a recognition of the degree of agency exercised by people using social work services and a commitment to using our own and our collective, creative (and political) imaginations to work in new ways. This means moving beyond traditional measures of involvement such as teaching assessment and interviewing to a wider concept of us all as drivers of the learning experience and creators of the curricula.

To this extent this paper should be seen as an exploratory discussion which raises important issues about the centrality of service user/carer involvement in social work education. As such it will provide the framework for a deeper evaluative study as to the efficacy and sustainability of such approaches.

References

Akcelrud Durao, F. (2006). Towards a model of inclusive exclusion: Marginal subjectivation in Rio de Janerio. *A Contra corriente, A Journal of Social History and Literature in Latin America, 3*, 88–106.

Allain, L., Cosis Brown, H., Danso, C., Dillon, J., Finnegan, P., Gadhoke, S., … Whitaker, F. (2006). User and carer involvement in social work education—A university case study: Manipulation or citizen control? *Social Work Education, 25*, 403–413.

Allman, P. (2001). *Revolutionary social transformation: Democratic hopes, political possibilities and critical education*. Westport, CT: Bergin and Garvey.

Anghel, R., & Ramon, S. (2009). Service users and carers' involvement in social work education: Lessons from an English case study. *European Journal of Social Work, 12*, 185–199.

Arnstein, S. (1969). A ladder of citizen participation. *Journal of the American Institute of Planners, 35*, 214–224.

Bennett, F., & Roberts, M. (2004). *From input to influence: Participatory approaches to research and inquiry into poverty*. York: Joseph Rowntree Foundation.

Beresford, P. (2013). Service user issues: Rights, needs and responsibilities. In B. Littlechild & R. Smith (Eds.), *A handbook for inter-professional practice in the human services: Learning to work together* (pp. 187–199). Harlow: Pearson.

Beresford, P., & Hoban, M. (2005). *Participation in anti-poverty and regeneration work and research: Overcoming barriers and creating opportunities*. York: Joseph Rowntree Foundation.

Boddy, J., & Statham, J. (2009). *European perspectives on social work: Models of education and professional roles*. London: Thomas Coram Research Unit, Institute of Education.

Burr, V. (1995). *An introduction to social constructionism*. London: Routledge.

Cacinovic Vogrincic, G. (2005). Teaching concepts of help in social work: The working relationship. *European Journal of Social Work, 8*, 335–341.

Cassell, P. (Ed.). (1993). *The giddens reader*. Basingstoke: Macmillan.

Castells, M. (2000). *End of the millenium*. London: Wiley.

Children's Rights Alliance and National Youth Council of Ireland. (2002). *Hearing young voices*. Dublin: The Open Your Eyes to Child Poverty Initiative. Retrieved February 16, 2015, from www.youth.ie/sites/youth.ie/files/HearingYoungVoices-Full.pdf

Davis, A., & Wainwright, L. (2005). Combating poverty and social exclusion: Implications for social work education. *Social Work Education, 24*, 259–273.

Department of Health. (2001). *Valuing people: A new strategy for learning disability for the 21st century*. London: HMSO.

Department of Health. (2009). *Valuing people now: A new three year strategy for people with learning disabilities*. London: Stationary Office.

Department of Health. (2010). *Personalisation through person-centred planning*. London: Author.

Dillon, M. (2009). Retrieved from www.youthmusic.org.uk

Dominelli, L. (2010). *Social work in a globalising world*. Cambridge: Polity.

Eischteller, G., & Holthoff, S. (2012). *The art of being a social pedagogue in practice: Examples of cultural change in children's homes in Essex*. Manchester, NH: ThemPra Social Pedagogy.

Eriksson, L., & Markstrom, A. M. (2003). Interpreting the concept of social pedagogy. In A. Gustavsson, H. E. Hermansson, & J. Hamalained (Eds.), *Perspectives and theory in social pedagogy* (pp. 9–22). Gotenburg: Bokforlaget, DaidLOS.

Fazzi, L. (2016). Are we educating creative professionals? The results of some experiments on the education of social work students in Italy. *Social Work Education, 35*, 89–99.

FEANTSA. (2009). *Homeless in Europe—Homelessness and the arts: Creativity, empowerment and social change, spring*. The magazine of the European Federation of National Working with the Homeless, AISBL, Spring. Retrieved February 16, 2015, from www.feantsa.org/spip.php?article1027&lang=en

Ferguson, I., & Woodward, R. (2009). *Radical social work in practice: Making a difference*. Bristol: Policy Press.

Fook, J. (2002). *Social work: Critical theory and practice*. London: Sage.

Foucault, M. (1980). *Power/knowledge: Selected interviews and other writings*. Brighton: Harvester Wheatsheaf.

Foucault, M. (1981). *Power/Knowledge: Selected interviews and other writings*. Brighton: Harvester Wheatsheaf.

Foucault, M. (1991). *Remarks on Marx*. New York, NY: Semiotext Books.

Freire, P. (1972). *Pedagogy of the oppressed*. London: Penguin.

Giddens, A. (1979). *Central problems in social theory*. Basingstoke: Macmillan Education.

Goodley, D. (2011). *Disability studies: An interdisciplinary introduction*. London: Sage.

Gramsci, A. (1971). *Selections from the prison notebooks of Antonio Gramsci*. (Q. Hoare & G. Nowell Smith, Eds. and Trans.). London: International Publishers.

Gray, M., & Webb, S. (2008). Social work as art revisited. *International Journal of Social Welfare, 17*, 182–193.

Gunther, K. H. (1993). *Freidrich Adolph Diesterweg (1790–1866)*. Retrieved December 3, 2012, from http://www.ibe.unesco.org/sites/default/files/diestere.pdf

Hacking, S., Secker, J., Spandler, H., Kent, L., & Shenton, J. (2009, Spring). The empowerment of people with mental health needs and other social exclusion impacts: Using arts participation: Evidence from the UCLAN/Anglia Research Project. *Homelessness in Europe*. Retrieved February 16, 2015, from www.feantsa.org/spip.php?article1027&lang=en

Hamalainen, J. (2003). The concept of social pedagogy in the field of social work. *Journal of Social Work, 3*, 70–80.

Hatton, K. (2001). Translating values: Making sense of different value bases – Reflections from Denmark and the UK. *International Journal of Social Research Methodology, 4*, 265–278.
Hatton, K. (2006). Europe and the undergraduate programme. In K. Lyons & S. Lawrence (Eds.), *Social work in Europe: Educating for change* (pp. 105–125). Birmingham, AL: BASW/Venture Press.
Hatton, K. (2013). *Social pedagogy in the UK: Theory and practice*. Lyme Regis: Russell House Publishing.
Hatton, K. (2015). *New directions in social work practice* (2nd ed.). London: Learning matters/Sage.
Hayden, C., Goddard, J., Gorin, S., & Van Der Spek, N. (1999). *State child care: Looking after children?* London: Jessica Kingsley.
Heikkila, M., & Junkunen, I. (2003). Obstacles to an increased user involvement in social services. In B. Munday (Ed.), *User involvement in personal social services*, University of Kent, with assistance of the Group of Specialists on User Involvement in Social Services (CS-US), Strasbourg: Council of Europe.
Hindess, B. (1996). *Discourses of power: From Hobbes to Foucault*. Oxford: Blackwell.
HM Government. (2009). *Valuing people now*. London: Stationary Office.
Humphreys, C. (2005). Service user involvement in social work education: A case example. *Social Work Education, 24*, 797–803.
Husen, M. (1996) *Det faelles tredje - om faellesskab og vaedier i det paedagogiske arbbejde, in B. Pecseli* (9 ed). Kulture & paedagogik, Kobenhavn: Socialpaedagogisk Bibliotek. Munsgaard/Rosinante.
Irvine, J., Molyneux, J., & Gillman, M. (2015). 'Providing a Link with the Real World': Learning from the student experience of service user and carer involvement in social work education. *Social Work Education, 34*, 138–150.
Jakes, S., & Cassidy, L. (n.d.). *Evaluating the national outcomes: Programme outcomes for communities, citizen development*. Retrieved February 16, 2015, from http://ag.arizona.edu/sfcs/cyfernet/nowg/cd_indicators.html
Jordan, B. (1996). *A theory of poverty and social exclusion*. Cambridge: Polity.
Jordan, B. (2006). *Social policy for the twenty-first century*. Cambridge: Polity Press.
Jordan, B. (2011). Making sense of the big society': Social work and the moral order. *Journal of Social Work (May)*, 1–7.
Jordan, B., & Drakeford, M. (2012). *Social work and social policy under austerity*. Basingstoke: Palgrave Macmillan.
Lathlean, J., Burgess, A., Coldham, T., Gibson, C., Herbert, L., Levett-Jones, T., … Tee, S. (2006). Experiences of service user and carer participation in health care education. *Nurse Education Today, 26*, 732–737.
Local Authority Circular/Department of Health. (2008). London: Department of Health.
Lorenz, W. (1994). *Social work in a changing Europe*. London: Routledge.
Lukes, S. (1975). *Power: A radical view* (2nd ed.). Basingstoke: Palgrave Macmillan.
Lukes, S. (2004). *Power: A radical view* (2nd ed.). Basingstoke: Palgrave Macmillan.
Lymbery, M. (2003). Negotiating the contradictions between competence and creativity in social work education. *Journal of Social Work, 3*, 99–117.
Marynowicz-Hetka, E. (2007). Towards the transversalism of social pedagogy. *Social Work and Society, International Online Journal, 5*, 3.
McLaughlin, H. (2009). What's in a name: 'Client', 'Patient', 'Customer', 'Consumer', 'Expert by Experience', 'Service User'—What's next? *British Journal of Social Work, 39*, 1101–1117.
Pauvels, L. (2010). Visual sociology reframed: An analytical synthesis and discussion of visual methods in social and cultural research. *Sociological Methods and Research, 38*, 545–581.
Payne, M. (2014). *Modern social work theory* (4th ed.). Basingstoke: Palgrave Macmillan.
Ramsden, S. (2010). *Practical approaches to co-production: Building effective partnerships with people using services, families and citizens*, prepared for the DoH, London: HMSO.
Robinson, K., & Webber, M. (2012). Models and effectiveness of service user involvement in social work education: A literature review. *British Journal of Social Work, 42*, 1256–1274.
Service User Inclusion Group. (2005). *Training service users to become actively involved in the new social work degree*. London: TOPSS England.
Shakespeare, T. (2013). *Disability rights and wrongs*. London: Routledge.

Skoura-Kirk, E., Backhouse, B., Bennison, G., Cecil, B., Keeler, J., Talbot, D., & Watch, L. (2013). Mark my words! Service user and carer involvement in social work academic assessment. *Social Work Education, 32*, 560–575.

Social Care Institute of Excellence. (2004). *Resource guide no 2: Involving service users and carers in social work education*. London: Author.

Social Care Institute for Excellence. (2013). *Co-production in social care: What it is and how to do it, SCIE guide 15*. London: Author.

Stepney, P., & Popple, K. (2008). *Social work and the community: A critical context for practice*. Basingstoke: Palgrave.

Tew, J. (2006). Understanding power and powerlessness: Towards a framework for emancipatory practice in social work. *Journal of Social Work, 6*, 33–51.

Townend, M., Tew, J., Grant, A., & Repper, J. (2008). Involvement of service users in education and training: A review of the literature and exploration of the implications for the education and training of psychological therapists. *Journal of Mental Health, 17*, 65–78.

Vygotsky, L. (2004). Imagination and creativity in childhood. *Journal of Russian and East European Psychology, 42*, 7–97.

Warren, J. (2007). *Service user and carer participation in social work*. Exeter: Learning Matters.

Waterson, J., & Morris, K. (2005). Training in 'Social' work: Exploring issues of involving users in teaching on social work degree programmes. *Social Work Education, 24*, 653–675.

Webber, M., & Robinson, K. (2012). The meaningful involvement of service users and carers in advanced – Level post-qualifying social work education: A qualitative study. *British Journal of Social Work, 42*, 1256–1274.

Wilson, A., & Beresford, P. (2000). 'Anti-oppressive practice': Emancipation or appropriation? *British Journal of Social Work, 30*, 553–573.

Expert by experience research as grounding for social work education

Petra Videmšek

ABSTRACT
This article is based on an investigation that involves five experts by experience in the field of mental health and eight students of social work. Both groups investigated the experiences of people with mental ill-health living in group homes. The article identifies the advantages if the researchers are expert by experience and the epistemological shift produced by the inclusion of people with the lived experience. Expert by experience research is a challenge to both experts by experience and for social work practice since it promotes the basic principle of social work as the science of doing. This study was based on the assertion that the real integration of theory and practice will not come from a rigid body of knowledge, but from the humility to learn from experts by experience.

Involving experts by experience into research

In the last two decades, we have witnessed a strong tradition of involving people with personal experience as active members of research teams (Beresford, 2000; Faulkner, 2009; McLaughlin, 2009; Ramon, 2003; Rose, 2009; Videmšek, 2009). An important source for the involvement of experts by experience into research was the rise of social movements like the feminist and peace movements and especially those led by service users and carers, particularly in the field of mental health, psychical and intellectual disabilities (Oliver, 1992; Rose, 2001; Videmšek, 2011, 2014; Winter & Munn-Giddings, 2001; Zaviršek & Videmšek, 2009). According to Thompson (2002) social movements played an important role in ensuring that service user's views were taken into account as relevant in the policy, practice development and implementation, as well as the evaluation of services.

Involvement in research is first recorded in the late 1960s when Mayer and Timms (1970) drew attention to service user perspectives; *The client speaks: working class impressions of casework*. The study was conducted in 1968 in London and included the perspectives of those who were satisfied and dissatisfied with the social services they received. Their research aim was to find the reasons which had led to the users' satisfaction or dissatisfaction with the service, and to present through a user perspective the ways users establish connections with existing services. In Slovenia the major shift towards expert by experience involvement was the result of disability activists who started to publish critical books, articles and daily news reports based on their own personal experiences with mental health services and with social workers. One of the first critical books on mental health was published by a professor and long term mental health survivor Tanja Lamovec in 1995 (Zaviršek & Videmšek, 2009). She also wrote about the phenomenological approach in research and the need for the involvement of experts by experience in research (Lamovec, 1995). She and others had pioneered a politically aware, user led organisation that had not only set up the first advocacy service along with a number of non-governmental organisations (NGO's) for and with people with mental health problems in Ljubljana, but also challenged the way knowledge was produced.

Not only social movements and activists, but also the development of new techniques of data collection and qualitative empirical material analysis provided conditions which enabled the inclusion of experts by experience into research as a researcher. Mesec (1998) states that in the past 40 years social work has witnessed a true renaissance of the so-called qualitative methods that used to accompany social work's first steps as a science (Mesec, 1998, p. 19). The review of these methods shows that changes in research in individual time periods were mainly due to researchers seeking to gain a better understanding of changes in society and to better represent the characteristics of people's actual problems.

Expert by experience involvement in research is an innovative topic. As Reason (1994) suggests, research should be done 'with' people, and not 'on' people—three levels of expert by experience involvement in research can be summarised as:

- Research within which users are members of the research team and are in the position of consultants—*consultation* (Barnes, 1993; McLaughlin, 2006, 2009);
- Research where users carry out research with the support of professionals—*collaboration* (Beresford, 2000, 2001; Humphries, 2001; Ramon, 2000);
- Research that is *user-controlled* and led (Ajduković, 2008; Beresford & Rose, 2009; Evans & Fisher, 1999; Videmšek, 2009; Wiltshire & Swindon Users Network, 1996).

All those levels speak about different points of involvement of service users. Consultation may be the first point of involvement but does not guarantee that any ideas, changes or issues raised by those who are being consulted will have any impact or influence whatsoever on outcomes (McLaughlin, 2009, p. 27). Collaboration implies that service users will be listened to and their ideas will have an impact upon research. Service user controlled research presents a challenge to traditional ways of research production. The history of service users involvement is defined with classifications and typologies started with Sherry Arnstein's (Arnstein, 1969) 'ladder of participation'. Arnstein (1969) defines eight levels of citizen participation. The eight types are arranged in a ladder pattern with each rung corresponding to the extent of citizens' power in determining the end product. This involvement ranges from non-participation to citizen power (Arnstein, 1969). The bottom rungs of the ladder are one Manipulation and two Therapy. These two rungs describe levels of 'non-participation'. Rungs 3 and 4 progress to levels of 'tokenism' that allow the 'have-nots' to hear and to have a voice: three Informing and four Consultation. When participation is restricted to these levels, there is no follow-through, no 'muscle', hence no assurance of changing the status quo. Rung 5, Placation, is simply a higher level tokenism. Further up the ladder are levels of citizen power with increasing degrees of decision-making influence. Rung 6, Partnership, enables them to negotiate and engage in trade-offs with traditional power holders. At the topmost rungs, 7 Delegated Power and 8 Citizen Control, citizens have become the major decision-maker and assumed full control. (Arnstein, 1969, p. 217–218).

McLaughlin (2015) defines four different models of service user involvement. These models move from viewing service users as objects to subjects, to social actors, to active participants (McLaughlin, 2015, p. 155). The main distinguishing feature of these models is the question of the degree of power. The above implies that inclusion of experts by experience in research represents a fundamental shift in power relations. Traditionally, an expert by experience in research was restricted to being the object of research. One of the biggest challenges was how to change this position. A review of the literature shows that service user's involvement in research represents a shift in power (Beresford, 2000; Beresford & Rose, 2009; McLaughlin, 2009; Powell, 2009), presents practical examples of service user's involvement (Beresford & Rose, 2009), introduced knowledge production (Lamovec, 1995, Powel, 2009, Beresford & Rose 2009), principles and concepts about service user research (Beresford, 2000; Faulkner, 2009). A number of different approaches can be recognised, such as consumerist approach, democratic approach. The first approach generally starts with policy and service system, the second is rooted to people's lives and their aspirations to improve the nature and conditions of their lives (Beresford, 2000; McLaughlin, 2009). Reading the published literature suggests how you can do the research and present principles and priorities of service user research. Literature review leads us to make practical use of the research and all this awareness. We wanted to add knowledge production and present whether there was a difference between the knowledge claims of research that is done by service users and the research that did not include service users.

With this research, I wanted to explore the knowledge production. I wanted to show, as noted by Jackie Powell (2009), that real integration of theory and practice will not come about through a ponderous, rigid body of knowledge, but from the humility to learn from practitioner's experiences (Powell, 2009, p. 325).

Methodology

In involving experts by experience[1] I sought to challenge traditional research and value the experience and knowledge of experts by experience.[2] I sought to find out if the involvement of experts by experience would lead to any changes in the context of research. For this study I undertook research with two groups of researchers, experts by experience and students of social work. Five experts by experience with whom I had cooperated previously on European mental health projects agreed to take part in the research along with 3rd year social work students.

Those two research teams were an educational experiment in which I wanted the student to understand better the nature of user led research, and to explore whether there were differences between the student's and expert by experience's research design. The study also wanted the student to reflect on what they had learned of the advantages and disadvantages of involving experts by experience in research. The main question was not just a question of 'what is different when the researchers are expert by experience?' but 'what can we learn from this process and how do we all, as researchers (student or expert by experience), shape knowledge production?' Efforts have been made to measure the extent to which researchers with different backgrounds conduct the investigations differently. I try to answer two research questions in this process:

- Can we perceive differences between experts by experience research and a trained researcher (trained student)?
- How can an expert by experience's perspective be identified through involvement in research?

Both groups of researchers had the same purpose: exploring group homes in Slovenia. The topic was chosen by experts by experience. The students also agreed to explore group homes for people with mental health difficulties in Slovenia. A sample of 20 interviews were undertaken, with 12 completed by experts by experience and 8 by students, covering a total of 5 different group homes. The research process followed two phases of research. The expert by experience researchers were involved in articulating the major issues they would like to explore. They chose to explore group homes in the field of mental ill health since three of them live in group homes.

We used qualitative methodology. The data collection technique used was semi- structured interviews that offered insight into individual experience, enabling us to explore user's narratives of experience and view of living in group homes. The semi structured interview were structured into four segments: (a) control; (b); social capital (c) choices (d) future perspective and used both open and closed questions.

In the second phase, the student researchers were asked to prepare a questionnaire on the same topic that had been previously chosen by the experts by experience. They were asked to define the research questions and to prepare the questions for the interview. They prepared their own questionnaire and chose the group homes where they undertook the data analysis. The students were also asked to record their critical reflections on their experience.

For exploring the main ideas and phenomena of expert by experience research, I used conceptual frameworks (Miles & Huberman, 1994). Conceptual frameworks help us to form a tentative theory of the phenomenon that we investigate (what is needed if the researchers are expert by experience, what is going on (in the existing services), what we have been able to see in two different research teams).

The analysis process followed a series of steps. Each researcher read all the interview transcripts and recorded their findings (perceptions, key statements and findings). In the group meeting we discussed the findings and related these to the literature review. We focused on the analysis of the qualitative interviews data in order to explore the differences between the two research groups. For both groups of interviews we added preliminary codes. Than we put those codes into a set of themes. After that we compared the themes, discussed them and compared the results, identifying similarities and differences.

Because the aim of the research was education, I used concept map tools. Concept maps are based on Ausubel's (1968) theory of meaningful learning. According to his theory, meaningful learning is based on a constructivist epistemology, which posits that human learning is based on cultural, religious and contextual situations and conceptualisations (Ausubel, 1968). Concept mapping, as developed by Novak and Gowin (1984), is unique because it makes concepts, and propositions composed of concepts, the central elements in the structure of knowledge and construction of meaning. The concept maps method helps us to understand and pictorially represent our thought patterns in an organised and structural process (Novak & Gowin, 1984) and I used grounded theory (Glaser & Strauss, 1967) to inductively develop key themes during the research process.

For the research proposed we did not need ethical approval or any ethical research governance since in Slovenia, we need ethical approval only if the research is done in an institution like a psychiatric hospital. Before we started the research we asked managers of the group homes for their agreement. We outline basic information about the research and its purpose and the right for participants to not participate whilst advising the staff we would be contacting them. We did consider all the potential risks to participants, and have procedures for how to continue with the work and for maintaining confidentiality. We have been aware that ethical issues are important in the research, especially if service users as researchers are involved. Before we started to do the research, we considered the need for support of service user researchers, respect for autonomy, anonymity and confidentiality, storing of data (all collected interviews have been stored at the Faculty in a the locked drawer whilst electronic data files have been password protected), rewards and recognition (two of service users choose to participate in an international conference and have been supported to do so, all others attended a local social work conference).

In the following text, I outline some of the key findings and examine what needs to be in place to promote and ensure experts by experience involvement.

What we can learn from our experiences?

The main purpose of the research was to show the knowledge production and differences between two different groups of researchers. From our experience we can outline some major differences that support involvement of experts by experience in research. Our findings 'demystify research' as a strictly professional form as said by Shula Ramon (2003) and contributes, as Maglajlić (2007) points out, to the 'development of theory, values and practice in a way which is not based on the premise that all theories are formed by dominant groups of people (Maglajlić, 2007, p. 57).

Based on the research, we can list some advantages for involvement of experts by experience in research:

(1) Experts by experience clearly define the problem because they understand the situation. They know what it feels like to undergo treatments and their various side effects, how it is to use the social services and be with those who you do not know or want to be with. Because of the aforementioned reasons, they have a good idea about what research questions should be asked and how questions might be asked differently. Beresford and Rose (2009) defines this as the uniqueness of experts by experience. In our experience students needed more time to identify the research problem and key research questions whilst experts by experience could identify these straight away.

(2) Questions are grounded in their life situation. Questions are simple, concrete and direct. In our situation that means that expert by experience researchers posed more direct questions than the students. For example, the experts by experience posed such questions as: Do you want to have a domestic animal in your group home? Do you like that the social worker is giving you the amount of cigarettes you can smoke? Do you want to have the bell on your door? Students however asked: How did you come to be in a group home? Do you have your own room?

Expert by experience research has proven that experts by experience pose different questions than those raised by other experts without experience, namely they are linked to concrete life situations, reflect knowledge of living conditions in the group and focus on specific changes which could be brought about through the research. As stated by Ramon (2003), users participating in user research apply their emphatic understanding as a research instrument with which to pinpoint the impact of important research questions vs. the less important ones (Ramon, 2003, p. 5). To affirm that experts by experience pose the right questions because they know the situation opens the issue of who can be called a service user researcher, as asked by McLaughlin (2009). He raises this question for further debate and consideration. In our experience we can assert that because experts by experience are recipients of the service, they add more to the process than those who are not, as it concerns then and is important to their life situation. One of the expert by experience interviewers said: 'Finally I haven't been asked the same questions as usually'. Experts by experience are able to see the policies and services both from the perspective of being a recipient of the policies and services but also from the point of view of what is required to make a difference in their life, as pointed out by McLaughlin (2009, p. 81).

(3) New topics are identified. Investigation shows that experts by experience open up new topics and give us evidence for new knowledge. McLaughlin (2009, p. 33) said that experts by experience are able to prioritise topic areas and this a recognition that their experience provides them with significant insights into the topics under consideration. In this research this included: suicide by people with mental health difficulties, a subject often overlooked in group homes, sexuality, forbidden visits and also questions of professional power (controlling the number of cigarettes, restrictions on domestic animals, access to internet etc.).

(4) The nature of the responses to interviews by experts by experience were different than those from student interviewers. The answers were more direct, personal, honest and open compared to those obtained by student researchers. Several researchers and service users report that (Beresford & Rose, 2009; Faulkner, 2009; Ramon, 2000; Rose, 2001). This can be explained by the fact that many people will only allow themselves to reveal their vulnerability, and allow others to approach them, in contact with a peer (Lamovec, 1995). The second reason unavoidably lies in the interviewee's relationship of dependence on the service (in our case the group home unit), and that is why respondents have difficulty revealing their true opinion of the service, while, when speaking to individuals with a similar experience, they can be more open in revealing their own experience. When service users feature as researchers, they are recognised by the respondents as equal interlocutors with whom they can speak more openly (without censorship). Power relations at the level of the relationship between the researchers and the object of the research are manifested in different ways. Researchers reveal their power by acting as specialists in their field, enjoying a reputation and having the possibility to ask questions, while the researched often have no power. In terms of power relations, it is all the more important that researchers be people with similar experience as those they are researching.

(5) If the needs and views of users are reflected in research, it is more likely to produce results that can be used to improve social work practice and articulate the answer to HOW to do it differently. In our case, experts by experience suggested, 'In the house it should be written that domestic animals are allowed and that the owner takes care of it'. 'Each of us decided by themselves about the amount of cigarettes. If we need help we will ask for it'. 'Risk is permitted'. I claim that expert by experience research represents the basis for the creation of services tailored to the individual. By entering the research field experts by experience are put in the position of co-creators of theory which is important for 'actionable knowledge'. Actionable knowledge in social work is knowledge that is shared with people, we jointly use it in a working relationship. (Čačinovič Vogrinčič, 2002, 2015). Experts by experience thus become part of looking for answers and co-creating solutions. From being passive service receivers, they obtain the position of active solution searchers.

The inclusion of experts by experience in research brings several advantages, not only in obtaining better results but also because expert by experience involvement in research can be used as a tool that actually brings empowerment to the expert by experience. In this research work, this occurred both on the individual and collective level. Experts by experience researchers have since continued with their own research.

(6) An important issue is in the creation of new knowledge. Humphries (2001). suggests that there is a need for research to generate different sorts of knowledge for understanding the complexity of social work practice. Humphries (2009) writes that participatory approaches open the space and recognise the knowledge of marginalised groups and the subjective elements of human experience, that is, the meanings attributed to events and behaviour by particular social actors. (Humphries, 2009, p. 313). Ramon (2003) pointed out that 'knowledge itself is powerful in providing a way to make sense, give meaning and predict reality … it provides a new way of looking at what has been taken for granted' (Ramon, 2003, p. 16). Knowledge as such is not monopolised and reserved for professionals but was shared and distributed to the participants in the research. Participation of the service users ensures reconstruction of knowledge and helps to develop more a 'democratic social science' as Oakley stated (1998, p. 725). Rose (2009) said that there is no 'universal knowledge produced' but only particular knowledge production through different standpoints. Different standpoints produce 'different truths' (Rose, 2009, p. 41).

This research shows that different sorts of knowledge helps us in understanding the complexity of social work practice. In our investigation new knowledge production lies in new themes that have been opened by experts by experience and also in the explanations of the existing services. From their questions and answers, we have been able to learn how important relationships in the group homes are for them (especially the relationship between them and social workers). The main model of working with them will be a partnership that is based on respect and that values life experiences. ('I am not sure if social workers see me somewhere else than here'). They raised the importance of time (how long people should stay in the group homes. What are the positive and negative sides of limitations on

> *Principles* and *values* of professional social work. We want to follow the principle of users' control over the whole process.
>
> *Philosophy* that is based on human rights and an awareness that there is more than one way to produce knowledge and more than one truth.
>
> *Orientation*, that leads social workers towards radical social work. Radical social work is not only about helping the individual to fit into the system, but also changing the system to fit the individual.
>
> *Moral courage*, to implement what we see and hear in the field work. With that, we enable that theories are not coming only from professional deduction but from the experience of experts by experience
>
> *Obligation* to be beyond existing practice and change it.
>
> *Moral vision* requires that we not only act within existing frames of understanding, but that we are able to see what should change or happen in response to our moral stance or professional values.
>
> A *process*, whereby we engage with experts by experience in respectful dialogue.

staying in the group homes etc.). Through our research experience, we are able to identify knowledge of what is an expert by experience perspective in social work.We can offer a deeper understanding of user perspectives to those who will always be without this component. User perspective in social work practice is:

(7) Experts by experience understand the system and have contact with other service users. In a way we can say that an expert by experience has easier access to data and interviewees. McLaughlin (2009) mentioned that people with mental ill health (and other stigmatised groups as well) are hard to reach groups. Experts by experience are more likely to know where others in similar circumstances or conditions congregate, thus providing greater access to the target population (McLaughlin, 2009, p. 33). From our experience, it was quite clear that interviewees would rather talk with someone with the same experience. If the researchers are expert by experience there is a more equal relationship. Lamovec (1995) pointed out that because an expert by experience has the same experience, people are more ready to talk with them without fear of what will happen afterwards. Easy access can also be explained by the fact that experts by experience know each other. Access to respondents is direct and not chosen by other people. (Students need to ask social workers to help them find some respondents).

Inclusion of experts by experience in research ensures that theories are also generated from experts by experiences and not only from professionally conceived deductions (Powell, 2009; Videmšek, 2009). As I have shown so far, by including people with lived experience in the research, we treated the expert by experience perspective as the starting point for our understanding of the work. We should also remember that some preconditions need to be obtained before involving experts by experience in research. I identified some preconditions that need to be settled before we do the research. Otherwise, we can face the danger that involving service users in research becomes merely propaganda and thereby undermines contributions to results.

Preconditions for involvement of experts by experience in research

Involvement of experts by experience in research connects with social work concepts such as empowerment, normalisation/social role valorisation, and also resonates with social work values: rights of equal citizenship and self advocacy. To enrich these values we need to address key questions.

Why do we want experts by experience involved in research?

Ostrer and Morris (2009) point out that it is more likely for academics to approach service users to take part in their research than vice versa. Researchers need to be aware that involving service users in their research will require them to be reflective and creative (Ostrer & Morris, 2009, p. 80). The first question to be resolved before any contact with experts by experience is to consider precisely why we want their involvement: is it merely to satisfy the requirements, or because it is in fashion, or is it because there is a considered and genuine belief in the value of user involvement? McLaughlin (2009) pointed out that it is quite clear that involving service users is justified in terms of making traditional knowledge claims (McLaughlin, 2009, p. 79). The reason for involvement should also lie in willingness to implement the main concepts of social work, such as: empowerment, co-creation, the ethic of inclusion etc.

In our case, I was clear that introducing an expert by experience perspective could positively influence the content of their research and make it more relevant to social work practice. I wanted to show that theory can be put into practice and that the involvement of experts by experience can be a tool for empowerment.

How will experts by experience be involved in the research process?

Experts by experience involvement in research may occur at many different levels as we have shown so far (Arnstein, 1969, Beresford & Rose, 2009; McLaughlin, 2009). In our case, experts by experience have been involved as researchers with full control over the process of research (from defining the topic, creating the questionnaire, undertaking the interviews, analysing the data and disseminating the findings).

How do we recruit experts by experience to become researchers?

One of the most productive ways of approaching experts by experience is through relationships that have already been established locally (e.g. with NGO's, with user groups). We can also invite them through less direct approaches (e.g. through posters or advertising in magazines, newsletters and papers). This approach may also be useful and might possibly recruit a wider range of users. In our case, the team knew each other, since we had cooperated on the European project Experience Involvement (EX-IN). When the project was finished some experts by experience expressed the wish for further cooperation. One member of the team also recruited new members through a presentation to NGO's.

I also asked experts by experience why they wanted to be involved. The answers obtained by our experts by experience researchers pointed to a combination of reasons, related to their mental ill health situation in combination with social services, as well as personal reasons (to be part of something new, to be away from the services) and also help to generate change.

What proposal should be prepared for presentation to experts by experience that want to join?

We need to explain why we would like to involve experts by experience in research. Once the decision to involve them has been made, a clear outline of the process and cooperation including training programme should be prepared and presented to experts by experience.

A genuine dialogue and trust needs to be developed if we want to capture the diversity of knowledge as a source of richness in understanding the perspective of life experience of service users, leading to a new formulation of 'social problems'.

However, the main problem that emerged was their lack of confidence in the research process. I have therefore set up a training programme with the aim of helping to increase confidence through training programmes. We also need to know that training programmes are not enough. We need to ensure that users are supported during the whole research process.

Training programme

Ramon (2003) stated, the research cannot be of high quality, if the researchers are insufficiently prepared to carry it out. Researchers need to be aware that 'professional researchers' are usually employed to do the research. They are skilled in their work. With this in mind, I prepared and developed the training programme for experts by experience; it was supported and led by me and one of the experts by experience. The training was divided into three parts. The first part of the training programme was an introduction (who we are; why they would like to do the research; our expectations. The second part included information about the research and a clarification of the purpose of the research, as well as a discussion on roles, responsibilities and ethical issues. The third part of the education programme addressed how field work is to be conducted, including actual examples (how to initiate an interview; self-presentation; handling difficult situations; listening; writing up). A lot of the time was devoted to self-presentation, to questions about handling difficult situations and to listening skills, writing up and dealing with one's own emotions. (Videmšek, 2009, p. 182).

Setting up research design

Who decided what the research is going to be is a key question of power and is also a question of funding. McLaughlin (2009) pointed out that involving service users in research is often written as if there were no costs and this is patently not the case. He said that involving service users in research is not a cost neutral situation and both those who are championing this approach, and those seeking to use it, need to first consider the implication of their choices, both in terms of benefits and costs (McLaughlin, 2009, p. 35). Our research was not financed and was done for educational purposes. During the research, I was able to cover the experts by experience travel costs and offer them some refreshment during the meetings. Beresford and Rose (2009) pointed out that one of the sharpest expressions of the inequalities of power affecting service users research is their unequal access to finding support (Beresford & Rose, 2009, p. 19).

It is not useful, however, that the academic researcher set out a precise proposal especially if we want to have joint research with a lot of apparent scope for expert by experience involvement. Our study came about directly as a result of expert by experience in the field of mental health interest about living in the group home. The topic was obviously relevant to them. The training programme helped every one of us to be involved in discussing the research design.

Doing the research and support during the interviewing

If we want experts by experience doing the research, we need to ensure supervision during the research process. Several reports have noted that practical, emotional and research support are critical ingredients of success (Delman & Lincoln, 2005; Faulkner, 2009; McLaughlin, 2009). McLaughlin (2009) suggested that during the research the lead researcher should also be sensitive to the needs of both service users co-researcher's and respondent's discomfort. (McLaughlin, 2009, p. 58). I ensured that we have regular group supervision and have been available for individual supervision when someone needs it during the research process.

Analysis

Experts by experience should also be involved in analysis. Although the type of data analysis may be fixed, the interpretations of data may vary considerably depending on who is doing the interpreting, since tables of data rarely come with their own explanations and no interpretation is value-free.

Working with different interpretations of the same data may provide new evidence and exciting lines of investigation, which had not been obvious at the beginning of the study.

Writing up the results, papers

If we want to ensure, that experts by experience have control over the whole process of the research, they should be supported also for writing up the results. In our investigation, we spent quite a lot of time on this discussion. We debated as to whether the expert by experience researcher wished to write the report and who would take the lead on that. Eventually, it was agreed that one expert by experience will start the write up and the rest of us will help. Not all of the research team wanted to participate at that stage. However, it was agreed in the group that all the names of researchers would be written on the report.

Dissemination

Research results are often disseminated in lengthy documents. Delmar and Lincoln (2005) demonstrated that research findings are more likely to have a policy impact if written up as brief summaries and without jargon and/or delivered orally. The involvement of experts by experience in dissemination is essential so that information is presented in an easily accessible and relevant form and any queries are addressed in an appropriate way. Research 'subjects' are often the last people to know the results of investigations in which they have participated, and are frequently left feeling used and unclear about how the research they have participated in will influence the practice.

The dissemination of research findings generally occurs in journals and during academic conference presentations. These usually have an impact only on a relatively small number of readers who are research-oriented. Dissemination occurred on a number of occasions. One member of the expert by experience research group attended several Gamian-Europe conferences. Experts by experience who have participated in research design, data collection and analysis, were in an excellent position to explain the research findings in a clear and thoughtful way. The most important dissemination for experts by experience was delivered at the Congress of Social Work in Slovenia.

Sustainability

Sustainability is demanding because such an involvement requires a continuation of the participatory process. In our case, experts by experience continued to be involved in research. Experts designed their own user led research. They managed to obtain funding for their own research from Ljubljana Municipality (2009). In user led research, they explored employment conditions for people with mental health difficulties. In 2010 the same group led their own research on living conditions for people with mental health difficulties (Videmšek, 2014).

Although I outline many advantages that are claimed for user involvement in research, their involvement is not without pitfalls.

Barriers to expert by experience involvement in research

Involvement of experts by experience in research also has some limitations or pitfalls. Rose (2009) pointed out that some criticisms revolve around the idea that user research is subjective, anecdotal and carried out by people over-involved in what they are doing. Such criticism is a counter-point to how mainstream researchers conceive what they are doing. That is, that their research is objective, produces ontological truths and that the position of science is neutral. Beresford and Boxall (2015) added that expert by experience research is still not seen as passing the test of positivist research.

Another criticisms lies in losing the objectivity of the research and its critical distance. People with experience are likely to have been or remain involved in practice and bring a greater awareness of the 'angry words' or feeling, but the question is how objective are they? How objective can people with experience that are living in the same circumstance be? Are they concerned with their interest or are they interested in social change? Participatory user led research seems to be too partisan and lacking objectivity and can be criticised as utopian, as relying on rational consensus and as being naive about group processes.

Barriers can also be dual relationship. In experts by experience research, we should think of the concept of dual relationship. We can understand double relationships as interconnection between different roles that people play (leader of self-help group, resident of group home, past resident of institution, etc.). A danger in this kind of relationship is in the risk of exploitation of the position. It is clearly known that experts by experience are very vulnerable and may have faced many traumas that happened to them over their lifecourse. We cannot assume that if someone is expert by experience in the field of mental health, they will necessarily be a good researcher. We need to be mindful of whether an expert by experience will necessarily be a good researcher.

Another potential drawback of participatory user research is its preoccupation for equalising of power between professional researchers and user researchers. The question is how we can ensure equality if inequality exists in the research (payment could be one of the unequal parameters), but this is the debate that is relevant for all research approaches that strive for participation of marginalised groups and needs to be discussed further.

Conclusion

The aim of this article was to present how students of social work can learn from the first hand experiences about different types of research and recognise how experts by experience knowledge can be a valued contribution to changing existing social services (Beresford & Rose, 2009; McLaughlin, 2009; Powell, 2009; Ramon, 2003). Going back to the beginning of the article, we were asked to consider whether we can perceive differences between experts by experience research and a trained researcher (trained student). The article leads towards the answer that yes, we can see the differences in involving service users in research and the experiment identified above has implications for social work education. Students recognised the value of experts by experience research and the place of first-hand experience as a source of knowledge. As Beresford (2009) notes, such experimental knowledge is seen as having key importance in survivor research (Beresford, 2009, p. 13). Students learned the importance of the experts by experience standpoint, that those who have been recipients of services have a different standpoint and produce 'different truths' as noted by Rose (2009, p. 41). From this experience, it can be shown that students can recognise the power imbalance between different researchers - experts by experience and academic researchers. This can be acknowledged through the different statuses that researchers have (paid/unpaid, high/low status in society). The students learned that experts by experience research is challenging and also valuable, not only for researchers but for the social services in general. They have learned that seeing experts by experience as only deficits or 'with problems' is a major cultural obstacle, which prevents the development of service users' involvement in research (Ramon, 2003). In the article I have highlighted some of the reasons why experts by experiences are getting involved in research.

Methodologically, without the inclusion of experts by experience, post-modern concepts of social work which are reflected in solution co-creation, the ethics of participation and power perspective, would be only abstract theories about social work rather than theories for social work. Experts by experience research contributes to the development of theory, values and practice that is based on the assertion that the integration of theory and practice will come from the contribution of both experts by experience alongside professionals knowledge (Powell, 2009).

Notes

1. An expert by experience is someone with experience of using social services now or in the past (read more about this in Haaster & Koster, 2007; McLaughlin, 2009). In our case experts by experience have been people who use services and who have done so in the past. I am very aware that an expert by experience can have a double identity (being a student and service user, or, academic and service user).

2. Expert by experience knowledge is in the literature also described as experimental or direct knowledge, as lived experience and as from experts by experience. The key point lies in the fact that people are experienced and it is learned from personal experience. This is not to deny the existence or validity of professionals' knowledge or the fact that they are based on direct experience. It means first-hand experience and reflection.

Disclosure statement

No potential conflict of interest was reported by the author.

References

Ajduković, M. (2008). Vloga doktorskega študija pri razvoju socialnega dela [The role of doctoral studies in the development of social work as a profession]. *Socialno delo, 47*, 269–279.

Arnstein, S. R. (1969). A ladder of citizen participation. *Journal of the American Institute of Planners, 35*, 216–224. Retrieved from http://lithgow-schmidt.dk/sherry-arnstein/ladder-of-citizen-participation.html

Ausubel, D. P. (1968). *Educational psychology: A cognitive view*. New York, NY: Holt, Rinehart and Winston.

Barnes, M. (1993). Introducing new stakeholders – User and researcher interests in evaluative research. A discussion of methods used to evaluate the birmingham community care special action project. *Policy and Politics, 21*, 47–58.

Beresford, P., & Boxall, K. (2015). Where do service user's knowledge sit in relation to professional and academic understanding of knowledge? In P. Staddon (Ed.), *Mental health service users in research* (pp. 69–87). Bristol: Policy Press.

Beresford, P., & Rose, D. (2009). Background. In A. Sweeney, P. Beresford, A. Faulkner, M. Nettle, & D. Rose (Eds.), *This is survivor research* (pp. 11–22). Herefordshire: PCCS BOOKS Rose- on Wye.

Beresford, P. (2000). Service user' knowledge and social work theory. *British Journal of Social Work, 30*, 489–503.

Beresford, P. (2001). Social work and social care: The struggle for knowledge. *Educational Action Research, 9*, 243–351.

Čačinovič Vogrinčič, G. (2002). Koncept delovnega odnosa v socialnem delu [Concept of working relationship in social work]. *Socialno delo, 41*, 91–96. Ljubljana: Fakulteta za socialno delo.

Čačinovič Vogrinčič, G. (2015). Researching co-created processes of help using the new language of social work. In D. Zaviršek (Ed.), *Re-visioning social work with individuals, collectives and communities: Social work research: Program book & book of abstracts* (p. 253). Ljubljana: Fakulteta za socialno delo. Retrieved from http://eswra.org/documents/ECSWR2015_book.pdf

Delman, J., & Lincoln, A. (2005). Service users as paid researchers. In J. Wallcraft, B. Schrank, & M. Amering (Eds.), *Handbook of service user involvement in mental health research* (pp. 139–153). Chichester, West Sussex: OxWiley Blackwell.

Evans, C., & Fisher, M. (1999). Users controlled research and empowerment. In W. Shera & L. Wells (Eds.), *Empowerment practice in social work: Developing richer conceptual foundation* (pp. 348–356). Toronto: Canadien Scholars' Press.

Faulkner, A. (2009). A rough guide to getting started. In A. Sweeney, P. Beresford, A. Faulkner, M. Nettle, & D. Rose (Eds.), *This is survivor research* (pp. 120–131). Herefordshire: PCCS BOOKS Rose- on Wye.

Glaser, B. G., & Strauss, A. L. (1967). *The discovery of grounded theory: Stategies fro qualitative research.* New York, NY: Aldine de Gruyter.

Haaster, van H., & Koster, Y. (2007). Philosophy of curriculum. In H. van Haaster (Ed.), *Training programme for people with experience in the mental health crisis to work as a trainer and peer supporter.* Retrieved from http://www.ex-in.info/produkte2.php?WEBYEP_DI=5.EX IN_Modules_Curriculum_engl.pdf file

Humphries, B. (2001, March 23–25). Putting participative research into practice. *Care Plan.*

Humphries, B. (2009). Critical social work research. In R. Adams, L. Dominelli, & M. Payne (Eds.), *Practising social work in a complex world* (pp. 308–321). Hampshire: Palgrave, Macmillan.

Lamovec, T. (1995). *Ko rešitev postane problem in zdravilo postane strup: Nove oblike skrbi za osebe v duševni krizi*. [When solution becomes a problem and the medicament becomes a poison: New forms of support for people in mental crisis]. Ljubljana: Lumi. Repinted 2006 by Fakulteta za socialno delo.

Maglajlić, R. A. (2007). *Cross National Co-operative inquiry of social work education in England and Bosnia and Hercegovina* (Doctoral disertation). Anglia Ruskin University, England.

Mayer, J., & Timms, N. (1970). *The client speaks: Working class impressions of casework*. London: Routledge.

McLaughlin, H. (2006). Involving young service users as co-researchers: Possibilities, benefits and costs. *British Journal of Social Work, 36*, 1395–1410.

McLaughlin, H. (2009). What's in a name: 'Client', 'patient', 'customer', 'consumer', 'expert by experience', 'service user' – what's next? *British Journal of Social Work, 39*, 1101–1117.

McLaughlin, H. (2015). Alternative futures for service user involvement in research. In P. Staddon (Ed.), *Mental health service users in research. Critical sociological perspectives* (pp. 153–169). Bristol: Policy Press.

Mesec, B. (1998). *Uvod v kvalitativno raziskovanje v socialnem delu* [Introduction to qualitative research in social work]. Ljubljana: Fakulteta za socialno delo.

Miles, B. M., & Huberman, A. M. (1994). *Qualitative data analysis. An expanded sourcebook*. Thousand Oaks, CA: SAGE.

Novak, J. D., & Gowin, D. B. (1984). *Learning how to learn*. New York, NY: Cambridge University Press.

Oliver, M. (1992). Changing the social relations of research production? *Disability, Handicap & Society, 7*, 101–114.

Ostrer, C., & Morris, B. (2009). First-hand experiences of different approaches to collaborative research. In A. Sweeney, P. Beresford, A. Faulkner, M. Nettle, & D. Rose (Eds.), *This is survivor research* (pp. 71–82). Herefordshire: PCCS BOOKS Rose- on Wye.

Powell, J. (2009). Developing social work research. In R. Adams, L. Dominelli, & M. Payne (Eds.), *Practising social work in a complex world* (pp. 321–330). Hampshire: Palgrave, Macmillan.

Ramon, S. (2000). Participative mental health research: Users and professional researchers working together. *Mental Health Care, 3*, 224–228.

Ramon, S. (2003). User research: Reflection and Action. In S. Ramon (Ed.), *Users researching health and social care: An empowering agenda* (pp. 11–26). Birmingham, AL: Venture Press.

Reason, P. (1994). *Human inquiry*. London: Macmillan.

Rose, D. (2001). *Users' voices: The perspectives of mental health service users on community and hospital care*. London: The Sainsbury Centre for Mental Health.

Rose, D. (2009). So what is Survivor research? In A. Sweeney, P. Beresford, A. Faulkner, M. Nettle, & D. Rose (Eds.), *This is survivor research* (pp. 38–44). Herefordshire: PCCS BOOKS Rose- on Wye.

Thompson, N. (2002). Social movements, social justice and social work. *British Journal of Social Work, 32*, 711–722.

Videmšek, P. (2009). From the Margin to the centre: Service users as researchers in social work practice. In V. Leskošek (Ed.), *Theories and methods of social work. Exploring different perspectives* (pp. 179–194). Ljubljana: Fakulteta za socialno delo.

Videmšek, P. (2011). Vpliv družbenih gibanj na razvoj socialnega dela v Sloveniji [Role of user's movement in changing control of expert by experience]. *Socialno delo, 52*, 129–138. Ljubljana: Fakulteta za socialno delo.

Videmšek, P. (2014). From definition to action: Empowerment as a tool for change in social work practice. In A. L. Matthies & L. Uggerhøj (Eds.), *Participation, marginalization and welfare services : Concepts, politics and practices across European countries* (pp. 63–76). Farnham: Burlington, Ashgate.

Wiltshire and Swindon Users Network (1996). *I am in control: Research into user's views of the wiltshire independent living fund*. Devizes: WCCUIN.

Winter, R., & Munn-Giddings, C. (2001). *A handbook for action research in health and social care*. London: Routledge.

Zaviršek, D., & Videmšek, P. (2009). Service users involvement in research and teaching: Is there place for it in Eastern European social work. *Ljetopis socialnog rada, 16*, 189–207. Zagreb.

From service-user to social work examiner: not a bridge too far

Hilda Loughran and Gary Broderick

ABSTRACT
The engagement of service-users in social work education has now become a recognised and accepted imperative. There are various ways in which this engagement can be formulated. This paper will address one such area that of developing a meaningful role for service-users in the assessment of social work learning. In partnership with a drugs rehabilitation centre in Dublin and University College Dublin (UCD), the authors worked with service-users in developing a curriculum and assessment method for a module on a Masters of Social Work programme. This paper describes how mixed-method research approach was used to engage both service-users and students in exploring and evaluating the assessment process. Both participant groups gave their informed consent to participate in focus groups, assignments, feedback and reflection activities. The findings indicated that service-users were keen to influence the way that social workers carried out assessments, and that social work students were, in turn, influenced by these views. The paper concludes with an appeal for such participatory approaches to social work education and learning where service-users can play meaningful roles in the important areas of student learning.

Introduction

Across a number of national and international contexts, progress has been made in recognising the important role of service-users in social work education. In the UK, this theme has become formalised in the requirements for professional social work and social care programmes (General Social Care Council [GSCC], 2012). Not so in Ireland. In fact the National Strategy for Service User Involvement in Health Services (2008) did not specify the inclusion of social work. While this might be seen to pose a risk that service-users would be less significant in social work education, in practice this is not the case. The imperative for inclusion of service-users in the Irish social work system is drawn from the Code of Practice guidelines of the Social Work Registration Board (CORU, 2010) and a commitment to these guidelines by programme providers. Gupta and Blewett (2008) and Smith et al. (2012) have discussed the challenges of engaging service-users in education. Concerns have been voiced that engagement may be tokenistic (Beresford & Boxall, 2012;

McLaughlin, 2010). As a result, many researchers may find it difficult to gather evidence to justify the inclusion of service-users in policy and practice (Taylor & Le Riche, 2006). The overall picture of service-user involvement in the education process appears to emphasise their role in informing students of the service-user perspective and in some cases playing a part in selecting prospective students. The terms service and user will be hyphenated in this article to emphasis the integrated use of the terms in this context and to avoid any misleading connotations that might be associated with the term user. Loughran and McCann (2015) in considering the state of knowledge in this area reiterated the concern identified by Beresford and Boxall (2012) that participation of service-users in research should be addressed if participation is to be achieved. Among the recommendations proposed by Duffy (2008, p. 14) was the call to develop an agreed definition of service-user and to find more creative ways of involving them. This question of defining service-user as a concept was also identified by McLaughlin (2009) and this problem informs the analysis of data collected from the current study.The idea that service-users have a role in assessment has been, to some extent, established more specifically in relation to assessment of practice placements. Edwards (2003) in reviewing this role for service-users, found much support for service-user's feedback. Included in this were suggestions about clarifying service-users understanding about student access to their comments. Edwards (2003, p. 345) also found that it was useful to maintain a separation between the task of providing feedback and that of assigning grades. This initiative adopted this separation focusing on developing a vehicle for feedback not grading. In discussing meaningful service-user involvement in social work education, the idea emerged that it would be interesting to create an opportunity for service-users to act in the role of examiners. This was informed by Edwards (2003) distinction between grading and feedback and Yorke's ideas of formative assessment. Yorke (2003, p. 479) noted that formative assessment can be provided by anyone and that it can be very occasional, yet still embody the essential supportiveness towards student learning.

Background to the study

The study now described had its origins in a collaborative initiative led by the university and drug prevention agency. Its key aim was to engage service-users in the assessment of a social work and addictions module delivered on a Masters in Social Work programme. This article describes the assessment initiative and present the findings from the research conducted to track the initiative. It will follow through with an analysis of the findings and consideration of the implications for enhancing service-user's engagement in assessment in social work education.

Before introducing the service-led assessment the Director of the SAOL Project (a support service for women with drug use issues) in conjunction with the university lecturer agreed to design and deliver the module. SAOL is committed to education and inclusiveness and was very enthusiastic about developing the assessment initiative. The Director checked to see if service-users would be interested. To support the initiative SAOL were prepared to provide any additional counselling or support that engagement with this project might demand and this was an important condition for research ethical approval. The already established partnership between the service and the university lecturer and the direct involvement of the Director of the service in the provision of the module greatly facilitated the process.

Following discussion it was agreed that conducting research on the process would provide much needed insight into expanding the role of service-users to incorporate an examining activity. Service-users themselves wanted the process to be recorded in some way. It was their view that writing about their involvement might have a better chance of influencing social work education into the future, and most of them were motivated to help social workers to understand drug use and the impact on service-users.

From the students' perspective, they were very familiar with reflective practice and the idea that 'through reflection as social workers we can change how we think, feel and behave to better meet the needs of service-users and carers' (Knott & Scragg, 2013, p. 54). This reflective approach was viewed as particularly important in light of the suggestion by Nelson (2012, p. 26) that social workers may find anti-discriminatory practice can be 'especially tricky if working with service uses who engage in illegal activities, like drug taking'. This concern makes reaching this often marginalised population of stabilising drug users all the more important. It can be challenging, and research on drug using parents confirms that there is limited evidence representing their views (Galvani, 2012, p. 93). This, in conjunction with concerns that social workers may feel a sense of inadequacy when working with drug use issues (Loughran, Hohman, & Finnegan, 2010) underpinned this initiative.

Methodology

This research was designed to provide data on the process of including service-users in an examining role in social work education over a two-year period on a social work masters module on social work and addiction. It sought to capture what that experience was like for students and service-users as well as the lecturers who had co-designed the module with the service-users. The research was not about the experience of the service-user as a service-user, but rather about their experience of contributing in this role to social work education. For the purposes of this research, no identifying information about students or service-users was necessary and only a summary profile to contextualise the data will be provided. The project had ethical approval from the lead author's Research Ethics Committee.

The service-user group changed over the two years. The first group had (n = 14) participants and the second group had (n = 13) aged from 19 to 43 with a median age of 29. Their involvement with the service ranged from 4 weeks to 22 months, three women participated in both years of the project. All but one has a history of opiate use and were on methadone and had some involvement with social work. Abstinence from street drugs is not a pre-requisite for engagement with SAOL and so was not a pre-requisite for involvement in this research but none of the service-users were under the influence of illicit drugs on the days they were engaged in this work. In the second cohort of service-users one of the group members chose not to participate in the activity. In gaining consent it was made clear to service-users that involvement was totally voluntary and that there would be no repercussions in choosing not to be involved. The number of service-users who attended varied from group to group but in each case at least two service-users and one staff or module provider sat in on the process of writing student feedback.

The two cohorts totalled n = 95 students of whom n = 64 (67%) participated in the research. Ages ranged from 22 to 36 years and 44 years respectively, with a median age for both of 26 years. Consistent with the gender profile of student social workers (Pease, 2011, p. 406) 12.5% of participants were male.

Study instruments and fieldwork

Both students and service-users were made aware that the purpose of the research was to advance understanding of service-user engagement in social work education. The letter assignment and the reflection statement would not impact on student grades nor would there be any impact on provision of service to the service-user.

Students' experience of the process was tracked by gathering data from: (1) a letter written to the fictional woman service-user in the case, 'Martha', which was additional to the essay assignment where they addressed a case on alcohol and drug related problems as designed by service-users, (2) a reflective statement on feedback on their work from the service-users, (3) class discussion. The research audited students' reaction to the feedback from service-users on how they addressed the issues in the case study by gathering the reflective statements from students.

Data regarding service-users' were gathered by recording, (1) discussion about the idea of engaging in social work education and the process of designing the case study for assessment, (2) discussion with service-users as they read the letters and decided on the feedback, (3) the written feedback to students, (4) focus group following the completion of the feedback task. Service-users decided that they would read the letters and give written feedback to each student. It was not part of the original plan that service-users would come in to meet students in person so this was not included in the research plan.

In relation to student information ethical approval directed that any additional research elements of the project had to be voluntary and separate from the module required assignment. This meant that we had access to all the letters submitted by students but submission of the reflections was voluntary.

A two track research methodology employed in this study is illustrated below. In this model the practice base that supported the education and research activity was viewed as an essential foundation to the process (Figure 1).

The two track module highlights the parallel steps in the design and implementation of the education initiative and the research of that initiative. It implies that from inception to completion activities around the research should be synchronised with the curriculum and assessment, in this case social work and addiction module. This model can be adapted to support other types of service user engagement.

Thematic analysis was employed. It is a method for identifying, analysing and reporting patterns (themes) within data (Braun & Clarke, 2006, p. 79). Data were read and reread to assist in identifying recurring themes from the written feedback of service-users and students' reflective statements. Themes were verified with service-users and through focus group and class discussion.

The assignment case

The service-users worked with the module providers in designing a case study which formed the basis of examining students in the module. Students would be assessed on writing an essay outlining the key issues in the case, discussing their intervention strategy and writing a letter to the service-user in the case. The module providers would assess the essay and assign a grade while the service-users' feedback was part of the formative assessment of the module.

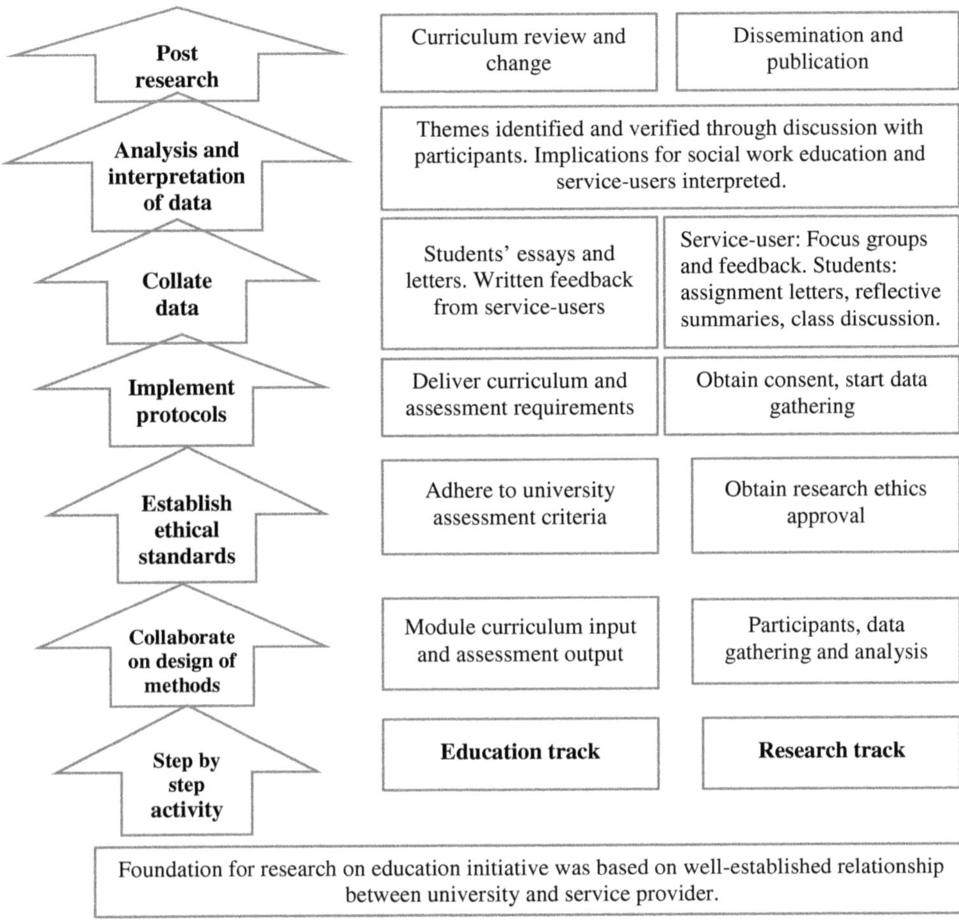

Figure 1. A step by step two track education and research service-user engagement methodology model.

The development of the case study itself raised many challenges for the module providers and the service-users which will be discussed later. The case, in brief, concerned Martha who was in early stages of dealing with her drug use, was on a relatively high dose of methadone, and was still providing some urine samples with traces of benzodiazepines and cannabis. She was having problems dealing with her teenage son, Jonathon. The involvement of the social worker was triggered when Jonathon over-doses on methamphetamine and is hospitalised. The police inform Martha and assess her to be under the influence of alcohol while in charge of her other two children. They remove the children from her care, giving them to their maternal grandmother. The children are returned to Martha shortly afterwards conditional on social work involvement. Martha is attending SAOL but is not keen to engage in a parenting support group which was recommended.

Findings

All the students in both cohorts (cohort 1 (n = 47) and cohort 2 (n = 48)) submitted the required assignment, essay plus letter. In the first cohort 23 students participated in the research by submitting reflections $n = 21$ (48%). This low response may have been due to delays in getting the feedback to students and attempting to gather the reflections in the last week of the semester. Improved timing of feedback and request for reflections and students positive views about the assignment from the previous year may have influenced the response of the second cohort as ($n = 41$) 85% submitted their reflective statements.

In both years, service-users spent up to five hours reading the letters and writing feedback. This in addition to 3–4 mornings spent on; finding out about the research, designing the case study and participating in discussions meant that engaging with the work took a lot of time and energy. Service-users reported that they enjoyed the process but did not like the repetitive nature of reading letters that had similar content. They also commented on the emotional response they had to the letters, for example feeling annoyed with some the assumptions made or being worried or sad for someone in that position. Many said they had received letters from social workers in the past; indeed most were still engaged with social workers and all their involvement was rooted in child protection issues. The service-users in year one requested to meet the students after the assignment was completed and the year two service-users did likewise. They wanted to meet the students so that they could talk to them face to face. The women felt this would help students to understand the impact they have on families and how important it is social workers to really listen to service users.

In year one two service-users came to talk to the students and in year two six visited the university. The smaller numbers who made the first visit may have reflected the time constraints as the visit happened on a day they were not on the SAOL programme. Even though the service-users initiated the meeting with students the actual visit raised some anxiety for the service-users. They were unfamiliar with the campus environment and most of them had no experience of talking to student groups. The stability of the group in terms of confidence and or relapse issues might also have been a factor. It is important to pay attention to these issues when asking active service-users to become engaged in activities such as research or contributing to education and training.

Developing the case

From the process of developing the case and subsequent discussion with service-users a number of themes emerged. These related to; the development of the case, the influences of their own experiences of social work and social care services and their stage of recovery from drug and or alcohol use.

The service-users worked with the Director to develop a case based on the service-users' ideas. The case they developed told the story of a women they called Martha who had a history of opiate use. Martha was engaged in the SAOL service and was stable on methadone. She had three sons aged 14 to 3 whom she was caring for with support from her mother. The case as initially presented had Martha overcoming her problems except that the social workers were still 'on her case'. The service-users focused on trying to get the social worker to accept that all was now OK and to let Martha get on with her life.

When module providers reviewed the case they realised that its focus was significantly different than that of the overall information contained in the module. The module adopted a risk and resilience framework and encouraged students to engage in assessment that looked at risk factors but also evaluated protective factors/resilience. This is in line with Allan's assertion (2014, p. 100) that although a person's problems need to be identified 'it is the positive elements in his life, his personal and environmental capital, which will support changed behaviour'. What became clear following the review of the first draft of the case was that the module curriculum addressed the risk aspects of drug use because it was felt that students needed this information. We had anticipated that the service-users would also want students to understand these dynamics. However, discussion with service-users revealed that their main concern was that social workers were not trained to recognise when service-users were doing well. So although the lectures espoused risk and resilience principles it may not have focused on recovery as much as service-users wanted.

To be consistent with the curriculum and address students' need to learn about assessment of drug use issues further discussion with service-users resulted in agreement to look at an earlier stage in Martha's life when it was more likely that she would have encountered social work services for the first time. The service-users agreed that they wanted to have a say in how Martha was treated from the outset and so amended the case to reflect this, having been given reassurances that we now appreciated that what we wanted to teach the students was not necessarily what they wanted students to learn. The next draft of the case allowed for development of an earlier intervention but also underlined the need to take account of the service-users' concerns. The implications of this will be discussed later.

Service-users' feedback to students

Service-user feedback on the letters was varied. A summary of key points was agreed with service-users from both cohorts and presented to the students in each of the years so that all could benefit from receiving the overall feedback in addition to each student received individual comments on their letter. The service-users offered constructive feedback and wanted to be as positive and encouraging as possible to the students. Table 1 provides a summary of the key points of feedback for both years identifying what the service-users liked about the content of the letters. It was decided to attempt to capture as broad a picture as possible rather than tabulate frequency as all comments are valuable.

Table 2 provides a summary of the key points of feedback for both years itemising what the service-users did not like about the content of the letters.

As can be seen in the tables, there was some disagreement among service-users on some points but overall across the two years, there was constant mention of some issues. A

Table 1. What service-users liked in the students' letters year one and year two.

Year one feedback	Year two feedback
• Clear introductions where role of social worker was explained and where there were contact details • The use of 'we' rather than 'I' • Recognition by the social worker of the positive things Martha was doing, but only if they were real • Ideas presented as possibilities not already formed plans • Acknowledgement that work needed to be done but also that Martha was trying • Shorter letters ... indicating that there would be consultation before deciding anything and safeguarding against anyone else reading their information • Very empathic and reassuring • Use of childrens' names • Expressions of concern for Jonathan • Including Martha's mother	• Enough information to know what was going to happen • Emphasis on working with service-user as a team • Positive but realistic • Good to know there would be a care plan agreed • Some mention of what they knew about Martha and where they got that information • Suggestion of meeting Jonathan and Martha together at some stage • Talk about supporting Martha • Making time to meet that would work for Martha

number of other points were discussed in both class and service-user groups including the issue of domestic violence which although inferred in the case was not commented on by students in the letter and by only one service-user in the feedback. This has implications for teaching social workers about dealing with domestic violence and drug use which will require further investigation.

Students' reflective summaries

Students' guidance for the reflective summary was to address the following: their thoughts about having service-users involved in this way; what if anything they learned that was different from other assignments; what was their reflection on the feedback they received; any other comments. The reflective statements were analysed and themes were identified across both cohorts of students. Table 3 presents a summary of the information from students' reflections on the feedback. The numerical value in the table represents the number of times that theme was mentioned.

Students' reflections varied in length and content. The numbers on the table indicate how many students referred to that specific theme. In cohort two, a number of students 24% ($n = 10$) commented on the usefulness of developing letter writing skills and some 15% ($n = 6$) took the opportunity to give general feedback on the module with little reference to their reflections regarding the interaction with service-users.

Some examples of specific reflections in first cohort of students: it helped me to identify gaps in my knowledge; made me realise I need to be more collaborative; I need to be more collaborative and not telling them what to do; it raised issues I would not have considered; gave me confidence and I think I might want to work in this field; raised my awareness of sounding judgemental. In the second cohort some examples were; using language that is collaborative is very important; the importance of not coming across as cold; some language

Table 2. What service-users did not like in year one and year two.

Year one feedback	Year two feedback
• In some grammar and spelling were bad ... did students not read over the letter? • Some incorrect information was included not in line with what they had been told about Martha • Some did not use the childrens' names or got them wrong which did not show respect • No introduction or intimidating or threatening introduction ... such as I am the Senior Social Worker • Use of 'I' not 'we' • Too official • Some sense of letter being judgemental • Too positive where social worker did not even know Martha well enough to know if it was true. Patronising if too friendly • Did not like the use of some words e.g.'despite', 'however'	• Where grammar and spelling were bad, it was demeaning • Incorrect information about what actually happened • Not personal enough • Too detailed, if it fell into the wrong hands • Not understanding the urine analysis e.g. showing prescription drugs • Too positive, patronising ... too much • Using authority figures e.g. referring to the Department (childrens' services) or the police was intimidating. One person against a whole department • Including comments like parenting capacity • Use of words e.g. collaboratively, biological, psychological, social-environmental, systemic, fortnight instead of two weeks. • Suggesting meeting son without his mother was not on • Expecting son to do all sorts of activities e.g. youth club, sports club when he won't even go to school • Having lists of possible thing Martha could do or could get involved in • Too short: like set letter. Too vague: don't know what's happening. Too detailed: decisions all made. Too official • Some judgemental tone • Appointments clashing with school • Use of 'chat' instead of 'meeting' or 'discuss'

Table 3. Student reflections themes and the number of students who raised the theme in their reflective commentary in each cohort.

Themes	Cohort one (n = 23) (%)	Cohort two (n = 41) (%)
Beneficial to have engagement with service-users	91	44
Specifically mentioned feedback was helpful	61	51
Increased awareness of use of language	35	15
Need to consider service-user e.g. be sensitive/respectful/ empathic	30	22
Found it practical/realistic	22	20
Helped ability to reflect	22	
Good opportunity for service-user to express their views	17	5
Were happy with grade and feedback	17	
Helped to emphasise need for collaboration	17	7
Found it artificial	13	
Increased awareness of power issues	9	
'Opened my eyes'	9	
More aware of confidentiality		15
Want more of this type of exercise		32

Note: The number of students who mentioned each theme is represented as a percentage of the total number of participants in each cohort.

used by social workers may be considered as normal but offensive to service-users; good to get service-user genuine feedback helps to empathise with them.

Although the first cohort had fewer respondents overall, they tended to focus more on reflecting on what they got from the experience. The response rate was increased with the second cohort by providing time for them to complete the reflective statement but this may have had the effect of including some who were less engaged in the process while in the first cohort those who responded had to make more of an effort to submit their reflections.

Discussion

What do we mean by service-user?

The experience of doing this research has led the authors to re-engage with the debate about the term 'service-user'. Any attempt to treat 'service-users' as a single, homogenous group is very unhelpful. In this instance it was found useful to distinguish between those who use social work services and those who felt that service was imposed on them. Most of the service-users had perception that social work was imposed and this had implications for the process, in particular the need to provide support during and after the process of reading and responding to the letters. Indeed, service-users processed their own feelings about social workers during the exercise and in thinking through how they would give feedback to the students. Despite some negative emotions regarding social work most of the service-users were concerned that the students might find the challenging or negative remarks disturbing. This led to a request to meet the students face to face. This was not originally planned but proved to be very impactful for both students and service-users. It also has led us to consider the need to develop further meaningful and manageable engagement with service-users across a range of experiences. It may be relatively easy to access service-users who have long standing and positive relationships with social work and social care services. In some cases service-users may not be just using the service but may have requested or invited engagement with the services. These service-users offer a distinctly different perspective than those who feel the service is imposed or who are in an early stage of dealing with their difficulties yet the views of all are equally important.

This research highlighted the ongoing debate as discussed by McLaughlin (2009) about what we mean by service-user. Does the term allow for distinctions between different stages of service use? Can we expect the same engagement for people who are currently dealing with crisis intervention by social workers rather than those who have long term established relationships with social workers and social care services or indeed are no longer actively using the service? This project highlighted some emotional and sometimes upsetting issues that can arise when asking current service-users to engage in this type of activity. However, not including service-users currently dealing with 'live' problems would undermine the integrity of the term service-user in this context. Duffy (2008) called for an agreed definition of service-users. This research identified further issues about such a definition and drew attention to describing different levels of involvement of service-users. How service-users themselves view the issue would also need to be considered. The following criteria might prove useful for social work educators when considering where service-users are situated in relation to these continua. One captures a spectrum for types of engagement with services and the second the stages of such engagement (Figure 2).

An ethical framework for service-user engagement practices

The influence of service-users own experiences came through the case they developed. Their ideas about the problems Martha had were built on their own issues as were their views of social workers. Across the two cohorts of women all but one had encountered social work services in relation to their drug or alcohol use and child care matters. Many of them had children taken into care and for some their children remained in care and were likely to

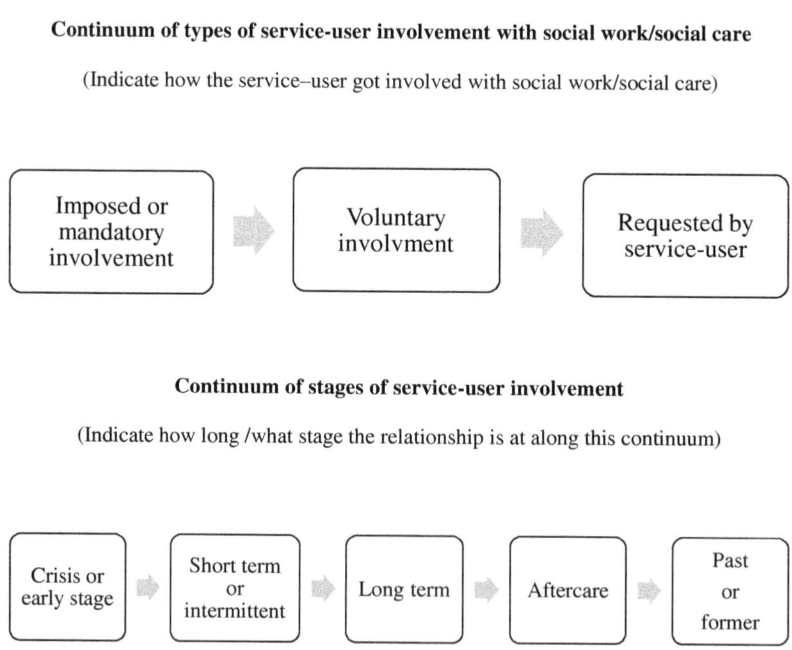

Figure 2. Defining service-user involvement with social work or social care.

do so for the foreseeable future. Some had social work involvement around other issues for example in general medical settings or their own time in foster care. The experiences outside child protection tended to be more positive and so this facilitated discussion about the varied role of social work. The case included a reference to an unsupportive and abusive partner and this too was reflective of some of their own experiences. The fact that the women were so knowledgeable about drug use, harm reduction, domestic violence and lone parenting meant that in some discussion of what they wanted social workers to know it was difficult for them to distinguish between a general standard of good practice and their own disappointment or even anger at the experiences they had with social work. The trust and confidence born of the long-standing relationship between the university lecture and the service providers were pivotal in successfully dealing with these often emotional discussions. The staff of the SAOL project were fully aware of these sessions and all service-users were asked if they needed follow-up support from their key-workers. While no one took up the option of immediate support, several discussed the session in planned key-working sessions afterwards. All spoke positively about the process while also acknowledging the sadness and anger it evoked for them. Four women spoke of their desire to use drugs after the sessions but all chose not to; in different ways all four reported that they did not want to risk their involvement in the process by taking drugs on the back of discussions. For the purposes of replicating this type of activity is worth noting that service-users availed themselves of the normal support within the service and no additional resources were required and discussions and feedback time were integrated into the educational programme of the service.

Arising from both the experiences around the visit to the university and more specifically the process of designing the case, it did become evident that the standards attached to gaining ethical approval for including service-users in research provided an invaluable guide. Research ethics demanded very details assurances for evidencing informed consent, providing additional support and acknowledging service-user vulnerability. This should include reflection by educationalists and researchers on power differentials experienced by participants. These should be instrumental in creating frameworks for defining ethical standards for service-user participation. In relation to this project, any anxiety on the part of service-users appeared to be replaced by immense pride. In both years, the women were delighted that they had represented their peers so effectively. The positive feedback they received from teaching staff and students was immensely important. There was no doubt that students benefitted and that service-users despite any upset, valued the engagement. It is important that educators provide a safe and meaningful space for this type of activity especially with service-users who may more typically have experiences of being excluded. The women involved stated that they did not feel their involvement was tokenistic a concern voiced by McLaughlin (2010).

A related theme was the importance of explaining the possible limitations of their influence. For example, service-users wondered if their current social worker would learn from their input. They became invested in helping social work students to understand drug use and their lives and wanted what they were doing to make a difference, something that we could not guarantee. An exploration of this issue continued in SAOL and led to a number of service-users making themselves available to speak at conferences and in public discussions; some moved on to SAOL Aftercare and have become involved in Peer Training programmes so that they can educate other service-users. While these actions cannot be exclusively attributed to their being involved in this research, such involvement played a part.

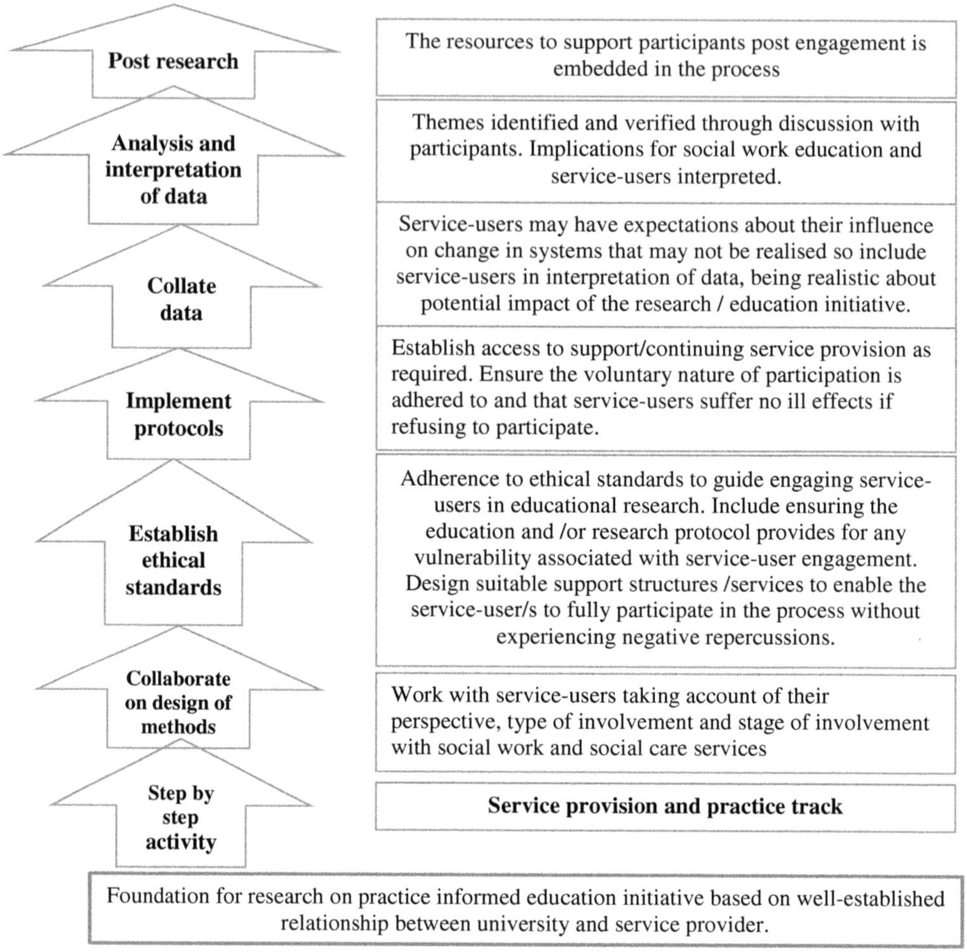

Figure 3. A step by step third track research, education and practice methodology model.

On reviewing, the process it would probably be more helpful to have designed this as a three track methodology. The addition of a third track as illustrated in Figure 3 below may help to explain some of the more complex aspects of education and practice based research as it shows the need to attend to needs of what ethical standard refers to as vulnerable participants. It underpins the importance of the research ethical standards adhered to in this research.

What educators want to teach and what service-users want social workers to learn

The themes that emerged for service-users from focus groups and their feedback revealed that what they wanted from social work was a sense of being worked with and not in Nelson's terms having social workers 'do social work to them'(2012, p. 23). Their clarity about wanting respect, empathy and sensitivity from social workers has strong resonance with what should be at the core of social work practices, building collaborative respectful relationships with service-users. They did not seem to be concerned about 'specialist' knowledge of drug use but did comment on how helpful it was that social workers were familiar with other services that might be accessed. This seems to contrast with the educators' concerns that students be knowledgeable in specialist drug use issues, in particular with regard to assessing the risks to children. As the process unfolded, this emphasis for service-users was more understandable. The service-users appeared to work from the view that 'social workers' are flawed in their understanding and therefore need help correcting their views. They read the letters from that position i.e. letters were probably going to be wrong. They did not expect to find good letters. By the end of the process though, they were more generous in their approach and stated regularly that they understood that their (social workers') job was a hard one and they had the needs of the children at the core of their work. In fact the second cohort identified 70% of the letters as being positive or good even though they felt it would be easier to deal with social workers if they paid more attention to the relationship with them as mothers who also cared about the good of their children.

The lesson that emerged from this for the educators was that in the struggle to have alcohol and drug issues recognised as essential to social work education (Dance, Galvani, & Allnock, 2016; Galvani & Allnock, 2016; Loughran et al., 2010) the importance of integrating this with core skills of relationship-building may have been under emphasised.

The educators had emphasised a risk and resilience model of assessment and yet the service-users had concerns that the focus was on risk at the expense of acknowledging the mother's attempts to deal with her problems. One might think 'that the service-users, given their close personal connection to Martha's story, may have been reluctant to be critical of her in any way. They were definitely concerned that social workers acknowledged that she was trying. This came out very clearly in designing the case initially. However, the service-users were not happy with Martha. They voiced that in the case they would have been concerned not so much about Martha having street drugs in her last urine sample but more that she was missing appointments and that in particular she was not prepared to accept parenting support. But they wanted it acknowledged that she was doing 'good enough' parenting and that she had 'good enough' recovery. They did want her to do more but empathised with her situation. They 'got' the fact that this was as good as could be expected given her current situation and that new action would need to be 'brought in' by social workers but not to expect Martha to do this by herself. The research supports Allan's (2014) acknowledgement of the importance of assessing positive elements in the lives of service-users. There needs to be further work done on applying the risk and resilience approach to drug using parents. Increased emphasis on harm reduction strategies can facilitate recognising resilience and small changes while not losing sight of substantive concerns.

Congruence between feedback and reflection

The aspiration for the education initiative was to generate a transformative change in the approach of social workers in engaging with drug using service-users. Such transformational reflection usually requires 'depth learning' (Knott & Scragg, 2013, p. 9). The analysis of the student reflective statements does provide some evidence that individual students demonstrated this deeper level of learning. Students reflected on their increased awareness of the impact of the language they use, for example recognising that mentioning authority figures might be intimidating and that use of terms such as parenting capacity might be viewed as judgemental. Students also developed an appreciation that they were perceived to be in a powerful position and that this by definition meant that service-users felt less powerful. During class discussion one student commented that from reading his feedback he felt he should apologise to the service-user. Across both cohorts of students 30 and 22% respectively highlighted that they needed to think more about being empathic, respectful and sensitive to service-users and that the exercise had assisted them in this endeavour. All these points were congruent with the feedback offered by the service-users.

What was somewhat disappointing was the number of students whose reflections consisted of appreciation for service-user input but without noting any specific learning. Almost everyone (83%) in cohort one and 44% of cohort two mentioned that the exercise was beneficial. A further 61% in cohort one and 51% of cohort two mentioned that they found the feedback helpful. However, the absence of detail in many of the reflective statements meant that it was not possible to get a sense of what these general comments mean in practice. While the value of the education initiative was confirmed by all participants the analysis of student reflection suggests that there is still much to be done in assisting students to apply reflective frameworks. Obvious changes would be making the reflective statement a requirement for the assignment and linking it to the feedback and providing follow on discussion. But there is more fundamental work to be done in assisting students to challenge themselves and in facilitating the development of the informed reflective practitioner (Knott & Scragg, 2013, p. 11) who can acknowledge their own prejudices and experiences and be informed by evidence.

This research supports the view that when appropriately engaged this service-user group have much to contribute to social work education. They can demonstrate to student social workers the importance of listening to parents, a key factor in building trusting relationships identified by Woolfall, Sumnall, and McVeigh (2008, p. 8). Further development and refinement of the process will be required to assess if that engagement has an impact on social work students in the longer term. These service-users often felt a sense of shame because of their drug use, they were rejected by family and community and felt guilty about perceived mistakes they have made. There was, therefore, tremendous excitement about being part of this process. To feel that their voice and experience could influence the way social workers of the future would meet and engage with their peers in better ways because of their involvement was hugely enticing, exciting and rewarding. Regularly service-users were to comment, 'It's great that we're doing this; other people don't get the chance'.

For further information on the SAOL Project visit: www.saolproject.i.e.

Acknowledgement

The service-users in the SAOL Project for their contribution to the research and also for their work on designing the case study, examining student's work, providing feedback and advice, and encouraging us to share their experiences by getting the work published.

Disclosure statement

No potential conflict of interest was reported by the authors.

References

Allan, G. (2014). *Working with substance users: A guide to effective interventions*. Basingstoke: Palgrave MacMillan.

Beresford, P., & Boxall, K. (2012). Service users, social work education and knowledge for social work practice. *Social Work Education, 31*, 155–167.

Braun, V., & Clarke, V. (2006). Using thematic analysis in psychology. *Qualitative Research in Psychology, 3*, 77–101.

CORU. (2010). *Code of professional conduct and ethics for social workers*. Social Workers Registration Board. Retrieved from http://coru.i.e./uploads/documents/typeset_Social_Worker_Code_Feb_2010.pdf

Dance, C., Galvani, S., & Allnock, D. (2016). The extent and nature of practitioners, encounters with alcohol and other drug use in social work and social care practice. In H. Loughran & W. Livingstone (Eds.), *Substance use in social work education and training: Preparing for and supporting practice* (pp. 5–20). Abingdon: Routledge.

Department of Health and Children & Health Service Executive. (2008). *National strategy for service user involvement in the Irish health service, 2008–2013, your service your say*. Dublin: Department of Health.

Duffy, J. (2008). *Looking out from the middle: User involvement in health and social care in Northern Ireland*. London: Social Care Institute for Excellence (SCIE). Retrieved from http://www.scie.org.uk

Edwards, C. (2003). The involvement of service users in the assessment of Diploma in social work students on practice placements. *Social Work Education, 22*, 341–349.

Galvani, S. (2012). *Supporting people with alcohol and drug problems: Making a difference*. Bristol: Policy Press.

Galvani, S., & Allnock, D. (2016). The nature and extent of substance use education in qualifying social work programmes in England. In H. Loughran & W. Livingstone (Eds.), *Substance use in social work education and training: Preparing for and supporting practice* (pp. 21–36). Abingdon: Routledge.

General Social Care Council. (2012). *General social care council: A decade of progress*. Author.

Gupta, A., & Blewett, J. (2008). Involving services users in social work training on the reality of family poverty: A case study of a collaborative project. *Social Work Education, 27*, 459–473.

Knott, C., & Scragg, T. (2013). *Reflective practice in social work*. London: Sage.

Loughran, H., Hohman, M., & Finnegan, D. (2010). Predictors of role legitimacy and role adequacy of social workers working with substance-using clients. *British Journal of Social Work, 40*, 239–256.

Loughran, H., & McCann, M. (2015). Employing community participative research methods to advance service user collaboration in social work research. *British Journal of Social Work, 45*, 705–723.

McLaughlin, H. (2009). What's in a name: 'Client', 'patient', 'customer', 'consumer', 'expert by experience', 'service user' – What's next? *British Journal of Social Work, 39*, 1101–1117.

McLaughlin, H. (2010). Keeping service user involvement in research honest. *British Journal of Social Work, 40*, 1591–1608.

Nelson, A. (2012). *Social work with substance users*. London: Sage.

Pease, B. (2011). Men in social work: Challenging or reproducing an unequal gender regime? *Affilia, 26*, 406–418.

Smith, M., Gallagher, M., Wosu, H., Stewart, J., Cree, V., Hunter, S., … Wilkinson, H. (2012). Engaging with involuntary service users in social work: Findings from a knowledge exchange project. *British Journal of Social Work, 42*, 1460–1477.

Taylor, I., & Le Riche, P. (2006). What do we know about partnership with service users and carers in social work education and how robust is the evidence base? *Health and Social Care in the Community, 14*, 418–425.

Woolfall, K., Sumnall, H., & McVeigh, J. (2008). *Addressing the needs of children of substance using parents: An evaluation of families first's intensive intervention final report*. Liverpool: Prepared for the Department of Health.

Yorke, M. (2003). Formative assessment in higher education: Moves towards theory and the enhancement of pedagogic practice. *Higher Education, 45*, 477–501.

What difference does it make? Findings of an impact study of service user and carer involvement on social work students' subsequent practice

Mel Hughes

ABSTRACT

This paper reports on a study which followed up a group of social work students to explore whether service user involvement in their education made any difference to their practice and whether there were different models or types of involvement which had a more significant impact than others. The findings showed that the impact was individual to each student. It was often specific encounters or 'light bulb moments' which led to increased awareness or insight into their own practice particularly when encountering similar situations or when pressures of practice led to them losing sight of service user perspectives. The paper shares these findings and considers the learning for educators in developing models of involvement which enhance impact on subsequent practice.

Research into service user involvement in social work education to date has focussed in many cases on evaluating specific activities or models of involvement at the time. Literature resulting from this has shown that students highly evaluate experiences which involve service users and carers; that involvement can motivate students and practitioners to implement changes to their practice in innovative ways (Khoo, McVicar, & Brandon, 2004); that involvement improves students' attitudes toward people with particular conditions or experiences (MacSporran, 2015) and can make educators reflect more deeply on the way they communicate (Perry, Gilbert, & Rawlinson, 2013). There is evidence that meaningful involvement can facilitate transformative learning (Mezirow, 2000) where students learn to critically question their own beliefs and views of the world and develop a more open and inclusive approach to their practice (Hughes, 2012; Rush, 2008). These are all outcomes which are congruent with the need for social work education to enable students to develop anti-oppressive practice and maintain professional values and standards and to prepare students for the complexities of the workplace where there may not be clear cut solutions.

From our own research at X University, we know that students value service user involvement and report it as being eye opening, humbling and inspiring to hear people's lived experiences and value their contribution to the design and delivery of their programme.

They identify how it has enabled them to relate more formal learning to their practice. In an evaluation of a first-year BA Social work unit which is service user led (Hughes, 2012) for example, one student said 'It wasn't until this unit that I really understood the importance of what we had been learning in Uni'. Members of our service user and carer partnership report that they feel listened to and feel that they are contributing to the future workforce and making a difference.

There is limited evidence however on what this difference might be. Carr (2004) for example, in a report for the Social Care Institute for Excellence (SCIE) identified that evaluations of service user involvement were more likely to focus on participation techniques, than on successful impact and outcomes. Morgan and Jones (2009) and Robinson and Webber's (2013) literature reviews (in health education and social work education, respectively) both concluded that whilst students and service users valued involvement in their education, there was little evidence in the literature of involvement changing behaviour in practice or in improving outcomes for service users. Studies which have sought to evaluate the impact on practice (MacSporran, 2015; Rush, 2008; Turnbull & Weeley, 2013), are based largely on current students and the immediate impact. A number of researchers and authors therefore continue to identify the need to develop evidence for the efficacy of different types of involvement (Robinson & Webber, 2013; Simons et al., 2006) and what impact different types of involvement has on student learning and their subsequent practice in the long term (Driessens, McLaughlin, & Van Doorn, 2016; Muir & Laxton, 2012; Rhodes, 2012; Terry, 2012; Turnbull & Weeley, 2013).

This paper reports on a study which followed up a group of social work students to explore whether service user involvement in students' education made any difference to their practice and whether there were different models or types of involvement which had a more significant impact on their practice than others.

Terminology

There is debate within the literature and in practice regarding the use of terminology for people who are the recipients of health and social work services or have a particular life experience from which students can learn. McLaughlin (2009) provides a useful critique of the most common terms and of how these represent the changing relationships within social work policy and practice (from client to consumer to service user to expert). In this paper, the terms 'service user' and 'experts by experience' are both used due to their common usage within UK policy, practice and literature and the preferences of our partnership group. It is acknowledged however that these terms are not without their problems. As McLaughlin (2009) suggests, the term service users 'neglects and denies the multiple socially constructed identities we all inhabit' whilst the term experts by experience fails to 'differentiate between the nature and types of experience'. Any term however that seeks to group together a diverse range of people and experiences will remain problematic. Attempts are made throughout this paper to provide more specific details so as not to generalise or to homogenise such a diverse group and to acknowledge the range of expertise and contributions individuals have made.

Context

The X University partnership group contributes to health and social work programmes across the Faculty of Health and Social Sciences and consists of over 90 active members (people who identify themselves as service users, carers or both). This is in addition to the contact students have with service users and carers whilst on placement; the involvement of service user-led organisations who contribute directly to teaching and assessment on social work programmes and the knowledge students draw on from their own life experiences. Our model includes service users and carers sharing experiences, expertise and insight to enable students and academics to think critically and to reflect on their personal and professional development but also moves beyond this to include people as consultants; reviewers; researchers; facilitators and assessors due to the expertise they have and the perspectives they can share. We recognise that terms such as service user, patient, carer or experts by experience will include people who are also students; practitioners, academics and professionals; people of many skills and backgrounds and multiple roles and identities. We seek to involve a wide range of people in many different ways, to reflect this diversity and to address the need identified in the literature to involve seldom heard voices (Duffy, 2013) and to explore different models and strategies to avoid tokenism (Simons et al., 2006). The types of involvement which students and graduates were asked to reflect on in this study therefore were diverse.

Methodology

The study adopted a narrative approach to seeking insight into the impact of service user involvement on social workers' subsequent practice. A narrative approach seeks to gather a range of personal stories and accounts regarding a particular experience and explores these in order to gain understanding of a central issue (Creswell, 2002). By listening to participants' stories, perspectives and critical reflections, we sought to increase our own insight and understanding and also facilitate the practitioners' own learning. Asking participants to share their own reflections, rather than to respond to a list of questions, placed more power with the individual participant and enabled them to identify what was significant for them. The open-ended narrative inquiry approach led to contributions that as a researcher, I may not have thought to ask for such as the learning from service users whilst on placement or during post qualifying programmes such as the Approved Mental Health Profession (AMPH) training.

The study invited final-year social work students and qualified social workers to reflect on whether service user involvement in their education made any difference to their practice and whether there were different models or types of involvement which had a more significant impact on their practice than others. Participants were invited to submit a written narrative or attend a focus group or individual interview where they could be supported to share their stories and reflections. Requests to participate were distributed to final-year social work students on the university's BA and MA Social Work programmes and to qualified social workers through our practice partners and the workforce development teams of four local authorities.

Ethics approval was gained through the University ethics procedure and involved providing potential participants with a participant information sheet which outlined the purpose and methods of the study; how their contributions would be used and of any disadvantages or advantages they might want to consider before choosing to take part. These included consideration of the impact of my dual role as researcher and senior lecturer on the qualifying programmes and my existing relationship with them. All participants were required to provide written consent for their contribution to be shared and for their anonymised narratives or excerpts from their narratives or contributions to be published.

The email requests resulted in the involvement of 20 participants; 6 students approaching the end of their qualifying programme; 2 newly qualified social workers undertaking their Assessed and Supported Year in Employment (ASYE); 6 social workers who had qualified within the last 10 years (since the implementation of the degree and the requirement for involvement in social work education) and six social workers who had qualified prior to 2005 on DipSW or CQSW programmes. Seventeen of the participants were on placement or working within local authority teams (8 in children's services and 10 in adults); 2 were working as freelance Practice Educators and independent social workers and one for an independent fostering agency. Thirteen of the participants were students or graduates of X University where I am practice lead and seven had graduated from other English Universities. Sixteen of the participants contributed to focus groups (two held at the university and one at the central offices of a local authority). One participant was interviewed individually at her workplace and three final-year students contributed written narratives.

Verbal narratives were recorded and transcribed and a thematic analysis (Braun & Clarke, 2006, 2013; Fugard & Potts, 2015) was then applied to the written narratives and transcriptions to identify key themes and patterns. Propositional statements were then generated from the research findings to foster further analysis and reflection. Propositional statements are suggestions which draw on ideas and theories generated by the knowledge gained so far (Hughes, 2012; Heron, 1996) and then shared with others for further consideration. As others apply their own meaning, further knowledge and insight can be generated. The propositional statements created from this study form the conclusion of this paper.

Findings and discussion

Of the 20 participants, all identified significant learning from the involvement of service users on their programme with the exception of three who recalled minimal involvement other than at the admissions stage. All 20 participants contributed examples of learning from service users in practice settings. Learning had come from different types of involvement and with participants identifying a number of ways that their learning had impacted on their subsequent practice. These were subsequently categorised under four key themes:

- Enhanced awareness of the lived experience.
- Taking on board suggestions of good practice from service users and carers.
- Developing a more critical 'real life' understanding.
- A culture of recognising service users and carers as experts.

Enhanced awareness of the lived experience

Within the data previously collected from students at the point of activity on my own programmes, the key area of learning for students was an enhanced awareness of the lived experience. This was still evident for students and practitioners reflecting on the impact of this involvement on their subsequent practice. One participant reflected on how some of the personal experiences shared in lectures had been very difficult to listen to. She remembered one person:

> she was in hospital for years and years and years and finally she'd been allowed out and it was like her whole life had been taken up by this institution, and I think just having someone to really delve deeper into that kind of experience – this is where I was, this is how I was feeling, this is what social services were telling me but this is actually the reality. She felt trapped and that no-one was listening to her. It was just really honest. Brutal stories can really help. I think for me they stick in my mind when I meet someone else I think oh yeah, I wonder if you're feeling like that right now.

One MA final-year student reflected on how an encounter with a family foster carer whilst on placement enabled her to gain better insight:

> She told me about how upset she was when she first started out as the training was the same for both the main stream foster carer and the family foster carers and how they were often referred to as 'cases' when they really were her grandson and family members that in reality were being talked about.
>
> It really helped me to understand the difficulties that were unique to family foster carers as they were also dealing with the breakdown of relationships in the family, disappointment, anxiety and fear, as these were all her loved ones.
>
> When I came to do my own Form F assessment on a family foster carer, I believe I was more prepared and could reflect this understanding of the carer's dilemmas when I provided an analysis in my assessment.

All of the participants who remembered involvement in lectures spoke positively about it. 'People coming in was a real highlight of our course' or 'we used to really look forward to those sessions'. One social worker commented on

> the courage it took for some of them to talk about something that was often a painful memory and quite personal to them but it helped me to gain insight into their life and also to think about what someone wants from their social worker.

One of the social workers explained how she considered it a privilege to hear about someone's lived experience.

Taking on board suggestions of good practice from service users and carers

Participants frequently referred to opportunities where they had been able to engage in discussions and consultations with service users and carers and ask questions about their experiences of social work and practitioner involvement. The significant factor in these examples was the level of interaction and engagement. A number of participants referred to specific sessions and people who had contributed, quoting them on suggestions or guidance they had offered. A newly qualified social worker now working in older people's mental health services said she had appreciated service users coming into lectures and talking honestly about what they thought of services. She referred to a mental health service user who had said she used to fear social services coming because of not being in control, not knowing what they were going to do and feeling ashamed about her continued self-harm.

> That for me helped my practice in the fact that I'm very mindful now that there are going to be people that don't want social services anywhere near them.

She explained how it made her more aware of how people react to the words 'social worker' or 'social services' and the need to 'come at it from a different angle and build a rapport first'. She explained how that single conversation had enabled her to manage expectations particularly around fear of social workers, particularly for older people in a mental health setting where she now works. She said

> some do genuinely think that they're going to end up in a straitjacket somewhere on lots and lots of pharmaceutical drugs and not seeing their families and that's quite scary for them.

She reflected on whether this lecture had felt so significant at the time: 'I don't think it did because I didn't want to work in mental health at the time but it obviously did stick with me'.

A number of participants identified examples which had become more significant once they encountered the situation for themselves in their practice and engaged in a double loop of the learning cycle having been able to put their learning into practice (Kolb, 1984). In one of the narratives, a final-year student explained how in her first year she had conducted an assessed role-play with someone who used substance use services.

> I did not know at the time, that I would end up in a drugs service, but my role play scenario was based around an addiction situation and as part of the feedback (the service user) talked to me a little about what it was like to work with people with addictions and I have since been able to reflect on the information he shared and how relevant it is to my current experiences working with addiction clients.

She goes on to explain that having the opportunity to learn from young people in her first placement setting with a range of experiences including Autism and mental health issues and the reading she then did to learn more about these experiences and what a diagnosis meant for different people, not only built her confidence but also 'enabled me to be more empathetic in my current role'.

A number of the participants identified aspects of their practice which had been informed by contributions on their course from service users and carers. A final-year MA student said

> We had an afternoon where we had lots of different service users come in and carers from all sort of different areas of social services. Having a conversation with a carer and with a service user who both really highlighted that the worst thing a social worker can ever do is to say 'I'll do something' and not do it.

The student reflected on how in one example, the worker had been off sick and there were understandable reasons but at the end of the day, what had been promised didn't get done.

> I think that by having that conversation with someone who had clearly been hurt a lot by lots of different team members you could see that actually that whole relationship could have been made better. Their whole care had been impacted by that and I think that for me, even if you do go off sick or something happens if you've made a promise you have to make sure that's going to be kept by the team.

A newly qualified social worker in the same focus group explained that as a result, she has learnt since not to make promises and to be much more open with service users by explaining when she hoped to have something done by and to phone them if there was a delay or to apologise when something doesn't get done.

> 'I've had a few crises in the last week, so I'm really sorry but your case didn't get the full attention it should and I'm sorry about that'. They do appreciate me being honest with them.

A newly qualified social worker in adult services remembered the same activity where a number of service users had come in to a lecture to share their experiences and suggestions. What she had remembered most was people's frustration at having to go through the same information again and again and then being very aware of the same frustrations being shared by service users in her subsequent practice.

> you could really see that, they were like 'why are you asking us the same questions that she asked me'? And the parents are like 'you've already gone through my direct payment like ten times, it's not changed, why am I doing it all over again, and again and again.

This reminded her of the discussion during her course and the need for openness and honesty. This was also identified as an example of learning in another focus group. An adult social worker said as a result she now always makes a point of summarising the case histories and explaining that she has done this to each service user so they don't feel they need to start from the beginning.

A number of participants identified the need to be honest and transparent with service users as being a key aspect of learning from their involvement in their course. One recounted a service user saying to her 'if you are not going to be able to offer me a service, just tell me so I can sort something else out'.

A newly qualified social worker in adult services said she still remembered one service user who had facilitated a group she was in during her first year (four years earlier) who talked about professionalism. She remembered him saying

> 'a lot of social workers are coming pretending to be my friends, and are there so casually, I have a lot of people who coming in jeans and leggings. I don't want them to be my friend I want my social worker to look like a social worker, so can you remember that', and I always remember that actually. I think you know depending on who I'm seeing I always make sure I have my badge and think about how I dress. I'll always remember that actually.

A number of the participants explained that having different views shared by service users helped them to reflect. Also on the topic of dress code, participants in one focus group said that they had received conflicting advice from service users on their course about whether to dress casually or smartly and how that had enabled them to realise that everyone is different. One student said how in practice she had learnt to adapt what she was wearing to different activities and people, as a result of conversations with service users:

> when I was working at a school and a social worker came in to assess a child and they were dressed in a suit and I sort of observed the social worker but from afar as I had the kids and I looked and the mother just said to me 'he can't even get down to play with him 'cos he's in a suit, how's he going to interact with her'.

In a different focus group, a social worker now working in a child health and disability team remembered a mother coming in to a lecture and saying that she has had social workers who have been to her house and not even acknowledged her daughter because of her level of communication needs. The social worker explained how this had significantly impacted on the student group at the time and led to a discussion about the need for basic communication.

A children's social worker said she always remembers a woman coming in who had survived domestic abuse.

> She had a huge impact on our student group especially when she said to us, 'don't ask us why we don't leave'. Now I say it to students and newly qualified workers – don't ask them that, they can't tell you'. That one statement was huge.

An experienced adult social worker said hearing people's views enabled her to think about what is important to the person which might seem small and be overlooked by others such as 'having Wheetos for breakfast or a spicy lunch because they find other food to be bland. 'I put things like that in the care plan'.

Whilst much of the learning related to developing good practice and upholding social work standards and professional values, many of the participants felt that service user involvement had enabled this to take place. One more experienced social worker who recalled there being minimal involvement on her qualifying programme said that without this, her current focus on involvement in her practice had only developed much later. 'It's far better that we now introduce this right from the start'.

Developing a more critical understanding

A number of the participants reflected on how opportunities to discuss issues or hear about people's experiences had enabled them to adopt a more critical approach to what they were reading and learning and an understanding of complexity which informed how they practice now. As with the examples above, this criticality often arose from service users presenting varied experiences or providing conflicting advice.

A BA final-year student said about a session in her first year:

> Service users from a day centre came to discuss their experiences. I found this highly beneficial, it enabled me to recognise that what is written in literature is slightly simplistic compared to reality. Although literature is fantastic, it does not have the same influence as a service user discussing their experiences, which almost makes the information we have learnt more real and applicable. I feel like I now question literature a lot more, and think how would this affect the service user? or what does this mean for the service user?

One participant, a mental health social worker who qualified five years ago at a university where she identified few examples of involvement, identified the risk to less-experienced students like herself, if different perspectives were not presented.

> I think at the time I used to take everything a service user said as universal. For a long time I thought this one woman's experience of post-natal depression was how it was for all women.

A culture of recognising service users and carers as experts

Having a range of involvement across the programme appeared to have successfully developed and promoted a culture for many of the participants in recognising service users as experts by experience and to value the opportunity to learn from them rather than 'do social work to them'. A newly qualified social worker said that she had taken this approach into her practice and now routinely explored a person's views on social care with them and sought to develop a relationship which was based on this level of mutual respect before focussing on the assessment.

A final-year MA student said that in her placement in a substance use team, she had organised a drop-in session for service users to share their experiences of services. She reflected on how powerful it had been to listen to people's experiences and their ideas on treatment services. It made her reflect on the importance of seeking meaningful feedback and engaging in conversations with people who are experts by experience.

> Before I was doing the course and I was working we used to give out feedback forms and it felt very hollow, it was kind of this thing that you said 'please bring this in and then send it back to the department' but when I did it used to feel like it was a way of criticising me if that makes sense, it didn't feel like useful feedback it was like a weird oh what if they say something but now feedback I get much more of the whole picture; the importance of it.

She explained that this had taken time. Students on my own programme are asked to identify a plan in each placement for how they are going to learn from the expertise of service users and then to review this at the end. When reflecting back on her first placement she said:

> I don't think I'd been in the placement long enough to really understand what I could learn from the people in the placement but I think this time round, because I already knew what things service users could potentially teach me I was more aware of the ways I could get taught those things by them.

Two of the more experienced participants who had qualified over 10 years ago, recognised this change of culture and said

> you see the difference in students now. They come in with an attitude toward service users of 'what can I learn from you'.

An experienced social worker who subsequently set up a new service said that involvement had been fundamental to her learning in her DipSW and that it just became the way she worked. 'It's absolutely fundamental, it underpins everything I do. Everything's in partnership'. She remembered recording interviews with children whilst on placement and how this had enabled her to focus on the voice of the child. She remembered having to write a narrative of the child's voice and explained how she still does that in her practice today.

Another participant identified experiences which had challenged concepts of 'them and us' such as one social worker who referred to a post qualifying session when they were participating in a lecture on mental health and it was only at the end that the lecturer disclosed their own mental health history. 'It breaks down stereotypes'.

Individual impact

Whilst there were some key themes in terms of what impact involvement had, the findings showed that the impact was individual to each student or practitioner. It was often specific encounters or 'light bulb moments' which led to increased awareness or insight into aspects of their own practice particularly when encountering similar situations or when pressures of practice led to them losing sight of service user perspectives. This was particularly evident in the reflections around professionalism and 'making promises' or not doing what you had said you would do because of a heavy case load or crisis.

> You try to do as much as you can because you don't want to let them down but in reality if a crisis comes in and you've had to drop everything you might have promised you'll call at three o'clock but you just have to accept it wasn't possible for you to do. You have to be honest and apologise.

A significant aspect of the findings were how even some years on, students and practitioners were able to identify specific encounters and conversations they remembered with service users and carers contributing to their course and how something they had said or what they themselves had learnt, had 'stayed with them'. 'I can picture them now' was a phrase used by a number of the participants. The memories were often in relation to advice on how to improve their own practice which they have since taken on board.

Learning from practice

Many of the participants including those who had qualified over 10 years ago remembered individual service users they had encountered on their practice placements and receiving feedback from them. Two of the social workers who qualified more than 10 years ago identified how much more important involvement had become in recent years and how much more meaningful it has become in their own practice.

> You are just stagnating if you are not constantly looking to your service users to develop the service. It's got to be meaningful; what's working, what's not working, can we do things differently? I've always found it quite inspiring and motivating to be sitting alongside a service user as an equal. It's about their lives so until you can get alongside them and understand their perspective, how can you improve?

A number of participants identified how much of their learning about service user perspectives had come from placement. One talked about being encouraged to immerse herself in deaf culture; another about how the nature of the 24 h family centre in which he was placed enabled him to gain a huge amount of insight into people's lives and to learn from them. 'The most meaningful conversations were at 2 am in the morning when they had just been on the phone crying to their mum'. When reflecting on the impact on his subsequent practice he said 'I learnt to listen'. Concern was expressed in this focus group as to whether opportunities to get alongside service users exist in current practice. Participants now working in children's services talked about the value of driving children to appointments. One said 'I've driven round three times on my way somewhere because of how much they were opening up'. Impromptu opportunities to have conversations with service users were valued by many of the participants over programme requirements to obtain feedback. Three of the participants questioned the value of having to obtain written feedback from service users whilst on practice which had been a requirement on their programme at the time. Those who were able to devise evaluation forms with service users or engage in other strategies such as interviews and conversations found this to be much more useful. Across all of the focus groups and narratives, the opportunity to engage with service users was identified as the most meaningful.

Limited impact

Particularly evident from the narratives were the types of involvement that were not mentioned or were perceived by the participants as being less significant in their learning or the shaping of their subsequent practice. A significant area of service user involvement across social work programmes and a requirement in England as stipulated by the Health and Care Professions Council (HCPC) is the involvement of service users and carers in the recruitment process. On my own programme, levels of involvement at the admissions stage are extensive as the carer and service user partnership group lead and assess a group activity which involves interviewees viewing a short film or documentary excerpt relevant to social work practice and discussing the service user perspectives within it. The carer and service user group then facilitate and provide feedback on a written activity where applicants are required to write a first person narrative from the perspective of one of the people within the film. In addition to assessing written skills, the aim of the activity is to evaluate the applicants' use of empathy. Marks and feedback from both of these activities and an interview with an academic and a social work practitioner, are then reviewed by the service user and carer coordinators and the admissions tutor to finalise offer decisions.

Despite this level of involvement, the only participants who referred to the interview day within their narratives, interview or focus groups were ones where the service users had been involved in the interview panel rather than a group or written activity. The responses to this involvement varied:

> My first experience of service user involvement on the course was my initial interview. This had two responses, initially I felt glad as the service user had experience of mental health services and this was the area I was discussing. At the time, I felt having service user involvement enabled me to express my interest in the particular field, to the point where I forgot I was in an interview. I think this benefited me personally, as it broke down the barriers of nervousness and I become more relaxed. Although, following the discussion I was apprehensive that I had not focused on the academic perspective enough.

Whilst another participant (a social worker who qualified five years previously) who remembered a service user being on the interview panel said

> They were just like another member of staff as they all took turns in asking questions. I suppose it did help when they asked me about my personal experience as I felt I could talk about that.

Another participant remembered there being a service user on the interview panel but wasn't sure if it had any impact on her directly 'I don't remember coming out thinking specifically oh yeah it was really good to have that service user in for that'.

On my own programme we have a number of activities where service users and carers assess students' work, which includes being on marking panels for assessed presentations; taking part and providing feedback on assessed role plays and in providing feedback on how effectively the service user voice is evidenced within students' practice portfolios. Of these activities, only the assessed role play which involves a high level of interaction and personal disclosure by the service user was recalled and explored in any depth by the participants. This was rated far more highly by current students and recent graduates who conducted assessed role plays with service users who had planned the activity and devised their own scenarios, than those who had conducted role plays within the student group with students taking on the service user role. Again, this was due to the activity being perceived as realistic, providing insight into the person's lived experience and students valuing the opportunity to discuss their 'practice' with the service user after it had ended. A social worker from a different university who had undertaken an assessed role play with service users questioned its value for those involved as she didn't feel there was this level of involvement or engagement and was left feeling concerned about the impact of multiple role-plays on the individual service users taking part; a concern also reported by Duffy, Das, and Davidson (2013) when reflecting on a similar activity.

Conclusions and implications for educators

The most common types of service user and carer involvement mentioned by participants were lectures and workshops where individuals shared their lived experience and their views on best practice; when gaining individual feedback on their assessed role-play; during a practice learning in the community unit where groups are facilitated by a service user; and when engaging in consultations of what makes a good social worker as part of their practice learning. All of these examples involved direct contact and provided opportunities for students to gain insight and engage in communicable learning where learners seek to understand (Mezirow, 2003).

Opportunities to engage in conversations with people who they considered experts by experience are well supported by a number of adult learning theories. Knowles (1990) argued that for adults, learning needs to be purposeful, to draw on previous experiences, to recognise their readiness to learn and their orientation to learning (what is relevant to their life) and to recognise what motivates them to learn. For most of the participants in this study, engaging with service users enabled them to see the relevance of what they had been learning elsewhere but also to learn directly from them and to use it to inform their own views of the world and their developing practice. It enabled them to gain insight and make sense of their wider experiences. In many cases, it enabled students to develop as empathic practitioners but also provided guidance on how to demonstrate this in their practice; how as well as why.

When exploring the lived experience, a number of the participants identified personal accounts which they had found 'shocking' or 'difficult to hear'. As one of the participants said however, 'brutal stories can really help'. This is supported by transformative learning theory where Mezirow (2003) places particular emphasis on perspective change and the transformation of beliefs, values and behaviour. Mezirow identified 10 phases of the transformative learning process which he argued occur as an adult seeks to clarify meaning, starting with 'a disorientating dilemma, self-examination of feelings and a critical assessment of assumptions' (Mezirow, 2003, p.4). Whilst others have argued that it requires a less linear process (Cranton, 2002; Merriam & Kim, 2008; Merriam & Ntseane, 2008; Walton, 2010), these elements were present for many of the participants reflecting on their learning from service users sharing these insights.

The lack of evidence within the narratives of lasting impact from involvement in admissions, assessment of students work and practice and curriculum design raises a number of questions. Further exploration is required to identify whether this reflects students and practitioners' perceptions of involvement only being when a person shares their story and lived experiences, rather than their expertise and judgement; whether the role of service users is well enough communicated during admissions or assessment processes; or whether the benefit of these types of involvement is in how it informs the decision-making process rather than the applicants' experience on the day or memory of it after. One of the service user and carer coordinators reflected on whether the high level of responsibility the service users have during admission and assessment processes, was in some ways 'too professional' in that the service users were perceived as staff and that role differed from what an applicant's expectations may be of a 'service user'. Anka and Taylor's (2016) review of service user involvement in social work assessments however, identified the presence of different power relations amongst those involved, with some students acknowledging that whilst they valued service user feedback, in summative processes, they perceived the academic or practice assessor's assessment as 'carrying more weight' (2016, p. 179). This could explain the limited recollection or impact identified by participants within this study.

A number of conclusions can be drawn from the research regarding the impact of service user and carer involvement on students' subsequent practice and the types of involvement that appeared to have more impact. In addition to the four themes identified from the participant stories, the following propositional statements were identified from the knowledge gained (Hughes, 2012; Heron, 1996). These are presented here by way of a conclusion to this paper and as recommendations for educators to foster further reflection and debate.

- The impact of different types of service user involvement on subsequent practice is unique to each student.
- Opportunities to hear personal experiences and the lived experience can have a long lasting impact on students and 'stays with them'.
- The most significant impact on subsequent practice often comes from service users advising students on best practice and what they want from a social work practitioner.
- Impact on subsequent practice is increased if the student experiences double loop learning (Kolb, 1984) for example, when going on to encounter a similar experience or scenario in their practice.
- Impact on subsequent practice is increased when students have the opportunity to engage and discuss issues with the service user. The impact comes from meaningful conversations.
- Having a diverse range of involvement and the opportunity to hear contrasting views and perspectives can be an effective catalyst for critical reflection.
- The reality of people's lives and their experiences of services and practitioner involvement can enable students to develop a less simplistic view of social work practice and a better understanding of complexity.
- For some students, it is only later when in practice that they recognise the significance of particular encounters and their learning from involvement.
- Opportunities for meaningful conversations with service users to support a student's learning and professional development can be facilitated in practice and university settings.

Disclosure statement

No potential conflict of interest was reported by the author.

References

Anka, A., & Taylor, I. (2016). Assessment as the site of power: A Bourdieusian interrogation of service user and carer involvement in the assessments of social work students. *Social Work Education: The International Journal, 35*, 172–185.

Braun, V., & Clarke, V. (2006). Using thematic analysis in psychology. *Qualitative Research in Psychology, 3*, 77–101.

Braun, V., & Clarke, V. (2013). *Successful qualitative research: A practical guide for beginners*. London: Sage.

Carr, S. (2004). *Has service user participation made a difference to social care services?* London: SCIE, Policy Press.

Cranton, P. (2002). Teaching for transformation. *New Directions for Adult and Continuing Education, 93*, 63–72.

Creswell, J. W. (2002). *Research design: Qualitative, quantitative and mixed methods design*. London: Sage.

Driessens, K., McLaughlin, H., & Van Doorn, L. (2016). The meaningful involvement of service users in social work education: Examples from Belgium and The Netherlands. *Social Work Education: The International Journal, 35*, 739–751.

Duffy, J. (2013). Service user involvement in teaching about conflict – An exploration of the issues. *International Social Work, 55*, 720–739.

Duffy, J., Das, C., & Davidson, G. (2013). Service user and carer involvement in role-plays to assess readiness for practice. *Social Work Education: The International Journal, 32*, 39–54.

Fugard, A. J. B., & Potts, H. W. W. (2015). Supporting thinking on sample sizes for thematic analyses: A quantitative tool. *International Journal of Social Research Methodology, 18*, 669–684.

Heron, J. (1996). *Co-operative inquiry: Research into the human condition*. London: Sage.

Hughes, M. (2012). Unitary appreciative inquiry (UAI): A new approach for researching social work education and practice. *British Journal of Social Work, 42*, 1388–1405. doi:10.1093/bjsw/bcr139

Khoo, R., McVicar, A., & Brandon, D. (2004). Service user involvement in postgraduate mental health education. Does it benefit practice? *Journal of Mental Health October 2004, 13*, 481–492.

Knowles, M. (1990). *The adult learner: A neglected species* (4th ed.). London: Gulf.

Kolb, D. (1984). *Experiential learning: Experience as the source of learning and development*. Englewood Cliffs, NJ: Prentice Hall.

MacSporran, J. (2015). A Mentor's PATH: Evaluating how service users can be involved as mentors for social work students on observational practice placements. *Social work and Social Sciences Review, 17*, 46–60.

McLaughlin, H. (2009). What's in a name: Client, patient, customer, consumer, expert by experience, service user – What's next? *British Journal of Social Work, 39*, 1101–1117.

Merriam, S. B., & Kim, Y. S. (2008). Non-western perspectives in learning and knowing. *New Directions for Adult and Continuing Education, 119*, 71–81.

Merriam, S. B., & Ntseane, G. (2008). Transformative learning in Botswana: How culture shapes the process. *Adult Education Quarterly, 58*, 183–197.

Mezirow, J. (2000). *Learning as transformation: Critical perspectives on a theory in progress*. San Francisco, CA: Jossey Bass.

Mezirow, J. (2003). *Epistemology of transformative learning*. Retrieved from www.transformativelearning.org/.../Mezirow_EpistemologyTLC.pdf

Morgan, A., & Jones, D. (2009). Perceptions of service user and carer involvement in healthcare education and impact of students' knowledge and practice: A literature review. *Medical Teacher, 31*, 82–95.

Muir, D., & Laxton, C. J. (2012). Experts by experience: The views of service user educators providing feedback on medical students' work based assessments. *Nurse Education Today, 32*, 146–150.

Perry, J., Gilbert, A., & Rawlinson, J. (2013). A systematic review of the evidence on service user involvement in interpersonal skills training of mental health students. *Journal of Psychiatric and Mental Health Nursing, 20*, 525–540.

Rhodes, C. A. (2012). User involvement in health and social care education: A concept analysis. *Nurse Education Today, 32*, 185–189.

Robinson, K., & Webber, M. (2013). Models and effectiveness of service user and carer involvement in social work education: A literature review. *British Journal of Social Work, 43*, 925–944.

Rush, B. (2008). Mental health service user involvement in nurse education: A catalyst for transformative learning. *Journal of Mental Health, 17*, 531–542.

Simons, L., Tee, S., Lathlean, J., Burgess, A., Herbert, L., & Gibson, C. (2006). A socially inclusive approach to user participation in higher education. *Journal of Advanced Nursing, 58*, 246–255.

Terry, J. (2012). Service user involvement in pre-registration mental health nurse education classroom settings: A review of the literature. *Journal of Psychiatric and Mental Health Nursing, 19*, 816–829.

Turnbull, P., & Weeley, F. M. (2013). Service user involvement: Inspiring student nurses to make a difference to patient care. *Nurse Education Practice, 13*, 454–458.

Walton, J. D. (2010). Examining a transformative approach to communication education: A teacher-research study. *College Student Journal, 44*, 157–177.

IDEA IN ACTION

Life at the other end: participatory film-making, power and the 'common third'

Yohai Hakak and Kevin Holmes

ABSTRACT

In this article, we will describe and analyse the production of the documentary film Life at the Other End (The documentary film Life at the Other End (2012) was screened at Picture This: International Disabilities Film Festival in Calgary, Canada; Steps-International Film Festival on Human Rights, Ukrain; at the Joint Social Work Education Conference, Royal Holloway University, London; Staffordshire Performing Arts Film Festival, UK and at the We Care Film Festival, New Delhi, India where it won the 2nd place as the best film on disability (up to 60 min category). The film can be watched on Youtube here: http://bit.ly/1O8zEqp). The film followed a group of experts-by-experience who are members in a Social Work Inclusion Group (SWIG) (SWIG or Social Work Inclusion Group is affiliated to the University of Portsmouth. For more details about SWIG please see here: http://swig.uk.net/) affiliated to the Division of Social Work at the University of Portsmouth. The film followed the group during a process of writing and performing a play based on their personal experiences in the social care system. The production process will be explored as a case study for the application of the 'common third' approach. The case will highlight some of the approach's strengths and will describe the circumstances in which it failed (This article is in memory of Andrew Chappell who chaired SWIG, took a central part in the play and film discussed here and passed away on 23 July 2016).

This article will analyse the process of producing a documentary film, in which the first author was the film's director and the second author was a participant and co-editor. While our approach is influenced by Nelson's (2013) 'practice as research', we have treated the process of producing the film also as ethnographic fieldwork which has allowed us to carefully explore the power relations between those involved in the production process, the interactions between them and the decisions they made. These will be the focus of our analysis which we will consider on the background of the wider context-of-production in which this film was created.

A growing number of artistic projects in different disciplines either result from or attempt to enhance the collaboration and partnership between marginalised groups and artists, social activists, social workers and therapists. Some of these collaborations result in artistic products, which give a unique insight into the marginalised communities involved, and can often challenge common stereotypes and promote social change. While there is rich literature analysing the prevalence of social stereotypes regarding a wide range of marginalised and minority groups, there is little research analysing the attempts of such groups to challenge such stereotypes and create more positive representations of themselves (Goris, Witteveen, & Lie, 2015). The current article will analyse such an attempt.

Goris et al. (2015) review the different key approaches to participatory film-making according to the centrality of artistic considerations compared to the centrality of the 'problem owners'—those with direct experience of the issues discussed—in making the film. As Goris et al. (2015) describe, very often when participants themselves hold the power and make the decisions, artistic considerations are marginalised and the films rarely reach wider audiences. In order to reach wider audiences, professional film-makers need to be involved and must be part of the decision-making. At the same time, we argue for more balanced power relations in participatory films between film-makers and participants. Adjusting a series of practices such as the consent and release forms, and sharing the planning as well as the editing stage—while it may entail some challenges—is likely to produce better films, not only ethically but artistically.

The power of art collaborations between 'problem owners' or experts by experience (service users) and social workers, therapists and artists goes beyond the empowerment of experts by experience. It also goes beyond the ability to promote social change or communicate more broadly the concerns of experts by experience to policy makers and politicians. It promotes the development of a different kind of relationship between experts by experience and professionals working with them. Such relations tend to be unidirectional and unequal, and focus on the service user and their problems. While helping-professionals who are engaged with experts by experience or other 'problem owners' are taught to develop their empathy, such a relationship commonly focuses on a problem owned by the experts by experience. The service user is thus defined and perceived by their problem and the professional's role is in helping to find the best way of dealing with or solving the problem. A relationship that is built around artistic collaboration that often brings together service-users, professionals and artists, changes such a dynamic. In such cases, the 'problem' has the potential of turning into a source of inspiration, ideas and stories which will be the essential building blocks for artistic activity. In addition, such collaborations shift the focus from the expert by experience into the participants' shared aim—the artistic activity. The 'Common Third' from Social Pedagogy describes exactly this shift of attention into a more neutral and equal locus of attention and effort (Bengtsson, Chamberlain, Crimmens, & Stanley, 2008). It creates a more positive interaction and thus better allows a process of learning, acquiring new skills and building confidence (Hatton, 2016). During certain parts of the process that will be described, the collaboration had indeed such an effect, while at other stages, this was hampered.

The context of production and the film

At the University of Portsmouth, social work students take part each year in a 'Create Day' during which they collaborate with experts by experience and artists in creating representations related to the lives and experiences of the experts by experience. The SWIG group includes a good range of confident and knowledgeable experts by experience, many of whom have expressed their interest in using artistic mediums with social work students. These collaborative sessions culminate in an afternoon when students and experts by experience present the outcome of their shared work (ie in drama, poetry, dance, music).

For the Create Day of 2009, SWIG members took on themselves to contribute the opening event and to collaborate, months in advance, with students from the Performing Arts department. They wanted to co-write and prepare a play based on their personal experiences and to present it to a group of 90 social work students.

Art as a medium played a central role for the group and created a unique dynamic that was full of humour, playfulness and joy which were inspiring and motivated us to try and capture some of it on film. The film structure we had in mind meant to use the process of producing the theatre production as its narrative structure. Part of the 'story' this film was hoping to tell, is the story of this process including its trials and tribulations. This was an opportunity to challenge common representations of service-users as 'passive', 'needy' and 'weak' recipients of services, through a case involving active, strong and confident individuals who improve social work education. We had an initial meeting with the group, in which the film idea was shared and gained their support. The university's media production unit agreed to help and provided us with the equipment, a camera and a sound technician, and later on also an editor.

Shooting the rehearsals

We started filming the rehearsals. One important and difficult decision we made early on was not to ask group members to sign Release Forms. These are forms that film-makers ask participants to sign, and in which participants declare they agree to being filmed and relinquish any right to influence the editing process. Since our initial intention was to break down power relations between experts by experience and artists we resisted this practice, not without creating great angst for the Head of the Media Production unit. While many of the people we consulted with, thought that this was putting the whole project in danger, we wanted to emphasise that this film will tell the participants' stories and will materialise only if they want it to. If participants don't agree with it at any stage they can and should say so, and they retain their ability to withdraw their participation at any stage.

The writing of the play and the rehearsals took place during a three-month period. The film captures the tension that arose between the participants during these rehearsals, and its resolution, but more than that it captures the creative, playful and humorous atmosphere that characterised the rehearsals. The different participants worked collaboratively with a shared aim. Filming these rehearsals was very easy and the camera's presence didn't create objections. We can assume that as long as the camera was following the rehearsals which included the whole group, participants felt relatively protected and were able to see and comment on what the film crew did. Things got more complicated later on.

After the rehearsals

As we didn't want to make a TV news item, we needed to focus on specific characters, and tell a story from their point of view. Out of 10 participants in the play, three were chosen already during an early stage of the rehearsals, based on their centrality in the group and in the play, and their willingness to participate.

Once the rehearsals were over and the play was performed successfully, we started filming the three key participants in their personal lives. We wanted to get to know them better and show how the contents of the play were shaped, reflected and affected by their personal lives. This stage was only slightly more difficult. Not all three were keen on being filmed and some fears and doubts were expressed at this stage, especially by one of the three. It is easy to assume that participants felt more exposed and less protected while being filmed on their own, and it was necessary to explain many times the film idea and rationale. Two out of the three leading participants had been filmed several times in the past, and were therefore more confident and open.

The editing

The rehearsals were shot from mid-January to mid-March 2009 and the additional filming was finished by the end of September 2009. The editing took almost three additional years and turned out to be the most challenging and difficult part of making the film.

After the shooting stage was over in Sept 2009, the film was scheduled to be screened six months later, on 15 March 2010, as the key event of the 2010 Create Day. At least some of the difficult events leading to, and on the day of this planned screening, were a result of the tensions building up towards that date. We should also mention that this was a relatively big editing project for the university's Media Production team with over 30 h of recorded footage. The project was competing over the editor's time with many other films that were queuing up to be edited by him. The fact that it was a very different film from the academic-educational films this team was used to complicated things further and delayed finishing the film.

The long period that SWIG members—the film's participants—had to wait for the film to be edited, combined with their high expectations, increased their tensions and anxiety. During a meeting at the end of January 2010, it became clear that the film will not be completed in time for the scheduled screening on 15 March 2010. After a heated debate the second author, who was one of the leading group members and a key participant in the film, suggested that he would edit the film on his own, in time for the event. Late in January he started a race against the clock.

We approached the date of the Create Day screening with two half-ready edits and a lot of frustration and stress among those involved. The edit prepared by the university's editor and the first author was seen as suspicious and derogatory. Being committed to the voice of experts by experience, we screened the version edited by the second author of this article, himself a leading member of the expert by experience group. Though the film was far from being completed, the film opened the 2010 Create Day and the responses were positive.

One of the contentious moments of that Create Day followed a short lecture given by the first author. This lecture aimed to deconstruct common stereotypical media representations of disability. But, the representations shown as part of this lecture were understood by one of the three key participants in the film, as an expression of the presenter's own perceptions about disability. This participant's comments about the lecture were very critical. Not only was the director unable to deliver a finished version of the film in time, his version was potentially negative and offensive and so was his lecture. These remarks were made in front of colleagues and students at an event that was planned to celebrate co-production with experts by experience.

The show had to go on and after some time for rest we went back to editing. The second author, as a representative of the experts by experience, joined the first author and we were assigned to a different editor. Though the editing process was long and exhausting—mainly due to the competing demands over the editor's time—and the film was only finished at the end of 2012, we had very few disagreements during that stage. The film was screened in several international film festivals and won the 2nd place for the best film on disability at the We Care Film Festival, New Delhi, India.

Conclusions

Producing a participatory documentary in a university context, especially one that is so much influenced by critical discourse, and the awareness of power relations between experts by experience and other professionals, couldn't materialise without sharing power. Things started going wrong during the editing stage when participants were not enabled to take part, and felt that power was not shared or that the information did not flow. These tensions were eased when a member of the group became a part of the editing team.

Making a participatory documentary involves working with participants and gaining their trust and cooperation. The more the film-maker/artist is able to create such a trusting relationship, the greater the likelihood that the participants will be open and allow access to different aspects of their life. Such increased access is more likely to provide rich material for the film. Ethically speaking, more equal sharing of power can only be positive. Therefore, we argue that sharing more of the power held by film-makers, while not relinquishing authorship completely, is likely to provide both artistic and ethical advantages to documentary film-makers, especially when working with discriminated against, and marginalised groups. Inclusion is a long process which involves learning new roles and new ways of doing things for all those involved. Practitioners and academics need to learn how to give up some of their power, and experts by experience need to learn how to adjust to a new reality and acknowledge when change has taken place. While suspicion is always useful, there is also a place to develop the ability to trust.

Disclosure statement

No potential conflict of interest was reported by the authors.

ORCID

Yohai Hakak http://orcid.org/0000-0002-8866-4324

References

Goris, M., Witteveen, L., & Lie, R. (2015). Participatory film-making for social change: Dilemmas in balancing participatory and artistic qualities. *Journal of Arts & Communities, 7*, 63–85.

Hatton, K. (2016). A critical examination of the knowledge contribution service user and carer involvement brings to social work education. *Social Work Education*. doi:10.1080/02615479.2016.1254769

Nelson, R. (2013). *Practice as research in the arts: Principles, protocols pedagogies and resistances*. Hampshire: Palgrave Macmillan.

Bengtsson, E., Chamberlain, C., Crimmens, D., & Stanley, J. (2008). Introducing social pedagogy into residential child care in England: an evaluation of a project commissioned by the Social Education Trust (SET) in September 2006 and managed by the National Centre for Excellence in Residential Child Care (NCERCC).

Index

Note: **Boldface** page numbers refer to tables and *italic* page numbers refer to figures. Page numbers followed by "n" denote endnotes.

For Product Safety Concerns and Information please contact our EU
representative GPSR@taylorandfrancis.com
Taylor & Francis Verlag GmbH, Kaufingerstraße 24, 80331 München, Germany

www.ingramcontent.com/pod-product-compliance
Ingram Content Group UK Ltd.
Pitfield, Milton Keynes, MK11 3LW, UK
UKHW050754180926
475701UK00007B/1050

* 9 7 8 0 3 6 7 5 9 2 7 9 0 *